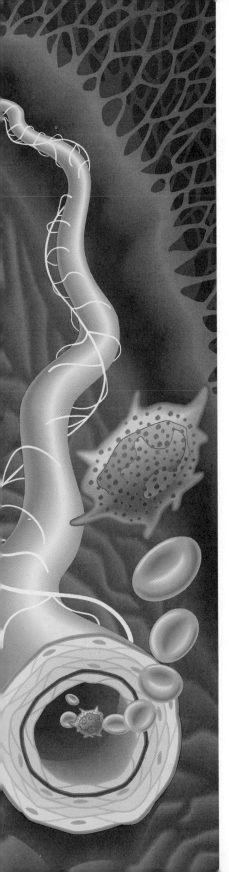

THE ELEMENTS OF
Medical
Terminology

April Applegate
Valerie Overton

Adapted from an original publication by
MedText, Inc.

Delmar Publishers Inc.™

I T P™

NOTICE TO THE READER

Cover illustration by Ted Polomis

Publishing Team

Acquisitions Editor: Adrianne C. Williams
Project Manager: John Pucillo
Developmental Editor: Helen V. Yackel
Project Editor: Megan A. Terry
Production Coordinator: Barbara A. Bullock

Art & Design Coordinator: Mary E. Siener
Book Designer: Dorothy Karaus
Medical Illustrator: Ted Polomis
Supplements Coordinator: Ralph S. Protsik

For information, address

Delmar Publishers Inc.
3 Columbia Circle, Box 15015
Albany, NY 12203-5015

Printed in the United States of America
Published simultaneously in Canada
by Nelson Canada,
a division of the Thomson Corporation

2 3 4 5 6 7 8 9 10 XXX 00 99 98 97 96 95 94

Library of Congress Cataloging-in-Publication Data
Applegate, April.
     The elements of medical terminology / April Applegate, Valerie Overton, John Pucillo.
        p.   cm.
     Includes index.
     ISBN 0-8273-6406-7
      1. Medicine—Terminology. 2. English language—Foreign elements.
    I. Overton, Valerie. II. Pucillo, John. III. Title.
      [DNLM: 1. Nomenclature. W 15 A648e 1994]
    R123.A67 1994
    610'.14—dc20
    DNLM/DLC
    For Library of Congress

93-32985
CIP

Table of Contents

Preface

Why Study Medical Terminology?

As a member of the biomedical and allied health professions, understanding and communicating medical information will be at the very heart of your work. On a day-to-day basis, your job will require you to understand terms related to anatomy, physiology, disease, diagnosis, and therapeutics. You must be able to see and hear the medical language used in your workplace and to process this information quickly and accurately.

This can be a challenging task. Medicine includes a seemingly limitless number of areas of specialization, each of which seems to have a language of its own. This text is designed to help you meet this challenge. You will learn the principles of medical terminology, build a working vocabulary of medical terms, and prepare yourself to master new terms in the future. You will be rewarded for your efforts with comfort and professionalism in the use of medical terminology.

What Will I Learn?

At first glance, medical terminology seems to be almost a foreign language, largely consisting of unpronounceable words with unfathomable meanings. But as you're about to discover in the pages that follow, medical terminology is not mysterious at all. You will see that medical terminology is actually quite logical and consistent. Once you learn the logic behind it, you should find medical terms easy to recognize, understand, and remember.

The goal of this text is to enable you to do more than simply memorize vocabulary words. You will learn skills that will enable you to _analyze_ medical terms by breaking them down into their basic components.

Understanding the _elements_ of medical terminology will not only help you master the terms in this book but will also help you decipher new medical terms that you encounter, even if you've never seen them before. This ability will give you additional confidence in performing your job effectively and professionally.

Acknowledgments

The authors and the project team at Delmar Publishers wish to express their appreciation to a dedicated group of professionals who reviewed and provided commentary on the manuscript at various stages.

Susan L. Berridge, RN, BSN, MA
Health Occupations Instructor
Jackson Area Career Center
Jackson, MI

Elsie G. Campbell, RN, MA
Professor Emeritus
Bakersfield College
Bakersfield, CA

Adrienne L. Carter-Ward, CMA, RMA, EMT
Instructor Trainer and Medical Assisting Instructor
National Headquarters NEC
San Bernardino, CA

Annalee Collins, RRA
Program Director
Health Information Administration Program
Northeastern University
Boston, MA

Barbara F. Ensley, RN, CMA-C
Haywood Community College
Clyde, NC

Janet L. Fisk
Medical Terminology Instructor
Department of Health Sciences
Santa Rosa Junior College
Santa Rosa, CA

Nancy Kiernan, MPT
Clinical Instructor
Department of Physical Therapy
Northeastern University
Boston, MA

Ralph S. Protsik
P.S. Associates, Inc.
Boston, MA

Yasmen Simonian
School of Allied Health Sciences
Weber State University
Ogden, UT

Jean Ternus, MS, RN
Nursing Instructor
Kansas City Kansas Community College
Kansas City, KS

Rules of Pronunciation

An important goal of this text is to guide you through the pronunciation of medical terms. The "see-and-say" guides provided throughout this book will help make pronouncing new terms easier. Nevertheless, you may feel uncomfortable pronouncing medical terms at first. Learning a few simple pronunciation rules will help:

Pronouncing g
- when followed by an **e** or **i, g** is usually pronounced like a **j** (e.g., geriatric and gingivitis)
- when followed by an **a, o, u,** or a consonant, **g** is usually pronounced like a "hard g" (e.g., gallbladder, gums, and glucose)

Pronouncing c
- when followed by an **e, i,** or **y, c** is usually pronounced like an **s** (e.g., cerebral, cirrhosis, and cyst)
- when followed by an **a, o, u,** or a consonant, **c** is usually pronounced like a **k** (e.g., cardiac, coronary, cut, and clot)

Pronouncing double consonants
- **p** is usually silent when it is followed by another consonant at the beginning of a word (e.g., pneumonia and psychiatry)
- **ph** is pronounced like an **f** (e.g., physiology)
- **rh** is pronounced like an **r** (e.g., rheumatoid)
- **ch** is pronounced like a **k** when it is followed by another consonant (e.g., chromosome)

Pronouncing o, a, and aw
The see-and-say pronunciation guides use:
- "o" for the "short o" sound as in *hot* (e.g., biopsy = BY-op-see)
- "a" for the "short a" sound as in *bat* (e.g., acne = ACK-nee)
- "aw" for the "aw" sound as in *saw* (e.g., palsy = PAWL-zee)

By following these rules and practicing the terms in this book, you should develop a comfortable, intuitive sense of how medical terms are pronounced.

Components and Features

To get the most out of this text, please take a few minutes to familiarize yourself with the major components and instructional features described on the following pages.

Unit 1
Basics of Medical Terminology

Much of the information you'll learn in these chapters will be essential to your understanding of later chapters.

Chapter 1 teaches you an approach for analyzing medical terminology. This approach will give you a "system" for learning and remembering new medical terms.

Chapter 2 presents word elements commonly used in anatomy and physiology. These word elements appear in terms pertaining to many different body systems – learning them now will help you master a vast array of medical terms.

Chapter 3 presents word elements that relate specifically to pathology, diagnosis, and treatment. These word elements are the principle building blocks of terms used in clinical settings.

Unit 2
Medical Terminology Relating to Body Systems

The chapters in this unit present medical terms in a methodical, system-by-system fashion.

Most basic root words pertain to specific body systems, usually to a particular anatomic part. You will find these root words and their related medical terms most meaningful and memorable if you learn them in the context of the body system to which they pertain. To help you do this, we have organized the chapters of Unit 2 around specific body systems.

Throughout this book, you will find a number of instructional features designed to enhance your learning. These features, and related study tips, are described on the following pages.

1 Learning Objectives

Learning objectives tell you what you should be able to do after successfully completing a chapter. Use these to structure your study of the chapter and to measure your mastery of its contents.

Upon completing this chapter, you should be able to:

- Describe the nervous system and explain the primary functions of its two major divisions
- Recognize, build, pronounce, and spell words that pertain to the nervous system
- Describe diseases, diagnostic tests, and surgical procedures that pertain to the nervous system

Overview

The nervous system functions as the body's master control center, coordinating all of the body's conscious and unconscious responses to environmental stimuli. As such, the nervous system includes some components that are responsible for detecting and interpreting changes in the environment, and others that enable the body to generate an appropriate response. The nervous system is also responsible for discriminatory functions, such as thinking and feeling.

2 Chapter Overviews

Chapter overviews give you the "big picture," explaining the main functions of the body system discussed in the chapter. Use the overview as a preview: as you study the rest of the chapter, think about how the facts and concepts you are learning fit into the "big picture."

3 Word Element Tables

These tables present key word elements that you will need to know. Study these tables to memorize the key word elements listed. To help you memorize key word elements, we have organized them by function or subsystem and have included examples of their use.

 RESPIRATION — These combining forms refer to respiration or breathing, the process by which oxygen is transported from the air to the tissues.

CF	Meaning	Example
ox/o	oxygen	hyp*ox*emia = reduced oxygen level in the blood
respir/o	breathing	*respir*ation = process of breathing
spir/o	breathing	*spir*ometry = measurement of breathing

4 Medical Illustrations

Medical illustrations help bring to life the structures and functions you are reading about. As you read each chapter, refer to the illustrations to locate the structures being discussed – and to visualize the physiologic events being described. For additional reference, see the full-color anatomical plates.

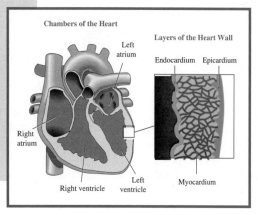

Chambers of the Heart

Layers of the Heart Wall

Left atrium

Endocardium Epicardium

Right atrium

Right ventricle Left ventricle

Myocardium

5 Word Elements

Word elements for many terms are called out in the margin. Reviewing these word elements as you read the text will help you associate specific word elements with their meanings. It will also help you to get a sense of how the word elements are used to build medical terms.

New Terms 6

New terms are highlighted in bold-faced letters and are defined within the text. Study these terms to assure that you feel comfortable with their meanings.

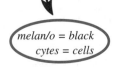

melan/o = black
cytes = cells

called the **basal** layer, consists of new and growing cells. In addition to squamous epithelial cells, the basal layer of the epidermis contains pigment-producing cells, called **melanocytes** (mel-LAN-no-sites). The pigment produced by these cells, called **melanin** (MEL-luh-nin), gives color to the skin. Unlike the dermis and subcutaneous tissue, the epidermis does not

7 See-and-Say Pronunciation Guides

These guides teach you how to pronounce new terms. The "see-and-say" approach is easier to use than the academic system you see in most dictionaries. For example, the pronunciation guide for **melanocytes** is mel-LAN-no-sites, which shows you exactly how to pronounce the word. In each term, the accented syllable is identified by capital letters. In terms with more than one accented syllable, the primary accent is identified by boldfaced capital letters and the secondary accent is identified by regular capital letters. For example, the pronunciation guide for **physiology** would be FIH-zee-**OL**-uh-jee.

Pathologic Conditions	Word Elements	Definition
tachycardia (TACK-ee-**KAR**-dee-uh)	tachy = rapid cardi = heart a = condition	abnormally rapid heart rate, usually defined as 100 or more beats per minute
thrombophlebitis (THROM-boe-fluh-**BIE**-tis)	thrombo = clot phleb = vein itis = inflammation	inflammation of a vein complicated by the formation of a blood clot within the vein
thrombosis (throm-BOE-sis)	thromb = clot osis = condition	condition in which a stationary blood clot obstructs a blood vessel at the site of its formation
valvulitis (VAL-vyoo-**LIE**-tis)	valvul = valve itis = inflammation	inflammation of a valve, particularly one of the valves within the heart

Terminology Tables 8

These tables present medical terms relevant to the body system under discussion. To help you learn these terms, we have divided them into categories: **pathologic conditions**, **diagnostic procedures**, and **therapeutic procedures**. We have also broken them down into their word elements so that you can learn to figure out their meanings without having to rely on memorization alone. Because it is not possible to introduce every term relating to every body system, these tables highlight the **key terms** that will be most useful in building your medical vocabulary; they are designed to help you become less reliant on a medical dictionary.

8. **Break Down and Define** the word elements within each of the following terms, and then define the term itself.

Example: a / mnesia   *without / memory*   *memory loss*

a. anesthesia

_____

b. electroencephalography

_____

c. meningitis

Exercises

Exercises within and at the end of the chapter allow you to practice applying the skills and information you've just learned and to monitor your own progress. Different types of exercises will reinforce different types of skills, including word analysis, word building, spelling, and so on. Be sure to work through all of the exercises in the chapter and review any concepts or terms with which you have trouble.

9

10 ## Audiocassette Exercises

Audiocassette exercises at the end of each Unit 2 chapter allow you to practice spelling key medical terms while you listen to their pronunciation on the audiotape cassettes that accompany this text. You can also use the audiotape cassettes to practice pronouncing the terms presented. Each term is followed by a pause for this purpose.

Listen to the section on your audiotape cassette that corresponds to this chapter and write the terms below. Be careful to spell each term correctly.

1. _____   6. _____
2. _____   7. _____
3. _____   8. _____
4. _____   9. _____
5. _____   10. _____

11 ## Appendices A-E

Appendices are located at the end of this book They provide additional information and reference tools essential to your training in medical terminology.

Body System	Class	Therapeutic Action
CARDIOVASCULAR	**anti-anginals** (beta blockers, calcium channel blockers, nitrates, vasodilators)	improve blood flow through the heart to alleviate angina
	anti-arrhythmics (beta blockers, calcium channel blockers, cardiac glycosides, quinidines)	restore normal heart rhythms by altering cardiac conduction or the heart's response to electrical impulses
	antihyperlipidemics	reduce cholesterol levels

A: *Pharmacology* – a glossary of pharmacologic terms that you are likely to hear in healthcare settings.

B: *Physicians and Allied Health Professionals* – a list of the major types of healthcare specialists and brief explanations of what they do.

C: *Abbreviations by Body System* – a list of commonly used medical abbreviations organized by body system.

D: *Alphabetical Abbreviations* – a list of the Appendix C abbreviations, as well as many additional medical abbreviations, in alphabetical order.

E: *Glossary of Word Elements* – an alphabetical, dictionary-style listing of the word elements presented throughout this book.

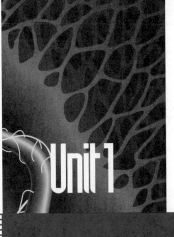

Unit 1

Basics of Medical Terminology

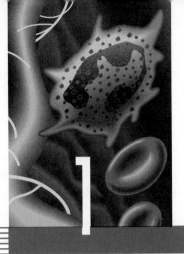

Principles of Word Building

Upon completing this chapter, you should be able to:

- Identify the three basic word elements used to build medical terms
- Explain the difference between a root word and a combining form
- Recognize when and when not to use combining vowels
- Explain how suffixes and prefixes are used to modify root words

Word Elements

Most medical terms can be broken down into two or more components or **word elements**. This text teaches you how to use this fact to your advantage, providing you with a basic approach for understanding unfamiliar medical terms. To define an unfamiliar term, you will simply:

1. identify its word elements,
2. analyze the meaning of each word element, and
3. put the meanings of all of the word elements together to define the word as a whole.

In order to use this approach, you will need to be familiar with the three basic types of word elements: root words, suffixes, and prefixes.

Root Words

The central meaning of a term is conveyed by a word element called the **root word**. It is the foundation to which other word elements are added to build a complete, meaningful word. All terms have at least one root word.

When being connected to other word elements, root words are converted into **combining forms**. A combining form is a root word to which a **combining vowel** has been added in order to link the root to a second root word or to a suffix. The most common combining vowel is **o**. Combining forms are typically represented by the root word, followed by a slash (/), followed by the combining vowel. Throughout this text, you will see combining forms represented in this way.

In medical terminology, root words (and their associated combining forms) usually refer to anatomic structures or physiologic concepts. Memorizing just a few will enable you to understand a wide variety of medical terms. Examples of combining forms for some common root words are listed in the table below.

Root Word	+	Combining Form	Meaning
cardi	o	cardi/o	heart
vascul	o	vascul/o	blood vessels
immun	o	immun/o	immunity
respir	o	respir/o	breathing
ren	o	ren/o	kidney
nephr	o	nephr/o	kidney
arthr	o	arthr/o	joint

NOTE: Most root words are derived from the Greek or Latin. Because of this dual origin, some anatomic structures are associated with two or more root words. For example, the roots **ren** and **nephr** both refer to the kidneys. In general, roots that refer to body organs originated from Latin words, while roots used in terms pertaining to organ disease are typically derived from the Greek. Thus, the Latin root **ren** is mainly used in anatomic terms, while the Greek root **nephr** is mainly used in terms related to kidney disease.

To form meaningful words, root words (or their combining forms) are combined with other word elements, such as suffixes.

Suffixes

A **suffix** is a word element added *after* a root word to modify the basic meaning of the word. To illustrate, let's look at a familiar medical term, cardiology. This term can be broken down into two word elements:

cardi/o = heart   **logy** = study of
combining form   *suffix*

The first word element is a combining form, **cardi/o**, which means *heart*. Note that **cardi/o** consists of a root word (**cardi**) to which a combining vowel (**o**) has been added in order to link it to a suffix that modifies its basic meaning. The suffix is **logy**, which means *study of*. Thus, **cardiology** is the *study of the heart*.

Let's look at another example, cardiac. This term can also be broken down into two word elements:

cardi = heart   **ac** = pertaining to
root word   *suffix*

The root word **cardi** means *heart*.
The suffix **ac** means *pertaining to*.
Cardiac is an adjective meaning *pertaining to the heart*.

Note that root word **cardi** is used rather than the combining form **cardi/o**. **Cardi** is connected *directly* to the suffix without a combining vowel because the suffix **ac** begins with a vowel rather than a consonant. In general, the combining vowel is added *only* when linking a root word to a suffix that begins with a consonant. When linking a root word to a suffix that begins with a vowel, the combining vowel is dropped. Thus, the correct term is cardiac, not cardioac.

Another example of this rule can be found in the term vasculitis.

vascul = blood vessels   **itis** = inflammation
root word   *suffix*

The suffix **itis** means *inflammation*. Because it begins with a vowel, the root word **vascul** is used rather than the combining form **vascul/o**. Thus, the correct term is vasculitis, which means *inflammation of the blood vessels*.

Many medical terms contain more than one combining form or root word linked to a suffix. For example, the term cardiovascular is composed of three word elements:

cardi/o = heart   **vascul** = blood vessels   **ar** = pertaining to
combining form   *root word*   *suffix*

As the breakdown above suggests, the term **cardiovascular** means *pertaining to the heart and blood vessels*. As you might expect, the first root word (**cardi**) is linked to the second root word (**vascul**) by a combining vowel (**o**). As in the previous two examples, however, **vascul** is connected to the suffix without a combining vowel, since the suffix **ar** begins with a vowel.

You should keep in mind that the rules for linking one root word to another are slightly different from the rules for linking root words to suffixes. Whereas the combining vowel is dropped when linking a root word to a suffix that begins with a vowel, the combining vowel is *always* used to link one root word to another, regardless of whether the second root begins with a vowel or a consonant. For example, consider the term cardioaortic.

cardi/o = heart   **aort** = aorta   **ic** = pertaining to
combining form   *root word*   *suffix*

As you can see, the combining vowel is used to link **cardi** to the second root word, even though the root **aort** begins with a vowel. A combining vowel is not used, however, to connect the root **aort** to the suffix, since the suffix **ic** begins with a vowel. Thus, the correct term is cardioaortic, not cardiaortic or cardioaortoic. The term means *pertaining to the heart and aorta*.

Prefixes

Virtually all medical terms contain root words and suffixes. Many contain **prefixes** as well. A prefix is a word element added *in front of* the root(s) to modify the basic meaning of the word.

For example, consider the term bradycardia.

brady = slow   **cardi** = heart   **a** = condition
prefix   *root word*   *suffix*

Bradycardia literally means *slow heart condition*; it is used to describe a condition characterized by a slow heartbeat.

Substituting one prefix for another can dramatically change the meaning of a term. For example, let's replace the prefix **brady** with the prefix **tachy**.

The term tachycardia is broken down as follows:

tachy = fast   **cardi** = heart   **a** = condition
prefix   *root word*   *suffix*

The prefix **tachy** means *fast*. The rest of the term is unchanged. Thus, **tachycardia** literally means *fast heart condition*, or a condition characterized by a fast heartbeat – the opposite of bradycardia.

Deciphering New Medical Terms

The three word elements we've discussed – root words, suffixes, and prefixes – are the basic building blocks of medical terms. After you learn the word elements most commonly used in medicine, you'll recognize them even in new combinations. This recognition will make it easier for you to understand new medical terms that you encounter in your work.

For example, the root word **cardi** appears in hundreds of medical terms pertaining to the heart: e.g., *cardiac, cardiovascular, cardiologist, cardiogenic,* and *cardiomyopathy.* Similarly, the suffix **logy** can be combined with a vast number of root words to describe the study of many different topics: e.g., *hematology, pulmonology, endocrinology,* and so forth.

Using the approach described in this chapter will enable you to break down and define even terms that look very intimidating. For example, consider the terms **electrocardiography** and **pericardiocentesis**.

electr/o = electrical   **cardi/o** = heart   **graphy** = recording
combining form   *combining form*   *suffix*

peri = surrounding   **cardi/o** = heart   **centesis** = puncture
prefix   *combining form*   *suffix*

Once you learn the common word elements that are presented in Chapters 2 and 3, you can easily figure out that electrocardiography is a procedure in which the electrical activity of the heart is recorded, while pericardiocentesis is a procedure in which the tissue (membrane) surrounding the heart is punctured with a needle. At this point, you will be well on your way to mastering medical terminology.

Review Exercises

1. **Match** the following.

    _b_   a word element added to the beginning of a word to modify its meaning

    _c_   a word element added to the end of a word to modify its meaning

    _a_   the foundation that conveys the basic meaning of a term

    _d_   a letter added to link two roots together or a root to a suffix that begins with a consonant

    a. root word

    b. prefix

    c. suffix

    d. combining vowel

2. **Break Down** each of the following terms into its word elements. As in the example below, draw a slash between the letters to indicate where you think the word should be divided, then identify each word element using the following abbreviations: RW = root word, CV = combining vowel, P = prefix, and S = suffix.

    Next to your breakdown, write a definition for the term. Feel free to refer to the table of root words and combining forms on page 4.

    Example: cardi / o / logy   *RW / CV / S*   *study of the heart*

    a. vascul|itis

    _____

    b. brady|cardia

    _____

    c. cardi|o|vascular

    _____

    d. immun|o|logy

    _____

    e. nephr|itis

    _____

    f. arthr|itis

    _____

3. **Fill in the blank.** The most common combining vowel is

_____ *o* _____.

4. **Circle** the choices that make each statement true.

   a. When combining two root words, (drop/keep) the combining vowel of the first root regardless of whether or not the second root begins with a vowel.

   b. When linking a root word to a suffix that begins with a vowel, (drop/keep) the combining vowel.

   c. When linking a root word to a suffix that begins with a consonant, (drop/keep) the combining vowel.

5. **Build** medical terms from the root words and suffixes provided. Using the rules listed in the previous exercise, you should be able to build these terms even though you do not yet know what they mean.

   Example: bronch + spasm (root word + suffix) *broncho / spasm*

   a. nephr + toxic
      (root word + suffix) _nephro / toxic_

   b. nephr + itis
      (root word + suffix) _nephr / itis_

   c. pyel + nephr + itis
      (root word + root word + suffix) _pyelo / nephr / itis_

   d. laryng + ectomy
      (root word + suffix) _laryng / ectomy_

   e. laryng + scopy
      (root word + suffix) _laryngo / scopy_

   f. oto + laryng + logy
      (root word + root word + suffix) _oto / laryngo / logy_

Answers to all review exercises can be found in the Answer Key, which begins on page 348.

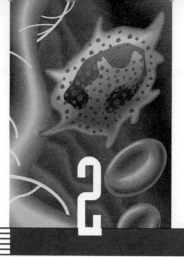

Word Elements Related to Anatomy and Physiology

Upon completing this chapter, you should be able to recognize and define the following word elements related to anatomy and physiology:

- Suffixes commonly used to form nouns
- Suffixes commonly used to form adjectives
- Suffixes commonly used to create singular and plural forms
- Prefixes commonly used to denote number or quantity
- Prefixes commonly used to describe normal function
- Prefixes commonly used to denote direction or location

Overview   As you study medical terminology, you will find that certain word elements can be applied to a wide range of anatomic structures and physiologic concepts, and are therefore present in a wide range of medical terms. For your convenience, we have gathered together the most common of these word elements in this chapter. If you learn these common word elements now, you will have a head start in being able to analyze and understand a vast array of medical terms.

To help you assimilate all of the word elements presented in this chapter, we have grouped them into categories by topic or meaning. We have also provided examples of medical terms in which they are used. In addition to studying the word elements themselves, pay attention to the use of combining vowels in these examples. This will help you not only remember the word elements, but also understand how they are combined to form meaningful words.

Many common root words, suffixes, and prefixes are related specifically to pathologic conditions, diagnostic techniques, and therapeutic or surgical procedures. These word elements are listed in the next chapter.

Common
Suffixes

As you may recall, a **suffix** is a word element added *after* one or more root words to modify the meaning of the root(s) and create a meaningful word. The suffixes most commonly used in medical terminology are presented in the tables below.

Suffixes Commonly Used to Form Nouns

The following suffixes are often added to root words to create nouns.

Suffix	Meaning	Example	Definition
-ation	process	vaccin*ation*	process of vaccinating (vaccin/o)
-blast	immature cell	osteo*blast*	immature bone (oste/o) cell
-cyte	cell	hepato*cyte*	liver (hepat/o) cell
-globin	protein	hemo*globin*	a blood (hem/o) protein
-is	forms noun from root word	derm*is*	middle layer of the skin (derm/o)
-ist	specialist	cardiolog*ist*	specialist in the study (log/o) of the heart (cardi/o)
-logy	study of	cardio*logy*	study of the heart (cardi/o)
-um	thing; structure	myocardi*um*	the structure formed by the muscle (my/o) tissue in the heart (cardi/o)

Suffixes Commonly Used to Form Adjectives

The following suffixes can be added to root words to create adjectives. You will probably recognize many of these suffixes, since they are used to create adjectives from non-medical as well as medical root words.

Suffix	Meaning	Example	Definition
-ac	pertaining to	cardi*ac*	pertaining to the heart (cardi/o)
-al	pertaining to	nas*al*	pertaining to the nose (nas/o)
-ar	pertaining to	muscul*ar*	pertaining to muscle (muscul/o)
-ary	pertaining to	pulmon*ary*	pertaining to the lungs (pulmon/o)
-ated	subjected to; having	myelin*ated*	having been covered with a myelin sheath (myelin/o)
-genic	producing	carcino*genic*	producing cancer (carcin/o)
-ic	pertaining to	gastr*ic*	pertaining to the stomach (gastr/o)
-ical	pertaining to	neurolog*ical*	pertaining to the study (log/o) of nerves (neur/o)
-ile	pertaining to	pen*ile*	pertaining to the penis (pen/o)
-ior	pertaining to	anter*ior*	pertaining to the front (anter/o)
-oid	resembling	muc*oid*	resembling mucus (muc/o)
-ory	pertaining to	audit*ory*	pertaining to sound (audit/o)
-ose	having the qualities of	varic*ose*	having the qualities of a twisted vein (varic/o)
-ous	pertaining to	ven*ous*	pertaining to a vein (ven/o)

Suffixes Commonly Used to Create Singular and Plural Forms

Because of their Greek or Latin origin, some medical terms use somewhat strange-looking singular and plural suffixes. Once you learn just a few of these forms, however, these terms will not seem intimidating.

Suffix (sing.)	Suffix (pl.)	Example
-a	-ae	vertebr*a* → vertebr*ae*
-en	-ina	lum*en* → lum*ina*
-is	-es	diagnos*is* → diagnos*es*
-nx	-nges	salpi*nx* → salpi*nges*
-on	-a	gangli*on* → gangli*a*
-um	-a	bacteri*um* → bacteri*a*
-us	-i	bronch*us* → bronch*i*
-x	-ces	appendi*x* → appendi*ces*

ex   ices

Review Exercises

1. **Match** the following suffixes with their definitions.

___d___ -globin   a. thing; structure

___f___ -logy   b. immature cell

___b___ -blast   c. cell

___a___ -um   d. protein

___e___ -ist   e. specialist

___c___ -cyte   f. study of

2. **Identify and Define** the four suffixes in this group that do NOT mean "pertaining to."

-ac	-genic	-oid	-al	-ic	-ous	-ar
-ical	-ory	-ary	-ile	-ose	-ated	-ior

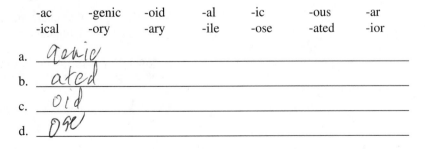

a. ___genic___

b. ___ated___

c. ___oid___

d. ___ose___

3. ***Convert*** each of the following from its singular to its plural form, using your knowledge of singular and plural suffixes.

a. conjunctiv*a* → *conjunctivae*

b. test*is* → *testes*

c. ov*um* → *ova*

d. alveol*us* → *alveoli*

As you learned in Chapter 1, a **prefix** is a word element added *before* one or more root words to modify the meaning of the root(s) and create a new word. Prefixes commonly used in terms related to anatomy and physiology are presented in the tables below.

Prefixes Commonly Used to Denote Number or Quantity

The following prefixes are commonly used to denote the number or quantity of anatomic structures or physiologic processes present. As you will see, they can be found in a wide variety of medical terms.

Prefix	Meaning	Example	Definition
bi-	two	*bi*ceps muscle	a muscle having two "heads" (-ceps)
di-	two	*di*arthric	pertaining to (-ic) two joints (arthr/o)
hemi-	one-half	*hemi*plegia	partial paralysis (-plegia) of one-half of the body, the right half or left half
mono-	one; single	*mono*nuclear	pertaining to (-ar) a cell having one nucleus (nucle/o)
multi-	many	*multi*gravida	a woman who has been pregnant (-gravida) more than once
nulli-	none	*nulli*para	a woman who has given birth (-para) to no living children
poly-	many	*poly*mor-phonuclear	pertaining to (-ar) having a nucleus (nucle/o) with many shapes (morph/o)
quadri-	four	*quadri*ceps muscle	a muscle having four "heads" (-ceps)

Prefix	Meaning	Example	Definition
semi-	one-half; partly	*semi*lunar valve	a valve resembling (-ar) a half moon (lun/o)
tri-	three	*tri*cuspid valve	a valve consisting of three pointed or tapered shapes (-cuspid)
uni-	one	*uni*lateral	pertaining to (-al) one side (later/o)

Prefixes Commonly Used to Describe Normal Function

The following prefixes are commonly used to describe normal anatomic structures and physiologic processes. As you will see, some of these prefixes are used to indicate normal functioning of a particular organ, while others are used to compare two or more structures or processes.

Prefix	Meaning	Example	Definition
eu-	good; normal	*eu*thyroid	having a normally functioning thyroid gland (-thyroid)
hetero-	different	*hetero*morphic	pertaining to (-ic) a different shape (morph/o)
homeo-	unchanging; same	*homeo*stasis	maintenance of an unchanging state (-stasis) or internal environment in the body
homo-	same	*homo*topic	pertaining to (-ic) the same place (top/o) on the body
iso-	equal; same	*iso*morphic	pertaining to (-ic) the same shape (morph/o)
normo-	normal	*normo*tension	normal blood pressure (-tension)

Prefixes Commonly Used to Denote Direction or Location in Time or Space

In anatomy and physiology, the location of one anatomic structure is typically described by comparing its position to that of another structure; similarly, the timing of one physiologic process is often described in comparison to the occurrence of another. The prefixes listed below are commonly used for this purpose and are found in numerous terms pertaining to anatomy and physiology.

Prefix	Meaning	Example	Definition
ab-	away from	*ab*ductor	a muscle that draws a limb (-ductor) away from the body
ad-	toward; near	*ad*renal	pertaining to (-al) a structure located near the kidney (ren/o)
ante-	before (in time); forward	*ante*version	forward tilting or turning (-version) of an organ from its usual position
contra-	against; opposite side	*contra*lateral	pertaining to (-al) something on the opposite side (later/o) of the body
dia-	through	*dia*rrhea	discharge (-rrhea) of abundant, watery feces through the anus
dis-	apart; away from	*dis*locate	to move (-locate) a structure away from its usual position, as in dislocating a bone from its joint
ec-	out; away from	*ec*topic	pertaining to (-ic) a structure out of place (top/o)
em-	in; inside	*em*pyema	a condition (-ema) characterized by the presence of pus (py/o) inside a body cavity, usually the chest cavity
en-	in; surrounded by	*en*demic	pertaining to (-ic) something that occurs in people (dem/o) in a particular geographic region
endo-	inside; within	*endo*metrium	the structure or tissue (-um) lining the inside of the uterus (metri/o)
epi-	on; over; above; outer	*epi*dermis	noun (-is) signifying the outer layer of skin (derm/o)
ex-	out; away from	*ex*hale	to breathe (-hale) out
exo-	outside	*exo*crine	secreting (-crine) to the outside surface of an organ rather than into the blood
hypo-	under	*hypo*thalamus	the gland located under the thalamus gland (-thalamus)
inter-	between; among	*inter*stitial	pertaining to (-al) the space (stiti/o) between tissue cells

Prefix	Meaning	Example	Definition
intra-	within; inside	*intra*venous	pertaining to (-ous) a process occurring inside a vein (ven/o)
ipsi-	same; same side	*ipsi*lateral	pertaining to (-al) something on the same side (later/o) of the body
para-	beside; beyond	*para*thyroid glands	the glands located beside the thyroid gland (-thyroid)
per-	through	*per*cutaneous	pertaining to (-ous) a process occurring through the skin (cutane/o)
peri-	around; surrounding	*peri*cardium	the structure or tissue (-um) that surrounds the heart (cardi/o)
post-	after (in time or place)	*post*partum	after labor or childbirth (-partum)
pre-	before (in time or place)	*pre*natal	pertaining to (-al) the time before birth (nat/o)
primi-	first	*primi*gravida	a woman who is pregnant (-gravida) for the first time
pro-	before (in time); in front of	*pro*lapse	sinking (-lapse) of an organ to a location in front of its usual position
retro-	backward; behind	*retro*version	backward tilting or turning (-version) of an organ from its usual position
sub-	under; beneath	*sub*cutaneous	pertaining to (-ous) a process occurring below the skin (cutane/o)
trans-	through; across	*trans*urethral	pertaining to (-al) a process occurring through the urethra (urethr/o)

Review Exercises

4. **Match** the following prefixes with the numbers or quantities they represent.

_d_	bi-	a.	none
_b_	hemi-	b.	one-half
_a_	nulli-	c.	one
_g_	poly-	d.	two
____	quadri-	e.	three
_e_	tri-	f.	four
_c_	uni-	g.	many

5. **Define** the prefixes in the following terms to complete their definitions.

   a. *Hetero*geneous means having ___different___ qualities or ingredients throughout.

   b. *Homo*geneous means having ___the same___ qualities or ingredients throughout.

   c. *Normo*topic refers to a structure that is located in its ___normal___ position.

   d. *Eu*trophic means pertaining to ___good___ nourishment or support.

   e. A *mono*cyte is a type of cell that has ___one___ nucleus.

   f. *Di*plopia is a condition of the eye characterized by ___double___ vision.

   g. *Multi*nodular refers to having ___many___ nodules.

   h. The *semi*circular canals in the ear are canals having the shape of ___one half___ circles.

   i. A *homeo*graft is a transplant from an organ donor who is of the ___same___ species as the transplant recipient.

   j. Two people who are *iso*geneic have the ___same___ genetic makeup.

6. **Match** the following prefixes with the locations they represent.

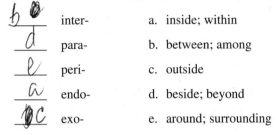

b inter-   a. inside; within

d para-   b. between; among

e peri-   c. outside

a endo-   d. beside; beyond

c exo-   e. around; surrounding

7. **List** the three directional prefixes meaning "through" that are used to describe substances or things passing through anatomic structures.

a. _per_

b. _trans_

c. _dia_

8. **Circle** the choices that will make each statement true.

a. An *ad*ductor is a muscle that draws a limb (away from/(toward)) the body.

b. *Ante*partum refers to events occurring ((before)/after) labor and childbirth.

c. *Hypo*dermic means pertaining to a process occurring (above/(under)) the skin.

d. *Intra*abdominal refers to structures ((inside)/outside) the abdomen.

e. *Post*operative refers to events occurring (before/(after)) a surgical operation.

f. *Pre*menstrual refers to events occurring ((before)/after) menstruation.

g. The *epi*cardium is the (inner/(outer)) layer of the heart.

h. The *sub*dural space is the space (above/(beneath)) the dura mater.

i. *Retro*grade urine flow is the ((backward)/forward) flow of urine.

9. **Define** the following prefixes.

a. pro-   _in front of_

b. ex-   _out_

c. ab-   _away from_

d. en- _in_

e. contra- _against_

f. primi- _first_

g. ipsi- _same_

h. ec- _out_

i. dis- _apart, away from_

j. em- _in, inside_

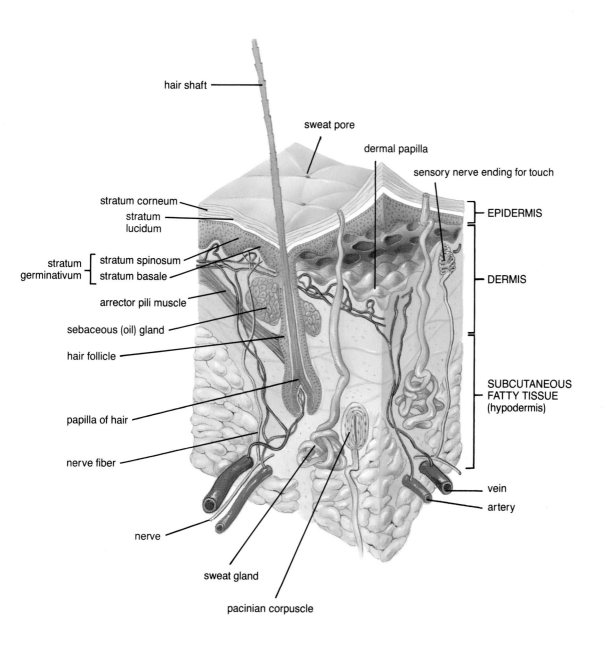

hair shaft

sweat pore

dermal papilla

sensory nerve ending for touch

stratum corneum

stratum lucidum

EPIDERMIS

stratum germinativum
- stratum spinosum
- stratum basale

DERMIS

arrector pili muscle

sebaceous (oil) gland

hair follicle

papilla of hair

SUBCUTANEOUS FATTY TISSUE (hypodermis)

nerve fiber

vein

artery

nerve

sweat gland

pacinian corpuscle

Plate 1 Cross Section of Skin

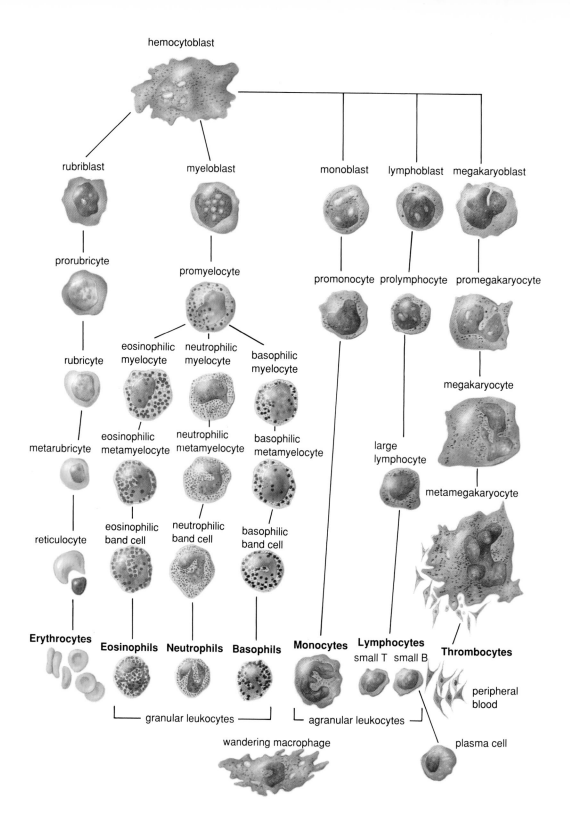

hemocytoblast

rubriblast

prorubricyte

rubricyte

metarubricyte

reticulocyte

Erythrocytes

myeloblast

promyelocyte

eosinophilic myelocyte

neutrophilic myelocyte

basophilic myelocyte

eosinophilic metamyelocyte

neutrophilic metamyelocyte

basophilic metamyelocyte

eosinophilic band cell

neutrophilic band cell

basophilic band cell

Eosinophils   **Neutrophils**   **Basophils**

granular leukocytes

wandering macrophage

monoblast

lymphoblast

megakaryoblast

promonocyte

prolymphocyte

promegakaryocyte

megakaryocyte

large lymphocyte

metamegakaryocyte

Monocytes   **Lymphocytes**

small T   small B

Thrombocytes

peripheral blood

agranular leukocytes

plasma cell

Plate 2 Blood Cells and Platelets

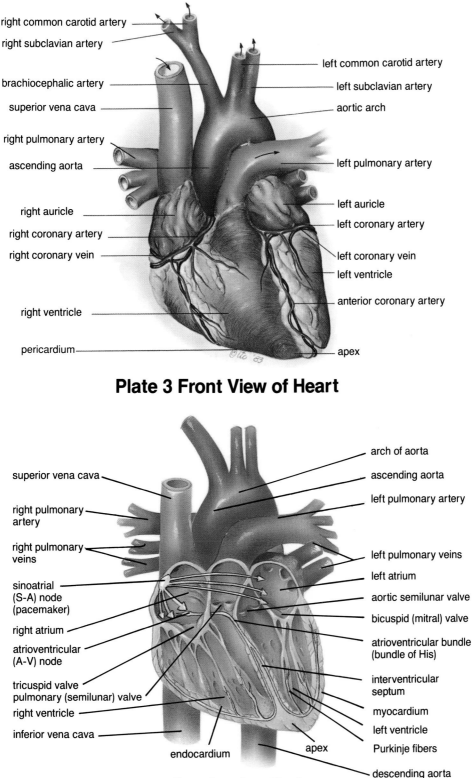

right common carotid artery

right subclavian artery

brachiocephalic artery

superior vena cava

right pulmonary artery

ascending aorta

right auricle

right coronary artery

right coronary vein

right ventricle

pericardium

left common carotid artery

left subclavian artery

aortic arch

left pulmonary artery

left auricle

left coronary artery

left coronary vein

left ventricle

anterior coronary artery

apex

Plate 3 Front View of Heart

superior vena cava

right pulmonary artery

right pulmonary veins

sinoatrial (S-A) node (pacemaker)

right atrium

atrioventricular (A-V) node

tricuspid valve

pulmonary (semilunar) valve

right ventricle

inferior vena cava

endocardium

apex

arch of aorta

ascending aorta

left pulmonary artery

left pulmonary veins

left atrium

aortic semilunar valve

bicuspid (mitral) valve

atrioventricular bundle (bundle of His)

interventricular septum

myocardium

left ventricle

Purkinje fibers

descending aorta

Plate 4 Conductive Pathways

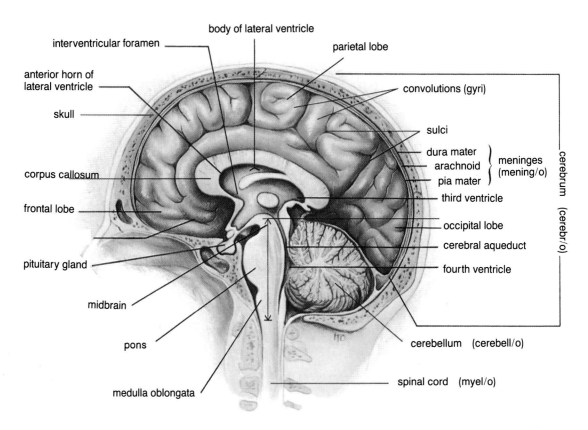

body of lateral ventricle

interventricular foramen

parietal lobe

anterior horn of lateral ventricle

convolutions (gyri)

skull

sulci

dura mater
arachnoid
pia mater
} meninges (mening/o)

corpus callosum

third ventricle

frontal lobe

occipital lobe

cerebral aqueduct

pituitary gland

fourth ventricle

midbrain

pons

cerebellum (cerebell/o)

medulla oblongata

spinal cord (myel/o)

cerebrum (cerebr/o)

Plate 5A Section of Brain

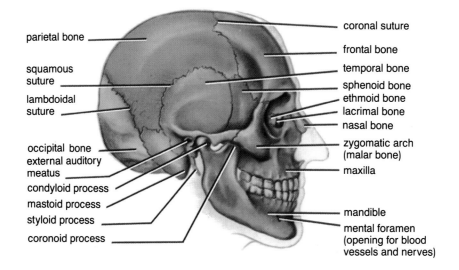

parietal bone

coronal suture

frontal bone

squamous suture

temporal bone

sphenoid bone

lambdoidal suture

ethmoid bone

lacrimal bone

nasal bone

occipital bone

zygomatic arch (malar bone)

external auditory meatus

maxilla

condyloid process

mastoid process

styloid process

mandible

coronoid process

mental foramen (opening for blood vessels and nerves)

Plate 5B Lateral View of Cranium

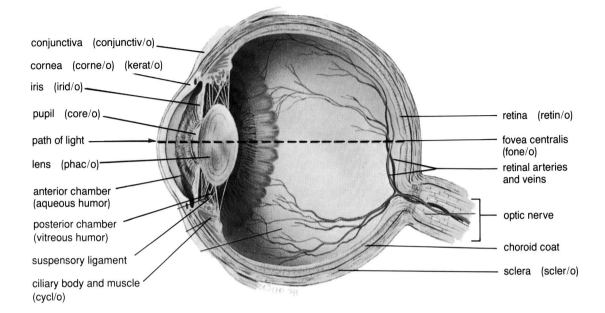

conjunctiva (conjunctiv/o)

cornea (corne/o) (kerat/o)

iris (irid/o)

pupil (core/o)

path of light

lens (phac/o)

anterior chamber
(aqueous humor)

posterior chamber
(vitreous humor)

suspensory ligament

ciliary body and muscle
(cycl/o)

retina (retin/o)

fovea centralis
(fone/o)

retinal arteries
and veins

optic nerve

choroid coat

sclera (scler/o)

Plate 6A Eye Structure

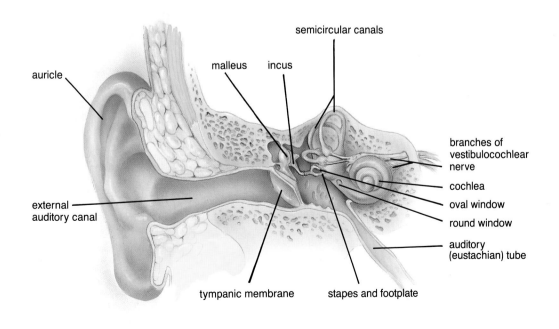

semicircular canals

malleus   incus

auricle

branches of
vestibulocochlear
nerve

cochlea

external
auditory canal

oval window

round window

auditory
(eustachian) tube

tympanic membrane   stapes and footplate

Plate 6B Ear Structure

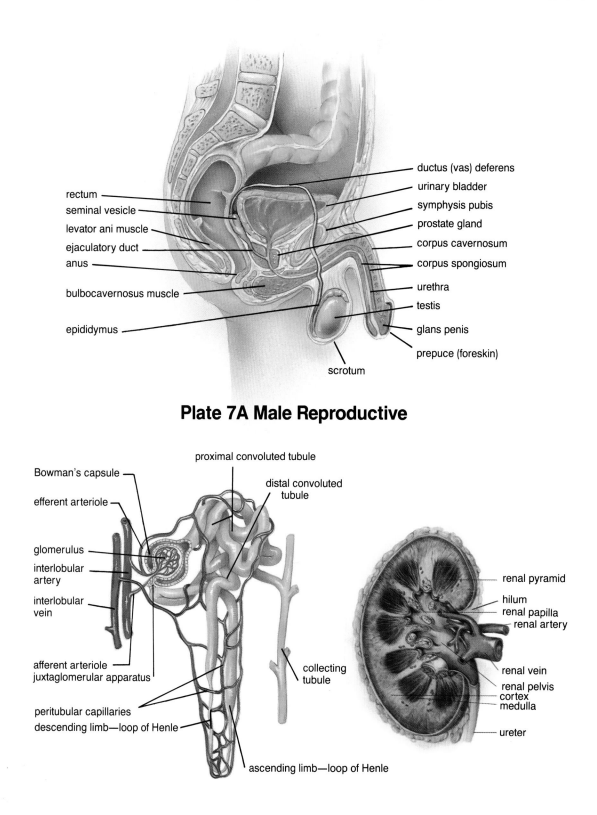

Plate 7A Male Reproductive

rectum
seminal vesicle
levator ani muscle
ejaculatory duct
anus
bulbocavernosus muscle
epididymus
scrotum

ductus (vas) deferens
urinary bladder
symphysis pubis
prostate gland
corpus cavernosum
corpus spongiosum
urethra
testis
glans penis
prepuce (foreskin)

Bowman's capsule
efferent arteriole
glomerulus
interlobular artery
interlobular vein
afferent arteriole
juxtaglomerular apparatus
peritubular capillaries
descending limb—loop of Henle

proximal convoluted tubule
distal convoluted tubule
collecting tubule
ascending limb—loop of Henle

renal pyramid
hilum
renal papilla
renal artery
renal vein
renal pelvis
cortex
medulla
ureter

Plate 7B Nephron and Cross Section of Kidney

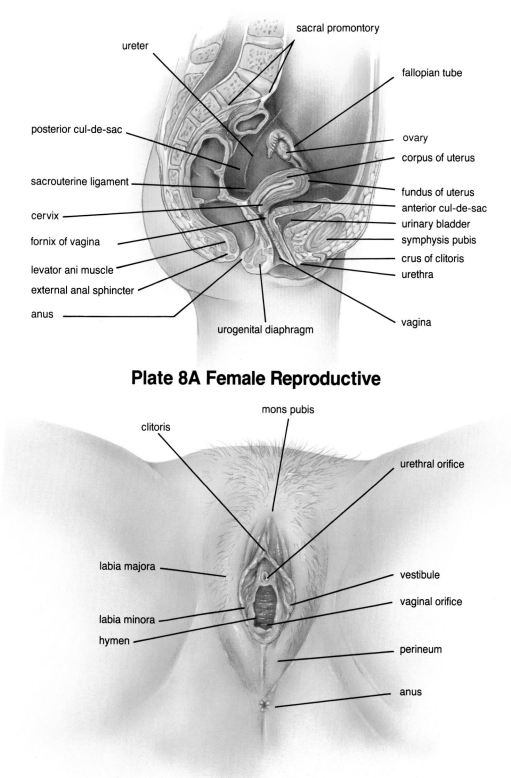

Plate 8A Female Reproductive

Plate 8B Female External Genitalia

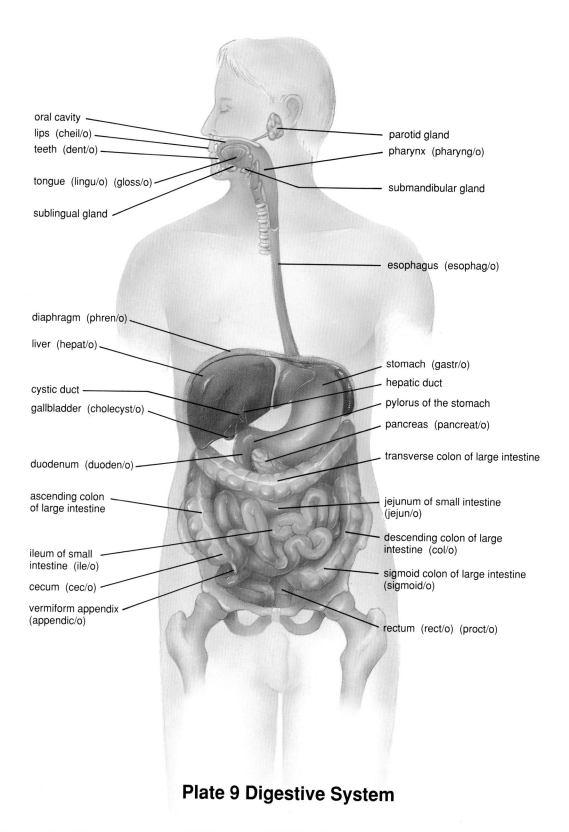

oral cavity

lips (cheil/o)

teeth (dent/o)

tongue (lingu/o) (gloss/o)

sublingual gland

parotid gland

pharynx (pharyng/o)

submandibular gland

esophagus (esophag/o)

diaphragm (phren/o)

liver (hepat/o)

cystic duct

gallbladder (cholecyst/o)

duodenum (duoden/o)

ascending colon
of large intestine

ileum of small
intestine (ile/o)

cecum (cec/o)

vermiform appendix
(appendic/o)

stomach (gastr/o)

hepatic duct

pylorus of the stomach

pancreas (pancreat/o)

transverse colon of large intestine

jejunum of small intestine
(jejun/o)

descending colon of large
intestine (col/o)

sigmoid colon of large intestine
(sigmoid/o)

rectum (rect/o) (proct/o)

Plate 9 Digestive System

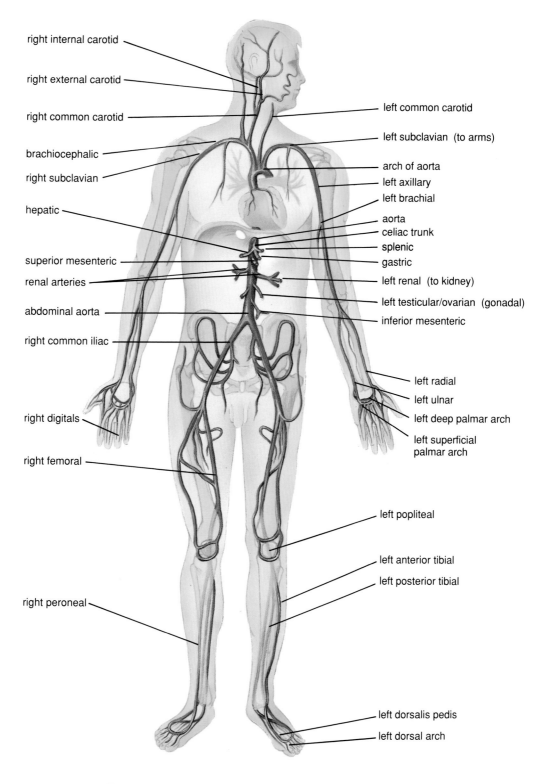

right internal carotid

right external carotid

right common carotid

brachiocephalic

right subclavian

hepatic

superior mesenteric

renal arteries

abdominal aorta

right common iliac

right digitals

right femoral

right peroneal

left common carotid

left subclavian (to arms)

arch of aorta

left axillary

left brachial

aorta

celiac trunk

splenic

gastric

left renal (to kidney)

left testicular/ovarian (gonadal)

inferior mesenteric

left radial

left ulnar

left deep palmar arch

left superficial
palmar arch

left popliteal

left anterior tibial

left posterior tibial

left dorsalis pedis

left dorsal arch

Plate 10A Arterial Distribution

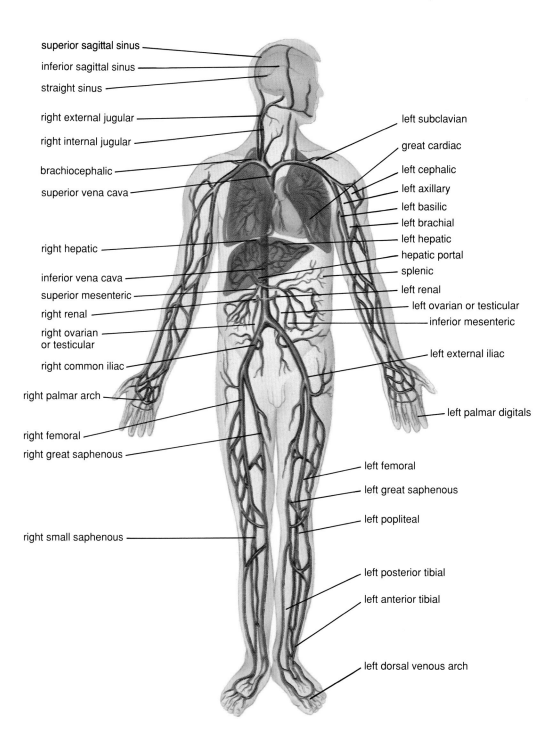

superior sagittal sinus

inferior sagittal sinus

straight sinus

right external jugular

right internal jugular

brachiocephalic

superior vena cava

right hepatic

inferior vena cava

superior mesenteric

right renal

right ovarian
or testicular

right common iliac

right palmar arch

right femoral

right great saphenous

right small saphenous

left subclavian

great cardiac

left cephalic

left axillary

left basilic

left brachial

left hepatic

hepatic portal

splenic

left renal

left ovarian or testicular

inferior mesenteric

left external iliac

left palmar digitals

left femoral

left great saphenous

left popliteal

left posterior tibial

left anterior tibial

left dorsal venous arch

Plate 10B Venous Distribution

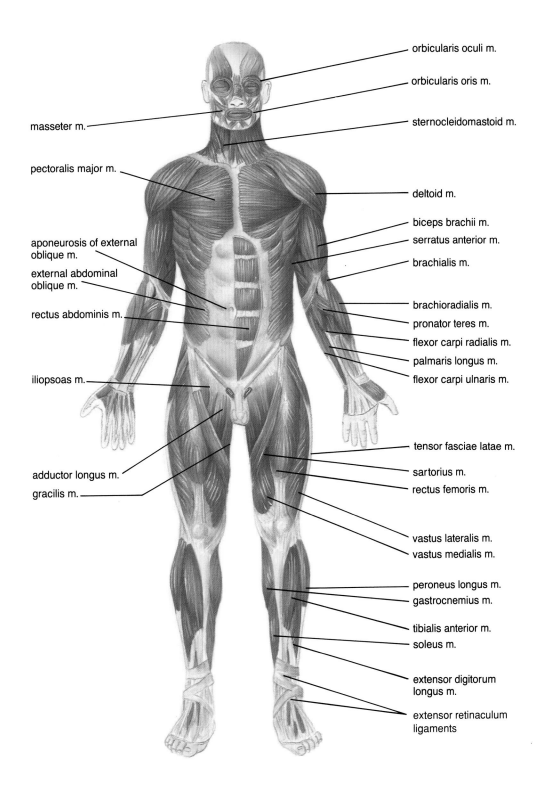

orbicularis oculi m.

orbicularis oris m.

sternocleidomastoid m.

masseter m.

pectoralis major m.

deltoid m.

biceps brachii m.

serratus anterior m.

brachialis m.

aponeurosis of external oblique m.

external abdominal oblique m.

brachioradialis m.

pronator teres m.

flexor carpi radialis m.

rectus abdominis m.

palmaris longus m.

flexor carpi ulnaris m.

iliopsoas m.

tensor fasciae latae m.

sartorius m.

rectus femoris m.

adductor longus m.

gracilis m.

vastus lateralis m.

vastus medialis m.

peroneus longus m.

gastrocnemius m.

tibialis anterior m.

soleus m.

extensor digitorum longus m.

extensor retinaculum ligaments

Plate 11A Muscular System, Anterior

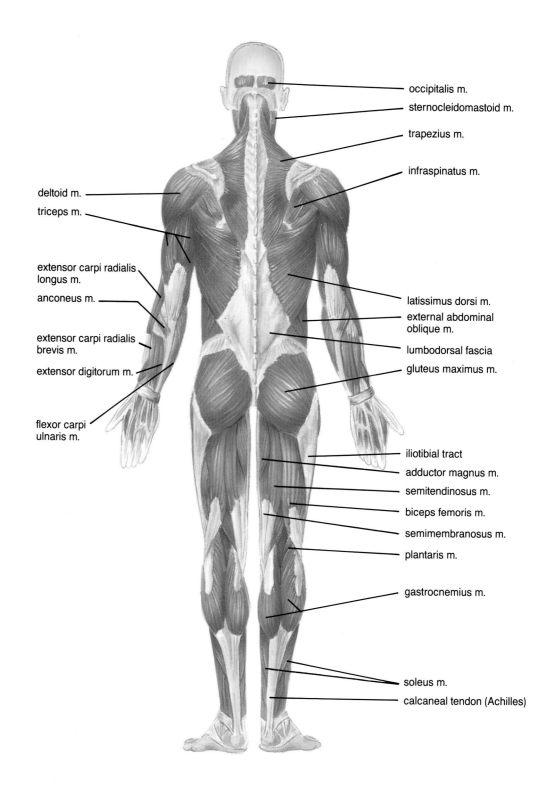

occipitalis m.

sternocleidomastoid m.

trapezius m.

infraspinatus m.

deltoid m.

triceps m.

extensor carpi radialis
longus m.

anconeus m.

extensor carpi radialis
brevis m.

extensor digitorum m.

flexor carpi
ulnaris m.

latissimus dorsi m.

external abdominal
oblique m.

lumbodorsal fascia

gluteus maximus m.

iliotibial tract

adductor magnus m.

semitendinosus m.

biceps femoris m.

semimembranosus m.

plantaris m.

gastrocnemius m.

soleus m.

calcaneal tendon (Achilles)

Plate 11B Muscular System, Posterior

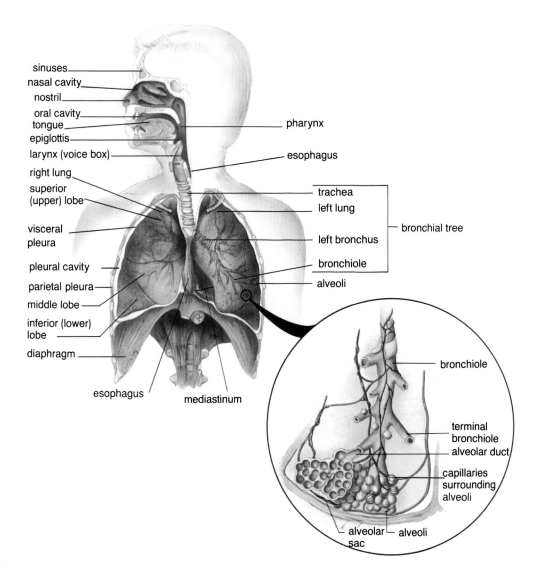

sinuses

nasal cavity

nostril

oral cavity

tongue

epiglottis

larynx (voice box)

right lung

superior (upper) lobe

visceral pleura

pleural cavity

parietal pleura

middle lobe

inferior (lower) lobe

diaphragm

esophagus

mediastinum

pharynx

esophagus

trachea

left lung

left bronchus

bronchiole

alveoli

bronchial tree

bronchiole

terminal bronchiole

alveolar duct

capillaries surrounding alveoli

alveolar sac

alveoli

Plate 12 Respiratory System

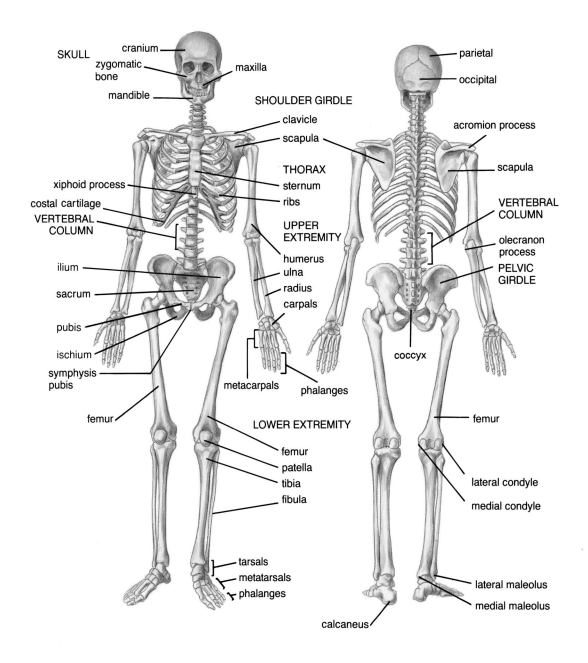

SKULL — cranium, zygomatic bone, maxilla, mandible

parietal, occipital

SHOULDER GIRDLE — clavicle, scapula

acromion process, scapula

THORAX — sternum, ribs

xiphoid process, costal cartilage, VERTEBRAL COLUMN

VERTEBRAL COLUMN, olecranon process, PELVIC GIRDLE

UPPER EXTREMITY — humerus, ulna, radius, carpals

ilium, sacrum, pubis, ischium, symphysis pubis, femur

coccyx

metacarpals, phalanges

LOWER EXTREMITY — femur, patella, tibia, fibula

femur, lateral condyle, medial condyle

tarsals, metatarsals, phalanges

lateral maleolus, medial maleolus

calcaneus

Plate 13 Skeletal System

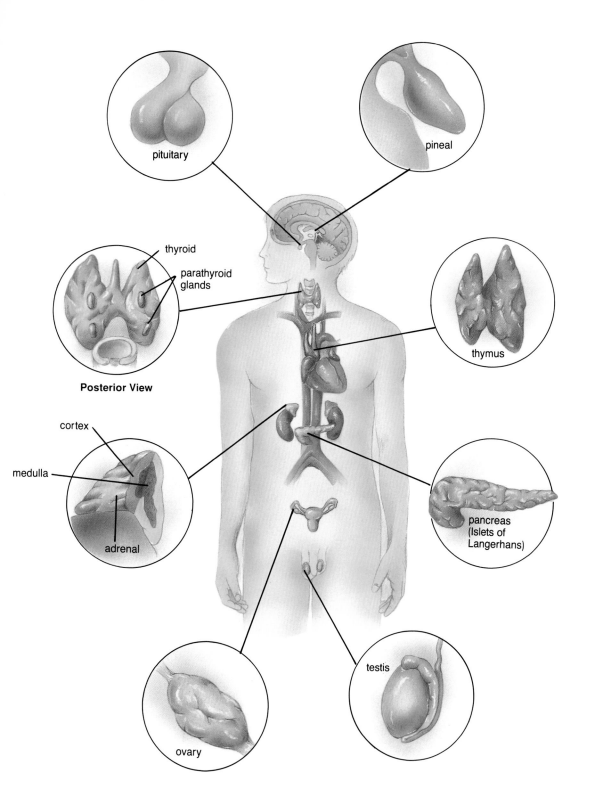

pituitary

pineal

thyroid

parathyroid glands

Posterior View

thymus

cortex

medulla

adrenal

pancreas (Islets of Langerhans)

ovary

testis

Plate 14 Endocrine System

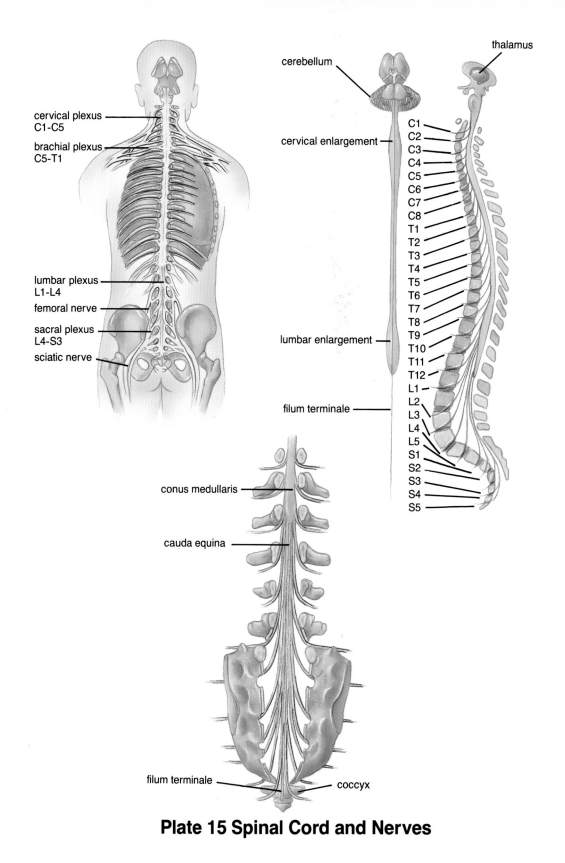

cervical plexus
C1-C5

brachial plexus
C5-T1

lumbar plexus
L1-L4

femoral nerve

sacral plexus
L4-S3

sciatic nerve

cerebellum

thalamus

cervical enlargement

lumbar enlargement

filum terminale

C1
C2
C3
C4
C5
C6
C7
C8
T1
T2
T3
T4
T5
T6
T7
T8
T9
T10
T11
T12
L1
L2
L3
L4
L5
S1
S2
S3
S4
S5

conus medullaris

cauda equina

filum terminale

coccyx

Plate 15 Spinal Cord and Nerves

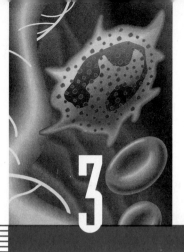

Word Elements Related to Pathology, Diagnosis, and Treatment

Upon completing this chapter, you should be able to recognize and define:

- Word elements commonly used to form terms related to pathology
- Word elements commonly used to form terms related to diagnostic procedures
- Suffixes commonly used to form terms related to therapeutic and surgical procedures

Overview In the preceding chapter, you were introduced to many suffixes and prefixes that are commonly used to build medical terms related to anatomic structures and physiologic processes. In this chapter, you will be introduced to word elements that commonly appear in terms describing pathologic changes in anatomic structures or physiologic functions. You will also be introduced to word elements that are commonly found in terms related to the diagnosis and treatment of pathologic conditions.

As in the preceding chapter, the word elements in this chapter are grouped into categories that reflect the context in which you will usually see them (i.e., pathology, diagnosis, or treatment). Also as in the preceding chapter, we have provided examples of medical terms using each of the new word elements.

Word Elements Related to Pathology

As you may already know from its word elements, pathology is a general term relating to the study (-logy) of disease (path/o). As such, medical terms related to pathology describe the signs and symptoms of disease. In many cases, these terms consist of one or more root words describing the body system(s) affected by a disease plus one or more suffixes and/or prefixes describing the kinds of changes that occur in that system as a result of disease processes.

Suffixes Commonly Used to Describe Pathologic Conditions

The following suffixes are commonly used to build words that describe the signs and symptoms of disease. In many cases, the suffix describes the nature or magnitude of the pathologic change. You may notice that some of the suffixes listed are actually compound suffixes, consisting of two or more word elements. For example, the suffix **-osis** is a general word element meaning condition, while the compound suffix **-sclerosis** refers to any condition (-osis) in which hardening (scler/o) of a structure or substance occurs. Compound suffixes are common in terms related to pathologic conditions.

Suffix	Meaning	Example	Definition
-a	condition	tachycardia	condition characterized by a fast (tachy-) heart (cardi/o) rate
-algia	pain	neuralgia	pain that follows the anatomic pathway of a nerve (neur/o)
-dynia	pain	otodynia	pain in the ear (ot/o)
-edema	swelling	lymphedema	swelling and accumulation of fluid in tissue due to blockage of the lymph (lymph/o) vessels
-ema	condition	emphysema	condition in which tiny air sacs in the lungs are destroyed as a result of excessive inflation (emphys/o)

Suffix	Meaning	Example	Definition
-esis	condition	diur*esis*	condition in which urinary (ur/o) output is abnormal (di-)
-ia	condition	pneumon*ia*	lung (pneumon/o) condition
-iasis	condition	nephro-lith*iasis*	condition characterized by the presence of stones (lith/o) in one or both kidneys (nephr/o)
-ism	condition	hyper-thyroid*ism*	condition characterized by excessive (hyper-) activity of the thyroid gland (thyroid/o)
-itis	inflammation	laryng*itis*	inflammation of the larynx (laryng/o)
-lytic	destroying; dissolving	thrombo*lytic*	related to or involving the destruction of a blood clot (thromb/o)
-malacia	softening	osteo*malacia*	softening and weakening of the bones (oste/o)
-megaly	enlargement	spleno*megaly*	enlargement of the spleen (splen/o)
-mycosis	fungal infection	oto*mycosis*	fungal infection of the external ear (ot/o)
-oma	tumor; growth	lymph*oma*	malignant tumor of the lymph nodes (lymph/o) or other lymph tissue
-osis	condition	mono-nucle*osis*	infectious condition characterized by abnormalities in the function of mononuclear cells (mononucle/o)
-pathy	disease	myo*pathy*	general term referring to any disease of muscle (my/o)
-penia	deficiency	leuko*penia*	deficiency of white (leuk/o) blood cells
-plasia	formation; growth condition	dys*plasia*	general term for abnormal (dys-) formation of any anatomic structure
-rrhagia (-rrhage)	profuse discharge of blood	meno*rrhagia*	excessive discharge of blood during menstruation (men/o)
-rrhea	discharge	otopyo*rrhea*	discharge of pus (py/o) from the ear (ot/o), usually as a result of bacterial infection
-sclerosis	hardening	arterio-*sclerosis*	hardening of the arteries (arteri/o)

Suffix	Meaning	Example	Definition
-sis	condition	necro*sis*	condition in which an area of tissue dies (necr/o) as a result of oxygen and nutrient deprivation
-spasm	sudden contraction	vaso*spasm*	sudden contraction of the muscular wall of a blood vessel (vas/o)
-stenosis	narrowing	uretero*stenosis*	narrowing of a ureter (ureter/o)
-toxic	poisonous	hepato*toxic*	damaging to the liver (hepat/o)
-trophy	nourishment; growth	dys*trophy*	tissue degeneration occurring as a result of poor (dys-) nourishment or prolonged disuse

Prefixes Commonly Used to Describe Pathologic Conditions

The following prefixes are commonly used to describe abnormalities in anatomic structures or physiologic processes. Note that, like the suffixes in the preceding table, many of these prefixes describe the degree or direction of change that occurs as a result of disease.

Prefix	Meaning	Example	Definition
a-	without; not	*a*taxia	condition characterized by an absence of or reduction in muscular coordination (-taxia)
an-	without; not	*an*esthesia	condition characterized by an absence or reduction in feeling or sensation (-esthesia)
ana-	without; not	*ana*cusis	without hearing (-cusis); deaf
aniso-	unequal	*aniso*coria	condition (-ia) in which the pupils (cor/o) of the eyes are unequal in size
atel-	incomplete	*atel*ectasis	incomplete expansion (-ectasis) of a lung; collapsed lung
brady-	slow	*brady*cardia	condition (-a) characterized by a slow heart (cardi/o) rate
de-	down; lack of; loss of	*de*mentia	loss of the ability to think clearly (-mentia)

Prefix	Meaning	Example	Definition
dys-	abnormal; painful; difficult	*dys*pnea	difficult or painful breathing (-pnea)
hyper-	excessive	*hyper*-glycemia	condition characterized by excessive amounts of sugar (glyc/o) in the blood (-emia)
hypo-	under; reduced	*hypo*-thyroidism	condition (-ism) characterized by underactivity of the thyroid gland (thyroid/o)
in-	not; without	*in*somnia	condition (-ia) characterized by an inability to sleep (somn/o)
macro-	large	*macro*-lymphocyte	a large lymph (lymph/o) cell (-cyte)
micro-	small	*micro*biology	the study of (-logy) very small living organisms (bi/o)
mio-	less; smaller	*mio*sis	condition (-sis) in which the pupils of the eye are constricted
neo-	new	*neo*plastic	general term pertaining to (-ic) the formation (plast/o) of new tissue; usually used to denote a cancerous growth or tumor
pan-	all	*pan*hypo-pituitarism	condition (-ism) in which the production of all pituitary (pituitar/o) hormones is reduced (hypo-)
presby-	old age	*presby*cusis	hearing (-cusis) impairment that occurs as a result of aging processes
pseudo-	false	*pseudo*cyesis	false pregnancy (-cyesis); condition in which signs of pregnancy occur in a person who is not pregnant
psor-	itching	*psor*iasis	condition (-iasis) characterized by scaling, itchy skin
tachy-	fast	*tachy*cardia	condition (-a) characterized by a fast heart (cardi/o) rate
un-	not	*un*myelinated	adjective (-ated) used to describe a nerve cell that is not covered by a myelin sheath (myelin/o)

Review Exercises

1. **Match** the following suffixes with their definitions.

_____ -megaly   a. enlargement

_____ -rrhagia   b. formation; growth condition

_____ -pathy   c. deficiency

_____ -algia   d. disease

_____ -plasia   e. tumor; growth

_____ -oma   f. sudden contraction

_____ -spasm   g. pain

_____ -penia   h. profuse discharge of blood

2. **Fill in the Blank.** All eight of the suffixes listed below mean

_____.

-a   -ema   -esis   -ia   -iasis   -ism   -osis   -sis

3. **Define** the following suffixes.

a. -dynia   _____

b. -edema   _____

c. -lytic   _____

d. -mycosis   _____

e. -toxic   _____

f. -trophy   _____

4. **Match** the following prefixes with their definitions.

_____ ana-   a. itching

_____ de-   b. without; not

_____ mio-   c. down; lack of; loss of

_____ psor-   d. less; smaller

5. **Define** the following prefixes.

a. dys- _____

b. pan- _____

c. pseudo- _____

d. atel- _____

e. neo- _____

f. aniso- _____

g. an- _____

h. tachy- _____

6. **Define** the word elements in the following terms to complete their definitions.

a. Hepato*megaly* is a condition characterized by _____ of the liver.

b. Tonsill*itis* refers to _____ of the tonsils.

c. *Presby*opia refers to a loss of vision occurring as a result of _____ _____.

d. Sebo*rrhea* is a condition characterized by excessive_____ of oil from the sebaceous glands.

e. *Brady*kinesia refers to movement that is unusually _____.

f. *A*kinesia means _____ movement.

g. *In*fertile means _____ fertile.

h. *Un*conscious means _____ conscious.

7. **Circle** the choices that will make each statement true.

a. Uretero*stenosis* is a condition in which one or both ureters are abnormally (narrowed/dilated).

b. (Myo*sclerosis*/Myo*malacia*) is a condition in which the muscles become abnormally hard, while (osteo*sclerosis*/osteo*malacia*) is a condition in which the bones become abnormally soft.

c. *Hyper*tension is (excessive/reduced) blood pressure, while *hypo*tension is (excessive/reduced) blood pressure.

d. A *micro*cyte is an unusually (large/small) red blood cell, while a *macro*cyte is an unusually (large/small) red blood cell.

Word Elements Related to Diagnostic Procedures

Diagnostic procedures include all of the various laboratory tests a physician may run to determine the cause and nature of a patient's illness. Because they are used to distinguish among various types of disease, some diagnostic tests are used by physicians in many different areas of medicine. Thus, most of the word elements in this section are used to build words that are related to a particular diagnostic approach rather than to a specific tissue or organ system.

Combining Forms Commonly Used to Describe Diagnostic Procedures

diagnostic = "pertaining to that through which one knows"

The following combining forms (CF) are used to build terms that refer to tests that a physician may order to identify the cause of a patient's complaint. In most cases, the root words in the table below refer to the *medium* used to generate information about the patient's illness.

CF	Meaning	Example	Definition
electr/o	electricity	*electro-*myography	recording (-graphy) of activity within a muscle (my/o) following the application of an electrical stimulus
radi/o	radioactivity	*radio*graphy	use of photographic plates to produce an image recording (-graphy) the absorption of x-rays by structures in the body
son/o	sound waves	*sono*gram	record (-gram) produced when high-frequency sound waves are used to generate an image using the process of ultrasonography
tom/o	section; layer (literally, "cut" or "incision")	*tomo*graphy	term used to describe any of several non-invasive diagnostic techniques in which specialized machines are used to produce a series of cross-sectional images recording (-graphy) the absorption of x-rays or the distribution of a radioactive substance in the body
ultrason/o	ultrasound; very high frequency soundwaves	*ultrasono-*graphy	general term for any of several non-invasive diagnostic techniques in which reflected ultrasound waves are recorded (-graphy) to generate an image of structures within the body

Suffixes Commonly Used to Describe Diagnostic Procedures

The following suffixes are commonly used to build words related to diagnostic tests. Note that, in many cases, these suffixes describe the *action* that a physician takes to obtain information for making or confirming a diagnosis.

Suffix	Meaning	Example	Definition
-alysis	separation into components; analysis	urin*alysis*	physical, microscopic, or chemical analysis of the urine (urin/o)
-assay	test; measure	radioimmuno-*assay*	test in which radioactive (radi/o) antibodies are used to measure blood levels of antigens recognized by the immune (immun/o) system
-centesis	puncture	amnio*centesis*	needle puncture of the amniotic sac (amni/o) surrounding a fetus to extract fluid that can be examined to determine whether various genetic disorders are present
-gram	record	electrocar-dio*gram*	record of the electrical (electr/o) activity in the heart (cardi/o)
-graph	recording instrument	electrocar-dio*graph*	instrument used to record electrical (electr/o) activity within the heart (cardi/o)
-graphy	recording	encephalo-*graphy*	any of several techniques used to record activity within the brain (encephal/o)
-metry	measurement	audio*metry*	measurement of an individual's ability to hear (audi/o) sounds of various frequencies
-scopy	visual examination	endo*scopy*	visual examination of one or more internal (endo-) organs using an instrument known as an endoscope

Prefix Commonly Used to Describe Diagnostic Procedures

The following prefix is commonly used in terms related to diagnosis.

Prefix	Meaning	Example	Definition
echo-	returned sound	*echo*cardio-graphy	non-invasive diagnostic technique in which reflected sound waves are recorded (-graphy) to generate an image of structures within the heart (cardi/o)

Review Exercises

8. **Match** the following word elements with their definitions.

_____	radi/o	a.	sound waves
_____	electr/o	b.	analysis
_____	-graphy	c.	section; layer
_____	-alysis	d.	radioactivity
_____	tom/o	e.	puncture
_____	son/o	f.	test; measure
_____	-centesis	g.	electricity
_____	-assay	h.	recording

9. **Define** the word elements in the following terms to complete their definitions.

a. *Echo*encephalography involves the use of _____ to generate an image of structures within the brain.

b. Opto*metry* is the _____ of visual acuity.

c. Broncho*scopy* is a procedure which involves _____ of the bronchial tubes.

d. *Ultrasono*graphy involves the use of _____ to generate an image of internal body structures.

e. An ultrasono*gram* is the _____ of the image created by ultrasonography.

f. An electroencephalo*graph* is a _____ used to record electrical activity in the brain.

Word Elements Related to Therapeutic and Surgical Procedures

Therapeutic and surgical procedures include all of the steps a physician may take to relieve the patient's distress and to cure the patient's illness. Like terms related to pathology and diagnosis, medical terms related to therapeutic and surgical procedures are built using a relatively small number of word elements.

Suffixes Commonly Used to Describe Therapeutic and Surgical Procedures

therapeutic = "pertaining to that which treats"

Suffixes are the main word elements used to build terms related to therapeutic and surgical procedures. In most cases, these suffixes describe an action that the physician takes; suffixes are generally attached to a root word that indicates the part of the body upon which the therapeutic action or surgical procedure is performed. Suffixes commonly used to form words describing therapeutic and surgical procedures are listed in the following table.

Suffix	Meaning	Example	Definition
-ectomy	surgical removal	append-*ectomy*	surgical removal of the appendix (append/o)
-lysis	dissolution; destruction	thrombo*lysis*	dissolution of a blood clot (thromb/o), usually by means of drug therapy
-plasty	surgical repair	valvulo*plasty*	surgical repair or replacement of a heart valve (valvul/o)
-rrhaphy	suture; stitch	hernio*rrhaphy*	stitching together of a tissue to correct or prevent a hernial protrusion (herni/o)
-stomy	surgical opening	ileo*stomy*	surgical creation of an opening between the ileum (ile/o) and the surface of the abdomen to allow the discharge of feces into a bag attached to the skin
-tomy	surgical incision	tracheo*tomy*	surgical incision through the neck into the trachea (trache/o) to gain access to an airway below a blockage
-tripsy	crushing	litho*tripsy*	crushing of a stone (lith/o) within the urinary bladder or urethra

Review Exercises

10. ***Match*** the following suffixes with their definitions.

_____ -lysis   a. suture; stitch

_____ -tripsy   b. dissolution; destruction

_____ -rrhaphy   c. crushing

11. **Build** medical terms which describe the following surgical procedures using the suffixes you have learned in this chapter.

a. surgical removal of the spleen (splen/o)

_____

b. surgical repair of a blood vessel (angi/o)

_____

c. surgical incision into a lobe (lob/o) of an organ

_____

d. surgical removal of the gallbladder (cholecyst/o)

_____

e. surgical creation of an opening between the colon (col/o) and the surface of the abdomen

_____

f. surgical repair of a joint (arthr/o)

_____

g. surgical creation of an opening in the eardrum (tympan/o)

_____

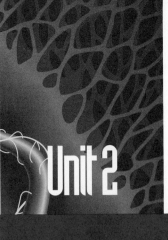

Unit 2

Medical Terminology Relating to Body Systems

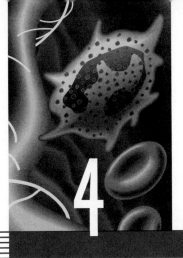

The Body as a Whole

Upon completing this chapter, you should be able to:

- List the main structural units of the body
- Define anatomic position
- Name and identify the three planes of the body
- Recognize, define, pronounce, and spell terms used to describe the location of body structures
- List and locate the four main cavities of the body
- List and locate the four quadrants and the nine regions of the abdominopelvic cavity

Overview   To recognize and use terms pertaining to specific body systems, it is necessary to understand the many general terms used to locate and describe structures within the body. To that end, this chapter provides an overview of the body as a whole. It explains the basic structural organization of the body and introduces terms used to describe the location of body structures. These terms are relevant to all body systems, so learning them will help you master the material presented in the remaining chapters of this book.

Word Elements

BASIC STRUCTURAL UNITS – The following combining forms (CF) refer to the basic structural units of the body. Together, cells and tissues make up the larger anatomic structures known as organs and organ systems.

CF	Meaning	Example
adip/o	fat	*adip*ose = having the quality of fat
chondr/o	cartilage	costo*chondr*itis = inflammation of a rib and its cartilage
cyt/o	cell	*cyto*logy = the study of cells
hist/o	tissue	*histo*logy = the study of tissues
nucle/o	nucleus	*nucleo*plasm = the fluid that fills the nucleus
sarc/o	flesh; muscle	*sarc*oma = tumor of muscular or fleshy tissue

PARTS OR REGIONS OF THE BODY – These combining forms refer to parts or regions of the body, such as the abdomen, chest, skull, and extremities.

CF	Meaning	Example
abdomin/o	abdomen	*abdomino*pelvic = pertaining to the abdomen and pelvis
acr/o	extremity (arm/leg)	*acro*megaly = enlargement of an arm or leg
crani/o	skull	*crani*al = pertaining to the skull
dactyl/o	finger or toe	*dactyl*edema = swelling of the fingers or toes
gastr/o	stomach	*gastr*itis = inflammation of the stomach
inguin/o	groin	*inguin*al = pertaining to the groin
lumb/o	loin; waist	*lumb*ar = pertaining to the waist
pelv/i	pelvis	*pelvi*metry = measurement of the pelvis
som/a	body	*som*asthenia = weakness of the body
somat/o	body	psycho*somat*ic = pertaining to the mind-body connection
thorac/o	chest	*thorac*ic = pertaining to the chest
umbilic/o	navel	*umbilic*al = pertaining to the navel
viscer/o	internal organs	*viscer*al = pertaining to the internal organs

LOCATION OF BODY STRUCTURES – These combining forms are used to describe the location of body structures. Although some can also be used to denote a structure, they are more often used to describe location.

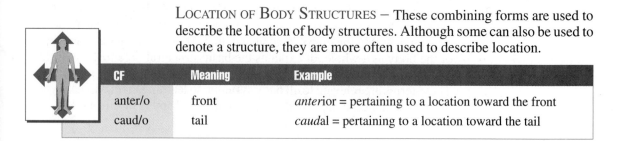

CF	Meaning	Example
anter/o	front	*anter*ior = pertaining to a location toward the front
caud/o	tail	*caud*al = pertaining to a location toward the tail

CF	Meaning	Example
cephal/o	head	*cephal*ic = pertaining to a location toward the head
dist/o	distant	*dist*al = pertaining to a distant location
dors/o	back	*dors*al = pertaining to a location toward the back
infer/o	lower; below	*infer*ior = pertaining to a location below
later/o	side	*later*al = pertaining to a location toward the side
medi/o	middle	*medi*al = pertaining to a location toward the middle
poster/o	back	*poster*ior = pertaining to a location toward the back
proxim/o	near	*proxim*al = pertaining to a near location
super/o	upper; above	*super*ior = pertaining to a location above
ventr/o	belly; belly-side	*ventr*al = pertaining to the belly (front side)

Structural Organization of the Body

The human body is made up of billions of cells. These cells do not all function independently; rather, they form many groupings. To understand the many functions of the body, it is useful to discuss the larger structural units formed by cells. The basic structural units of the body are cells, tissues, organs, and systems (see Figure 4-1).

Figure 4-1: Structural units of the body.

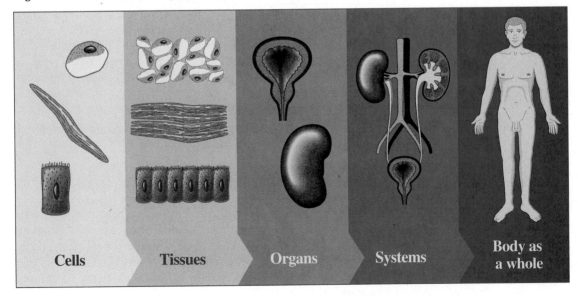

Cells   Tissues   Organs   Systems   Body as a whole

Cells

The **cell** is the smallest structural and functional unit of life. All living organisms, from tiny one-celled bacteria to plants to humans, are made up of cells. Cells have many shapes and sizes, but they share three main parts:

cyt/o = cell

- cytoplasm, the fluid that fills the cell and contains everything needed for cell metabolism

nucle/o = nucleus

- the nucleus (NOO-klee-us), which contains genetic material (the chromosomes, which are made up of many genes that provide instructions for cell reproduction and production of vital cell molecules and nutrients)

- a cell membrane, which surrounds and encloses the cytoplasm and nucleus

The human body contains many different types of cells, many of which have specialized functions. Important types of cells include epithelial (EH-pih-**THEEL**-ee-ul) cells, muscle cells, nerve cells, fat cells, and bone and cartilage cells. You will learn more about these cell types in later chapters.

Tissues

hist/o = tissue

Groups of cells that are structurally and functionally similar are called **tissue.** Different types of cells form different types of tissue, each of which has specialized functions. The four main types of tissue are:

- epithelial tissue, designed to protect body surfaces

- muscle tissue, designed for contraction

- nerve tissue, designed for the transmission of electrical impulses

adip/o = fat
chondr/o = cartilage

- connective tissue, designed to support and connect other types of tissue; connective tissues include adipose (AD-dih-pose) or fat tissue, bone, and cartilage

sarc/o = flesh;
muscle

Together, the soft tissues of the body make up what is commonly referred to as "flesh."

Organs

viscer/o = internal organs

Groups of tissue that work together to perform a specific activity are called **organs.** Organs are usually easy to identify, since they take on characteristic shapes as well as characteristic activities. For example, the stomach and the heart are two organs that are easily distinguishable based on their different shapes and functions. Most organs, like the stomach and heart, are internal organs (located inside the body). The skin is a large external organ that serves as a protective covering for the body.

Systems

Groups of organs that are interconnected or that contribute to the same larger activity are called **body systems.** For example, the kidneys, ureters, urinary bladder, and urethra each have different specific functions, but together they act to eliminate wastes from the body in the form of urine. Thus, they form the urinary system. The main systems of the body include the cardiovascular, blood, lymphatic, immune, respiratory, digestive, urinary, nervous, endocrine, reproductive, skeletal, muscular, skin, and special sensory systems. These systems will be described in the remaining chapters of this book.

Location and Orientation of Body Structures

To describe the location of body structures, it is helpful to have a point of reference. To describe the location of the heart, for example, most people would say something like "it's in left part of the chest." There are several ways to organize and orient the body to make describing the location of body structures easier. Common reference points include the position of the body, body planes, and other structures.

Body Position

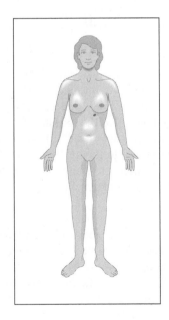

Figure 4-2:
The anatomic
position.

The body, of course, can be in many different positions – standing, kneeling, lying down, etc. To assure uniformity in descriptions of location, the **anatomic position** is used as the reference point when describing the location or direction of body structures. In the anatomic position, the body is standing erect, with the arms at the side and the palms facing forward (see Figure 4-2). The locations of body structures are always described as if the body were in this position, regardless of how a patient is actually positioned at any given time. For example, patients are usually in the **supine** (lying face up), **prone** (lying face down), or other **recumbent** (lying down) position when being examined, but the location of their body structures are still described as if they were in the anatomic position.

Planes of the Body

A **body plane** is an imaginary flat surface that divides the body into two sections. Different planes divide the body into different sections: front and back, left side and right side, and top and bottom. These planes serve as points of reference for describing the direction from which the body is being observed. Refer to Figure 4-3 while you read the following paragraphs.

The **frontal plane,** also called the **coronal** (kor-OH-nul) **plane,** is a vertical plane that divides the body into front and back portions. The terms **anterior** and **ventral** are used to refer to locations toward the front, while the terms **posterior** and **dorsal** are used to refer to locations toward the back. For example, the abdomen is anterior to the spine, and the spine is posterior to the abdomen.

anter/o = front
ventr/o = belly; belly-side
poster/o and dors/o = back

Figure 4-3: Body planes.

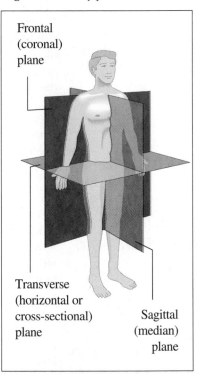

Frontal (coronal) plane

Transverse (horizontal or cross-sectional) plane

Sagittal (median) plane

medi/o = middle

The **sagittal** (SAJ-jih-tul) **plane,** also called the **median plane,** is another vertical plane; it divides the body into left side and right side. If the plane is exactly in the middle of the body and divides the body into two equal halves, as in Figure 4-3, it is called the **midsagittal plane.** The term **lateral** is used to refer to locations toward the side (either side), while the term **medial** refers to the middle or to locations toward the middle of the body. For example, the ears are lateral to the nose, and the nose is medial to the ears. Similarly, the little toes are lateral to the big toes, and the big toes are medial to the little toes.

later/o = side

trans- = through; across

super/o = upper; above
cephal/o = head
infer/o = lower; below
caud/o = tail

The **transverse plane,** also called the **horizontal** or **cross-sectional plane,** is a horizontal plane that divides the body into upper and lower portions. The terms **superior** and **cephalic** (seh-FAL-lick) refer to locations above or toward the upper portion, while **inferior** and **caudal** (KAW-dul) refer to locations below or toward the lower portion. For example, the brain is located superior to the throat, while the lungs are inferior to the throat.

Directional Terms

The directional terms introduced so far are summarized in the following table. Note that some of the terms used interchangeably above are not precisely synonymous. Although they are commonly used interchangeably, you should be aware of the distinctions between these terms.

Term	Word Elements	Definition
anterior	anter = front ior = pertaining to	pertaining to the front or to a location toward the front
ventral	ventr = belly; belly-side al = pertaining to	pertaining to the belly or to a location toward the belly or front
posterior	poster = back ior = pertaining to	pertaining to the back or to a location toward the back
dorsal	dors = back al = pertaining to	pertaining to the back or to a location toward the back
lateral	later = side al = pertaining to	pertaining to the side or to a location toward the side
medial	medi = middle al = pertaining to	pertaining to the middle or to a location toward the middle of the body/structure
superior	super = upper; above ior = pertaining to	pertaining to a location above or toward the upper portion
cephalic	cephal = head ic = pertaining to	pertaining to the head or to a location toward the head or upper portion
inferior	infer = lower; below ior = pertaining to	pertaining to a location below or toward the lower portion
caudal	caud = tail al = pertaining to	pertaining to the tail or to a location toward the tail or lower portion

Figure 4-4: Directional terms.

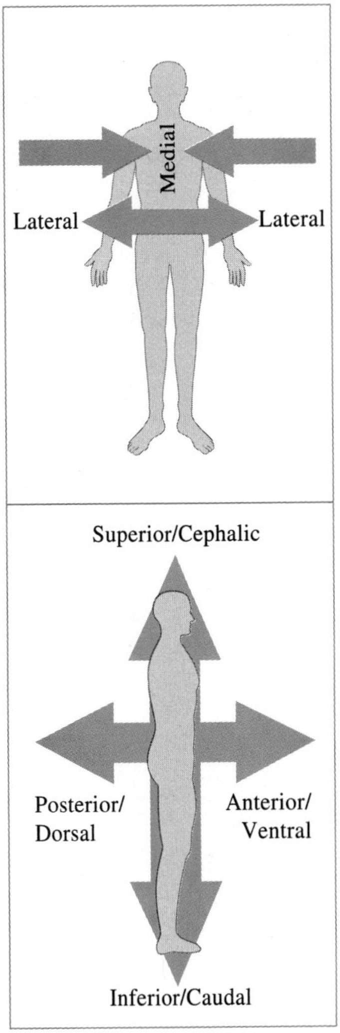

Other Directional Terms

proxim/o = near
dist/o = distant

peri- = around;
surrounding

The location of a structure can also be described in relation to some defined center or reference point. For example, **proximal** (PROCK-sih-mul) refers to something closer to a point of interest, while **distal** (DIS-tul) refers to something farther from the point of interest. Likewise, **central** refers to something in the center of the item of interest, while **peripheral** refers to something away from the center of the item of interest. Unless otherwise specified, the center is assumed to be the torso of the body. The proximal end of the thigh is the part near the hip and torso, for example, while the distal end of the thigh is the part near the knee. In neurology, on the other hand, the brain and spinal cord are considered to be the center of the nervous system; therefore, the term "central nervous system" refers to the brain and spinal cord, while "peripheral nervous system" refers to nerves located away from the brain and spinal cord.

Some locational terms refer to the depth of a structure in the body. For example, structures inside the body are called **internal,** while those on the outside of the body are referred to as **external.** Similarly, structures located close to the surface are described as **superficial,** while those located far beneath the surface are referred to as **deep.** The term **parietal** (per-RYE-uh-tul) refers to structures that line body cavities.

Keep in mind that the directional words introduced in this chapter can be used in several ways:

- to describe the location of a whole structure in relation to another structure or point of reference (as in the examples given above)
- to identify a portion of a structure (e.g., the anterior aspect of the stomach is the front portion of the stomach)
- to name or distinguish two similar structures (e.g., the superior rectus muscle is located above the eye, while the inferior rectus muscle is located below the eye)

Body Cavities

thorac/o = chest
abdomin/o = abdomen
pelv/i = pelvis

Medical personnel sometimes locate structures of interest by referring to the body cavity in which they can be found. A **body cavity** is a hollow space in the body that contains internal organs. There are four cavities in the body: two ventral cavities and two dorsal cavities. These cavities are illustrated in Figure 4-5.

As you should expect, the two ventral cavities are located in the front part of the body. They are the **thoracic** (ther-RASS-ick) **cavity**, which contains the heart and lungs, and the **abdominopelvic** (ab-DOM-ih-no-**PEL**-vick) **cavity**, which contains organs of the digestive and reproductive systems. The thoracic and abdominopelvic cavities are separated by a thick muscular

Figure 4-5: *The four major body cavities.*

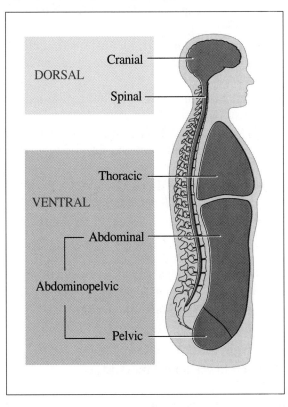

Figure 4-5: *The four major body cavities.*

wall called the diaphragm. As Figure 4-5 indicates, the abdominopelvic cavity is made up of two subcavities, the abdominal and pelvic cavities. Subdivision of the abdominopelvic cavity into the abdominal and pelvic cavities is useful because of the different types of organs present in each (digestive versus reproductive). There is no dividing wall between them, however, so they are actually one large cavity (the abdominopelvic cavity).

The two dorsal cavities are located in the back part of the body. They are the **cranial cavity** (cranio = skull), which contains the brain, and the **spinal cavity** (also called **spinal canal**), which contains the spinal cord. The spine can be further subdivided into several regions. These regions are discussed in *Chapter 16: Skeletal System.*

As you can see, three of the body cavities lie within the main part of the body (i.e., in the torso), and one body cavity is located in the head. There are no body cavities in the extremities (the arms and legs) or the fingers and toes.

Divisions of the Abdominopelvic Cavity

The abdominopelvic cavity contains by far the greatest number of organs of any of the body cavities. To describe the location of organs within the abdominopelvic cavity, it is useful to divide the cavity into regions or quadrants.

By convention, the abdominopelvic cavity is divided into nine regions for the purpose of identifying the location of internal organs. These nine regions are created by superimposing an imaginary "tic-tac-toe" board over the abdominopelvic cavity (see Figure 4-6). Starting with the top row, these regions are named:

chondr/o = cartilage

- **right hypochondriac** (HI-poe-**KON**-dree-ack), the upper right region located under the cartilage of the ribs

gastr/o = stomach

- **epigastric** (EH-pih-**GAS**-trick), the upper middle region located over the stomach

- **left hypochondriac,** the upper left region located under the ribs

Figure 4-6: *The nine regions of the abdomino-pelvic cavity.*

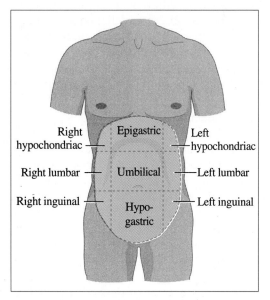

- **right lumbar** (LUM-bar), the middle right region located near the waist (lumb/o = loin; waist)
- **umbilical** (um-BIL-lih-kul), the middle region located in the area of the navel (umbilic/o = navel)
- **left lumbar**, the middle left region located near the waist
- **right inguinal** (ING-wuh-nul), the lower right region located near the groin (inguin/o = groin)
- **hypogastric** (HI-poe-**GAS**-trick), the lower middle region located under the stomach
- **left inguinal,** the lower left region located near the groin

Instead of nine regions, the abdominopelvic cavity can be divided into four quadrants:

- **right upper quadrant (RUQ)**
- **left upper quadrant (LUQ)**
- **right lower quadrant (RLQ)**
- **left lower quadrant (LLQ)**

Figure 4-7: *The four quadrants of the abdomino-pelvic cavity.*

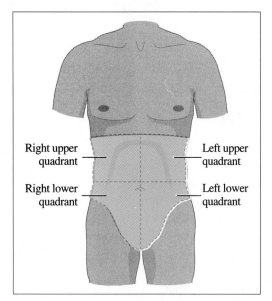

In contrast to the region system, which is used mainly to identify the placement of internal organs, the quadrant system of subdividing the abdominopelvic cavity is generally used for clinical examination and reporting. For example, a clinician might note that a patient's abdomen is tender in the RUQ (right upper quadrant), signalling different clinical possibilities than if the tenderness were observed in the LLQ (left lower quadrant). In a detailed report on an operation, on the other hand, a physician might describe the location of a structure or injury according to its location in an abdominopelvic region. A physician might refer to the surgical approach taken to correct a left inguinal hernia, for example.

Note that in both schemes for subdividing the abdominopelvic cavity, the designations of right and left refer to the *patient's* right and left, not to the observer's right and left.

Review Exercises

1. **Define** the following combining forms.

   a. som/a   _body_

   b. nucle/o _____

   c. cyt/o _____

   d. somat/o _____

   e. hist/o _____

   f. adip/o _____

   g. viscer/o _____

   h. sarc/o _____

2. **Define** the following body positions.

   a. anatomic _____

   b. supine   _lying face up_

   c. prone   _lying face down_

   d. recumbent _just lying down_

3. **Label** the body planes shown on the illustration.

   a. _____

   b. _____

   c. _____

4. **Define** the term and state its opposite for each of the following.

   a. distal _____

   b. internal _____

   c. superficial _____

   d. peripheral _____

5. *Match* each body plane with the descriptions of how it divides the body.

_____ left side and right side   a. frontal (coronal)

_____ front and back   b. sagittal (median)

_____ upper and lower   c. transverse

_____ anterior and posterior   (horizontal, cross-sectional)

_____ cephalic and caudal

_____ lateral and medial

_____ dorsal and ventral

_____ superior and inferior

6. *Match* the following combining forms with their definitions.

_____ anter/o   a. side

_____ poster/o   b. front

_____ later/o   c. upper; above

_____ super/o   d. back

_____ infer/o   e. lower; below

7. *Define* the following combining forms.

a. ventr/o   _____

b. dors/o   _____

c. medi/o   _____

d. cephal/o   _____

e. caud/o   _____

f. proxim/o   _____

g. dist/o   _____

h. thorac/o   _____

i. abdomin/o   _____

j. pelv/i   _____

k. crani/o   _____

l. acr/o   _____

m. dactyl/o _____

n. inguin/o _____

o. umbilic/o _____

p. lumb/o _____

q. gastr/o _____

r. chondr/o _____

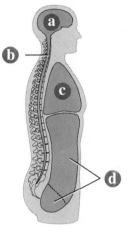

8. *Label* the four body cavities shown on the illustration and indicate which are ventral and which are dorsal.

    a. _____

    b. _____

    c. _____

    d. _____

9. *Identify* the body cavity in which each organ is located.

    a. the brain _____

    b. the heart _____

    c. the spinal cord _____

    d. the stomach _____

    e. the intestines _____

    f. the lungs _____

10. *Label* each of the four quadrants of the abdominopelvic cavity shown on the illustration.

    a. _____

    b. _____

    c. _____

    d. _____

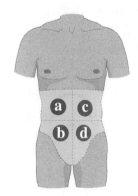

11. **Label** the nine regions of the abdominopelvic cavity shown on the illustration.

a. _____

b. _____

c. _____

d. _____

e. _____

f. _____

g. _____

h. _____

i. _____

12. **Break Down and Define** the word elements within each of the following terms, and then define the term itself.

Example: postero / later / al   *back / side / pertaining to*   *pertaining to a location toward the side and back*

a. inferomedial

_____

b. anteroposterior

_____

c. dorsoventral

_____

d. anterosuperior

_____

e. somatomegaly

_____

f. dactyledema

_____

g. abdominothoracic

_____

h. cytogenic

_____

Case Study. Read the case notes below. For each boldfaced term, provide a brief definition and indicate whether the term is spelled correctly; if it is misspelled, provide the correct spelling.

Example:

corronal plane: *vertical plane dividing the body into front and back*

Spelled correctly? ☐ Yes ☑ No *coronal plane*

Patient presented as a 20-year-old male athlete with a right knee injury. Ordered magnetic resonance imaging of the knee. Three sequences were performed in the **corronal**, **sagital**, and **tranverse** planes. The ligaments of the knee were intact, although the **anterier** ligament was slightly thickened. The **lateral** meniscus of the joint was normal. The **medial** meniscus showed evidence of a major tear, with greatest signal on the **posterior** aspect of the medial meniscus. Patient underwent surgery to remove the medial meniscus. Two incisions were made in the knee: an **anteromedial** and an **anteriolateral** incision. The tear in the medial meniscus extended 3 mm from the midsection to the posterior aspect. This portion was removed. No other significant damage was noted.

a. sagital plane: _____

   Spelled correctly? ☐ Yes ☐ No _____

b. tranverse plane: _____

   Spelled correctly? ☐ Yes ☐ No _____

c. anterier: _____

   Spelled correctly? ☐ Yes ☐ No _____

d. lateral: _____

   Spelled correctly? ☐ Yes ☐ No _____

e. medial: _____

   Spelled correctly? ☐ Yes ☐ No _____

f. posterior: _____

   Spelled correctly? ☐ Yes ☐ No _____

g. anteromedial: _____

   Spelled correctly? ☐ Yes ☐ No _____

h. anteriolateral: _____

   Spelled correctly? ☐ Yes ☐ No _____

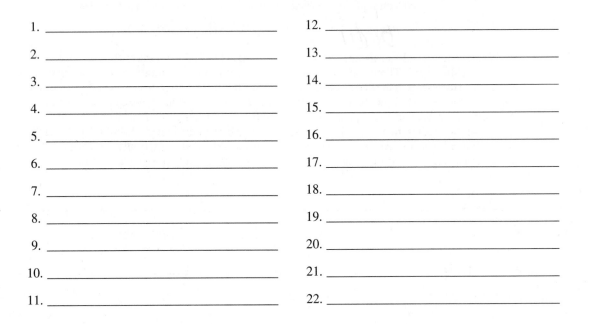

Listen to the section on your audiotape cassette that corresponds to this chapter and write the terms below. Be careful to spell each term correctly.

1. _____

2. _____

3. _____

4. _____

5. _____

6. _____

7. _____

8. _____

9. _____

10. _____

11. _____

12. _____

13. _____

14. _____

15. _____

16. _____

17. _____

18. _____

19. _____

20. _____

21. _____

22. _____

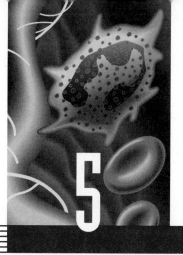

5

Cardiovascular System

Upon completing this chapter, you should be able to:

- Describe the cardiovascular system and explain the primary functions of its organs
- Recognize, build, pronounce, and spell words that pertain to the cardiovascular system
- Describe diseases, diagnostic tests, and therapeutic procedures that pertain to the cardiovascular system

Overview   The cardiovascular system is responsible for distributing nutrients to cells and tissues throughout the body and for transporting waste products from the tissues to the organs of elimination. Exchange mechanisms in the digestive organs and lungs supply the circulating blood with the oxygen and other nutrients required for normal cellular function. The cardiovascular system transports these substances throughout the body, delivering them to even the most remote cells and tissues. At the same time, the circulating blood extracts byproducts of cellular metabolism from the tissues and transports these substances to the organs responsible for eliminating wastes. Gaseous waste products such as carbon dioxide are delivered to the lungs for exhalation, while non-gaseous metabolites are carried to the kidneys for elimination in the urine.

Word Elements

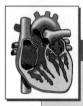

THE HEART – The following combining forms refer to the heart, including structures within the heart and the pulse created by the beating of the heart.

CF	Meaning	Example
atri/o	atrium	*atri*al = pertaining to the atria
cardi/o	heart	*cardi*ology = the study of the heart
sphygm/o	pulse	*sphygm*oscopy = examination of the pulse
valvul/o	valve	*valvul*itis = inflammation of a valve
ventricul/o	ventricle	*ventricul*ar = pertaining to the ventricles

THE VASCULATURE – These combining forms pertain to the vasculature. Some are general and refer to any type of blood vessel; others refer to specific types of blood vessels.

CF	Meaning	Example
angi/o	vessel	*angi*ography = visualization of the blood vessels
aort/o	aorta	*aort*ic = pertaining to the aorta
arteri/o	artery	*arteri*ostenosis = narrowing of the arteries
arteriol/o	arteriole	*arteriol*ar = pertaining to the arterioles
phleb/o	vein	*phleb*itis = inflammation of a vein
vas/o	vessel	*vas*oactive = acting on the blood vessels
vascul/o	vessel	*vascul*ar = pertaining to the blood vessels
ven/o	vein	*ven*ous = pertaining to the veins
venul/o	venule	*venul*ar = pertaining to the venules

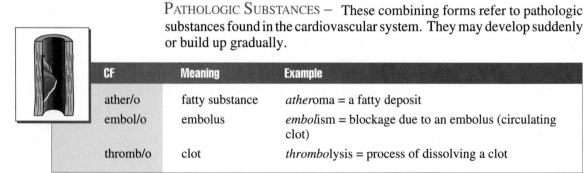

PATHOLOGIC SUBSTANCES – These combining forms refer to pathologic substances found in the cardiovascular system. They may develop suddenly or build up gradually.

CF	Meaning	Example
ather/o	fatty substance	*ather*oma = a fatty deposit
embol/o	embolus	*embol*ism = blockage due to an embolus (circulating clot)
thromb/o	clot	*thromb*olysis = process of dissolving a clot

SUFFIXES — The following suffixes pertain to the cardiovascular system. They are used to describe cardiovascular structures and processes.

Suffix	Meaning	Example
-cuspid	tapered; pointed	tri*cuspid* = having three points
-lunar	moon-shaped	semi*lunar* = having the shape of a half moon
-sclerosis	hardening	arterio*sclerosis* = hardening of the arteries
-spasm	sudden contraction	vaso*spasm* = sudden contraction of the muscles in a blood vessel
-tension	tautness; blood pressure	hyper*tension* = elevated blood pressure
-version	turning	cardio*version* = turning the heart to a normal beat by applying an electrical shock

Anatomy and Physiology

The cardiovascular system consists of the heart and all of the blood vessels in the body. These structures are described below.

The Heart

cardi/o = heart
mediastin/o = in the middle

The heart is a hollow, muscular organ located in the **mediastinum** (ME-dee-uh-**STY**-num), the area of the chest between the lungs. Although it weighs less than a pound and is only about the size of a clenched fist, the heart acts as a highly efficient pump, ejecting blood into the blood vessels with enough force to assure its distribution to all parts of the body.

endo- = within
my/o = muscle
epi- = above
peri- = surrounding

As Figure 5-1 shows, the walls of the heart consist of three distinct layers: an inner membranous layer called the **endocardium** (EN-doe-**KAR**-dee-um), a muscular middle layer called the **myocardium** (MY-oh-**KAR**-dee-um), and an outer layer called the **epicardium** (EH-pih-**KAR**-dee-um). The heart is enclosed in a fibrous sac called the **pericardium** (PEHR-ih-**KAR**-dee-um). Fluid in the space between the epicardium and the pericardium lubricates both tissues and reduces friction as the heart beats.

atri/o = atrium
ventricul/o = ventricle

inter- = between
septum = dividing wall

Inside, the heart is divided into four chambers: two upper chambers called **atria** (AY-tree-uh), and two lower chambers called **ventricles** (VEN-trih-kulls). The atria function as "holding tanks" for blood returning to the heart between beats; the ventricles are responsible for pumping blood out of the heart, back into the circulation. The right and left atria are separated by a muscular wall called the **interatrial septum** (IN-ter-**AY**-tree-ul SEP-tum). Similarly, the right and left ventricles are separated by a structure known as the **interventricular** (IN-ter-ven-**TRIH**-kyoo-ler) **septum**.

Figure 5-1:

The four chambers of the heart (frontal view) and the three layers of the heart wall (cross section). By convention, drawings of the heart are made from the perspective of the patient. Thus, the right atrium and right ventricle appear on the left side of the drawing, and the left atrium and left ventricle appear on the right.

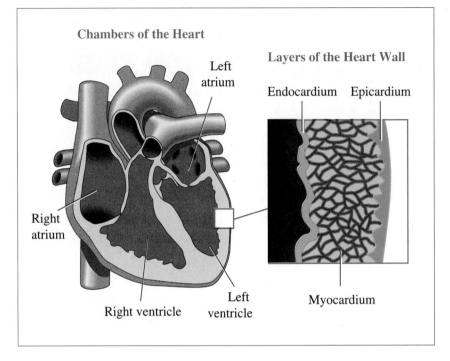

sin/o = sinus; cavity

Electrical signals are conducted through the heart muscle by a specialized system of fibers and tissues known collectively as the **cardiac conduction system** (see Figure 5-2). Electrical impulses are initiated in the upper part of the right atrium, in an area of specialized tissue called the **sinoatrial** (SIE-no-**AY**-tree-ul) or **S-A node**. Because it determines the normal rhythm of the heart, the S-A node is sometimes referred to as the heart's **pacemaker**. Similarly, the normal rhythm of the heart is referred to as the **sinus rhythm**.

Electrical impulses originating in the S-A node spread through both atria, causing them to contract and eject blood into the ventricles. As the atria contract, the electrical signal spreads to a second area of specialized tissue at the base of the right atrium called the **atrioventricular** (AY-tree-oh-ven-**TRIH**-kyoo-ler) or **A-V node**. From the A-V node, the signal passes to a collection of fibers known as the **bundle of His** (HISS) or, less commonly, as the A-V bundle. This bundle of fibers enters the interventricular septum and divides into two segments called the right and left **bundle branches**. The bundle branches, in turn, give rise to a network of fibers that spread over the ventricular walls. These fibers, called the **Purkinje** (purr-KIN-jee) **fibers**, stimulate the ventricles, causing them to contract and pump blood out of the heart. After a brief rest period, a new signal is generated by the S-A node and the process is repeated.

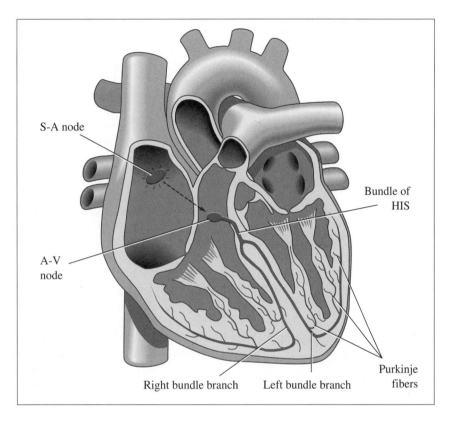

S-A node

Bundle of
HIS

A-V
node

Right bundle branch   Left bundle branch

Purkinje
fibers

electr/o = electricity
-gram = record

Electrodes placed on the skin can detect patterns of electrical activity within the heart from outside the body. An instrument records the activity detected by the electrodes, producing a tracing called an **electrocardiogram** (ih-LECK-troe-**KAR**-dee-oh-gram), which is commonly referred to as an ECG or EKG. A normal ECG tracing produces a characteristic shape that reflects the spread of electrical excitation through the heart; this shape has three components (see Figure 5-3):

- a P wave, which corresponds to the electrical activity that causes the atria to contract

- a QRS complex, which corresponds to the electrical activity that causes the ventricles to contract

- a T wave, which roughly corresponds to the return of the ventricles to their resting (non-electrically stimulated) state

Deviations from this pattern can provide important evidence of cardiovascular dysfunction or disease.

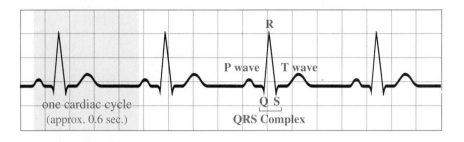

Figure 5-3:
A normal ECG
tracing.

The Vasculature

vascul/o, vas/o, and
angi/o = vessel

The blood vessels in the body are collectively referred to as the **vasculature** (VAS-kyoo-luh-tyer). Different types of blood vessels vary both in their structural features and in the circulatory functions they perform.

arteri/o = artery

The large vessels that carry blood away from the heart are called **arteries** (AR-ter-reez). The walls of arteries are thick and muscular, enabling them to withstand the high pressure under which blood is ejected from the heart. Most of the arteries in the body are named for the organs or systems they supply with blood; the arteries that deliver blood to the kidneys are known as the renal arteries, for example, while the artery supplying blood to the liver is called the hepatic artery. Farther from the heart, arteries divide into smaller branches called **arterioles** (ar-TEER-ee-ohlz). Due to its highly oxygenated state, blood in the arteries and arterioles has a bright red color.

Figure 5-4: Blood vessels (cross-sectional and long-itudinal views).

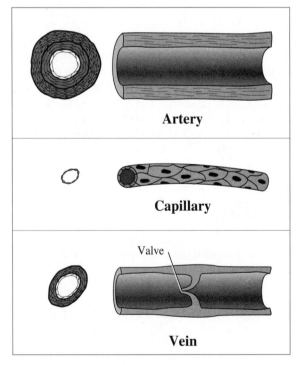

Artery

Capillary

Valve

Vein

Within the tissues, arterioles divide into even smaller vessels known as **capillaries** (KAP-ih-lehr-reez), which are the sites of exchange between the blood and the tissues. In contrast with the muscular walls of the arteries and arterioles, capillary walls are exceedingly thin, consisting of only a single layer of cells. As a result, oxygen and other nutrients are able to pass freely from the capillaries into the tissues. In exchange, carbon dioxide and other waste products of cellular metabolism move into the capillaries for removal from the tissues.

Blood leaving the capillary beds enters slightly larger vessels called **venules** (VEN-yools). Venules (venul/o = venule), in turn, merge to form larger vessels called **veins**, which are responsible for carrying blood back to the heart. Because most of its oxygen has been replaced

ven/o = vein

by carbon dioxide and other waste products, blood in the veins and venules is darker in color than the blood in the arteries. Blood in the veins is also under far lower pressure than that in the arteries. Because of this, the veins must rely on mechanisms other than the pumping action of the heart to move blood. The walls of veins are thinner and less muscular than arterial walls, which allows the skeletal muscles to assist in propelling the blood through the veins. In addition, veins contain specialized structures called **valves**, which prevent the backflow of blood into the tissues.

valvul/o = valve

Circulation

Blood returning from tissues other than the lungs enters the heart by way of the **venae cavae** (VEE-nee KOV-ee), the two largest veins in the body. Blood returning from the upper portion of the body enters by way of the **superior vena cava** (VEE-nuh KOV-uh), while blood from the lower portion of the body enters through the **inferior vena cava**. The venae cavae empty into the right atrium. When the atria contract, blood in the right atrium is forced through the **tricuspid** (try-KUSS-pid) **valve** into the right ventricle. When the ventricles contract, blood in the right ventricle is forced through the **pulmonary semilunar** (PULL-muh-nehr-ee SEH-me-**LOO**-ner) **valve** into the **pulmonary artery**; at the same time, the tricuspid valve closes to prevent the backward flow of blood into the atrium. Blood that enters the pulmonary artery is carried to the lungs. There it undergoes **oxygenation** (OCK-sih-juh-**NAY**-shun), a process in which carbon dioxide (a waste product of cellular metabolism) is exchanged for oxygen from the environment (see Figure 5-5).

super/o = upper; above
infer/o = lower; below

tri- = three
-cuspid = tapered; pointed
pulmon/o = lungs
semi- = half
-lunar = moon-shaped

Oxygenated blood returns to the heart by way of the **pulmonary veins**, which empty into the left atrium. Atrial contractions force blood from the left atrium through the **mitral** (MY-trul) **valve**, also called the **bicuspid** (bi-KUSS-pid) **valve**, into the left ventricle. When the ventricles contract, blood in the left ventricle is forced through the **aortic** (ay-OR-tick) **semilunar valve** into the **aorta** (ay-OR-tuh), the body's largest artery, for distribution to the tissues.

mitral = "shaped like a miter or turban"
bi- = two
aort/o = aorta

Functionally, then, the heart acts as a pump for two distinct circulatory pathways. The pathway mediated by the right side of the heart, which pumps blood to the lungs for oxygenation, is called the **pulmonary circulation**. The pathway mediated by the left side of the heart, which pumps oxygenated blood to the tissues, is called the **systemic** (sis-TEH-mick) **circulation**. In both the systemic and pulmonary circulations, arteries always carry blood away from the heart, while veins always carry blood to the heart.

Figure 5-5: *The pulmonary and systemic circulations (frontal view).*

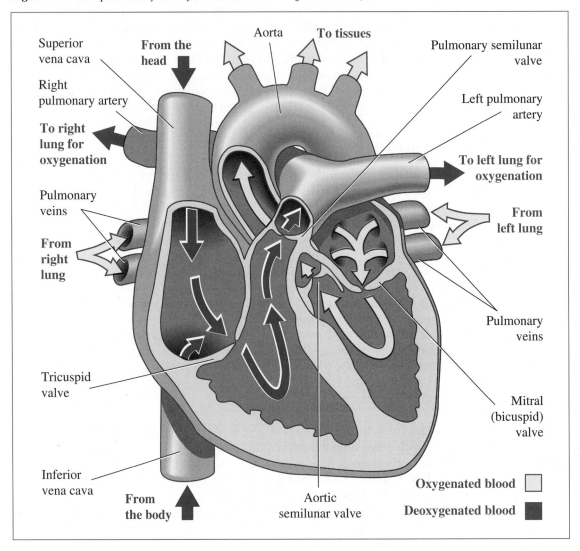

coron/o = heart; crown

Like other organs in the body, the heart muscle itself needs a constant supply of oxygen and nutrients. This need is met by the **coronary** (KOR-uh-nehr-ee) **arteries**, a pair of vessels that branch off from the aorta and form a crown-like network of vessels around the ventricles (see Figure 5-6). Abnormalities in these vessels can lead to cardiac dysfunction and even to death by disturbing the oxygen supply of the heart muscle.

Figure 5-6:
The coronary arteries
(frontal view).

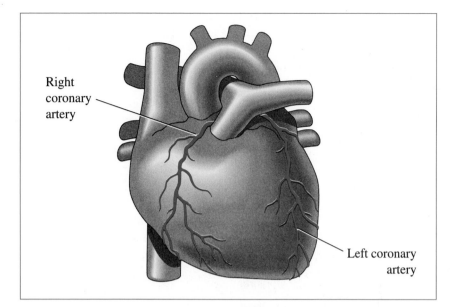

Right
coronary
artery

Left coronary
artery

Blood Pressure

systole = contraction

diastole = expansion

The sequence of events occurring during each beat of the heart is called the **cardiac cycle**. The phase of the cardiac cycle in which the ventricles contract, ejecting blood into the circulation, is called **systole** (SIS-tull-lee). The phase in which the heart muscle relaxes, allowing the ventricles to refill with blood from the atria, is known as **diastole** (die-ASS-tull-lee). Each cycle of systole and diastole lasts less than a second, enabling the heart to beat 70-90 times each minute and to pump more than 75 gallons of blood each hour.

Blood pressure refers to the force exerted by blood on the walls of the arteries. This pressure varies over the course of the cardiac cycle, increasing when blood is ejected from the heart (during systole), and decreasing as the heart relaxes (during diastole). Blood pressure is usually written as a fraction, with **systolic** (sih-STALL-ick) **pressure** in the numerator and **diastolic** (DIE-uh-**STALL**-ick) **pressure** in the denominator. A blood pressure recording of 120/80, therefore, indicates a systolic pressure of 120 millimeters of mercury and a diastolic pressure of 80 mm Hg.

Review Exercises

1. **Match** the following suffixes with their definitions.

_____	-sclerosis	a.	moon-shaped
_____	-tension	b.	tautness; blood pressure
_____	-cuspid	c.	turning
_____	-version	d.	hardening
_____	-spasm	e.	tapered; pointed
_____	-lunar	f.	sudden contraction

2. **Match** the following combining forms with their definitions.

_____	ven/o	a.	aorta
_____	atri/o	b.	heart
_____	arteriol/o	c.	vein
_____	vas/o	d.	clot
_____	cardi/o	e.	atrium
_____	thromb/o	f.	vessel
_____	aort/o	g.	arteriole

3. **Define** the following combining forms.

a. ventricul/o _____

b. angi/o _____

c. venul/o _____

d. arteri/o _____

e. sphygm/o _____

f. vascul/o _____

g. valvul/o _____

h. embol/o _____

i. phleb/o _____

j. ather/o _____

4. **Match** the following cardiovascular structures with their functions.

_____ coronary arteries

_____ valves

_____ atria

_____ venae cavae

_____ ventricles

_____ aorta

_____ S-A node

a. serves as the electrical "pacemaker" of the heart

b. deliver deoxygenated blood to the right atrium

c. prevent the backward flow of blood in the veins and between chambers of the heart

d. receives oxygenated blood from the left ventricle for delivery to the tissues

e. supply oxygen and nutrients to the heart muscle

f. serve as "holding tanks" for blood returning to the heart

g. eject blood received from the atria into the pulmonary and systemic circulations

Terminology

The following are selected terms that pertain to pathology of the cardiovascular system and to related diagnostic and surgical procedures. As you will see, most of the disorders listed involve either changes in the rate and force of cardiac contractions or changes in the ability of the blood vessels to deliver oxygen and nutrients to the tissues. Keeping this in mind will help you to understand other terms you may hear as well as the rationale behind treatment of cardiovascular disorders.

Pathologic Conditions	Word Elements	Definition
aneurysm (AN-nyer-iz-um)	an = backward eurysm = "to widen"	balloon-like sac formed when weakening of the arterial wall leads to a localized dilation, introducing a risk of rupture of the wall
angina pectoris (an-JIE-nuh or AN-jih-nuh PECK-ter-us)	angina = "to choke" pector = chest is = thing	severe chest pain and a feeling of suffocation resulting from inadequate blood flow to the heart muscle
angiospasm (AN-jee-oh-SPAZ-um)	angio = vessel spasm = sudden contraction	sudden contraction of the smooth muscle in a blood vessel wall, which can temporarily interrupt blood flow
aortostenosis (ay-OR-toe-steh-NO-sis)	aorto = aorta stenosis = narrowing	narrowing of the aorta, congenitally or as a result of disease; also called aortic stenosis
arrhythmia (ay-RITH-me-uh)	a = without rrhythm = rhythm ia = condition	any irregularity in the heart beat
arteriosclerosis (ar-TEER-ee-oh-sklur-OH-sis)	arterio = artery sclerosis = hardening	diminished elasticity in arterial walls, usually due to normal aging processes; also referred to as hardening of the arteries

Pathologic Conditions	Word Elements	Definition
atheroma (ATH-er-**OH**-muh)	ather = fatty substance oma = tumor; growth	fatty deposit that obstructs blood flow through a vessel, usually an artery; also referred to as an atherosclerotic plaque (ATH-er-oh-sklur-**OT**-ick PLACK)
atherosclerosis (ATH-er-oh-sklur-**OH**-sis)	athero = fatty substance sclerosis = hardening	condition in which fatty deposits within a blood vessel obstruct blood flow and reduce the elasticity of the vessel
bradycardia (BRAY-dee-**KAR**-dee-uh)	brady = slow cardi = heart a = condition	abnormally slow heart rate, usually defined as 60 or fewer beats per minute
cardiac arrest	cardi = heart ac = pertaining to arrest = stop	cessation of cardiac function, usually due to non-synchronous muscular contractions
cardiomyopathy (KAR-dee-oh-my-**OP**-uh-thee)	cardio = heart myo = muscle pathy = disease	general term referring to any disease of the heart muscle
coarctation (KOE-ark-**TAY**-shun)	co = together arcta = "to tighten" tion = process	narrowing of a blood vessel due to a congenital malformation; most commonly seen in the aorta
congestive heart failure	congest = "to heap together" ive = pertaining to	condition in which the ability of the heart to pump blood is impaired, causing fluid to back up in the lungs and other tissues; also referred to as CHF
coronary artery disease	coron = heart; crown ary = pertaining to	any disease process that impairs the ability of the coronary arteries to deliver an adequate supply of blood to the heart muscle
embolism (EM-bull-lih-zum)	embol = embolus ism = condition	sudden blockage of an artery by a clot or other particle circulating in the blood
endocarditis (EN-doe-kar-**DIE**-tis)	endo = within card = heart itis = inflammation	inflammation of the membrane lining the interior of the heart (the endocardium), usually due to infection
essential hypertension	hyper = excessive tension = blood pressure	type of hypertension in which the cause of elevated blood pressure is unknown
fibrillation (FIH-brul-**LAY**-shun)	fibrilla = "small fiber" tion = process	irregular, quivering contractions of ventricular muscle resulting from desynchronization of electrical impulses in the heart

Pathologic Conditions	Word Elements	Definition
flutter	flutter = "to fly about"	condition characterized by rapid but regular contractions of the atria or ventricles; heart rate may exceed 250 beats per minute
heart block	no word elements	disturbance in the transmission of electrical signals through the cardiac conduction system
hypertension (HI-per-**TEN**-shun)	hyper = excessive tension = blood pressure	consistently elevated blood pressure; usually defined as blood pressure equal to or greater than 140/90 on at least two separate occasions
hypotension (HI-poe-**TEN**-shun)	hypo = reduced tension = blood pressure	abnormally low blood pressure
infarction (in-FARK-shun)	infarct = area of tissue death ion = process	area of tissue death (necrosis) occurring as a result of oxygen deprivation; also refers to the process by which such a lesion is formed
ischemia (iss-KEE-me-uh)	isch = "to suppress" emia = blood condition	temporary oxygen deficiency due to an interruption of blood flow to a tissue or organ
left ventricular hypertrophy (ven-TRIH-kyoo-ler hi-PER-troe-fee)	hyper = excessive trophy = nourishment; growth	enlargement of the left ventricular wall, usually occurring as a result of chronic hypertension
malignant hypertension	hyper = excessive tension = blood pressure	condition of dangerously high blood pressure which is sustained over time, causing damage to the vasculature
mitral stenosis (MY-trul steh-NO-sis)	mitral = "turban-shaped" (valve) stenosis = narrowing	narrowing of the opening between the left atrium and left ventricle, with obstruction of blood flow between them
mitral valve prolapse (MY-trul VALV PRO-laps)	mitral = "turban-shaped" (valve) pro = in front of lapse = "falling; sinking"	condition in which a flap of the mitral (bicuspid) valve collapses into the left atrium during systole
murmur (MER-mer)	no word elements	soft blowing sound heard between normal beats of the heart, usually resulting from vibration in a valve
myocardial infarction (MY-oh-**KAR**-dee-ul in-FARK-shun)	myo = muscle cardi = heart al = pertaining to infarct = area of tissue death ion = process	condition in which delivery of oxygen to a portion of the heart muscle is impaired, resulting in death of the tissue in that area; also referred to as a heart attack or as an MI

Pathologic Conditions	Word Elements	Definition
myocarditis (MY-oh-kar-**DIE**-tis)	myo = muscle card = heart itis = inflammation	inflammation of the muscular layer of the heart wall (the myocardium), usually due to infection
palpitation (PAL-pih-**TAY**-shun)	palpitat = "to throb" ion = process	an unusually rapid or strong heart beat that is perceptible (and often frightening) to the patient
pericarditis (PEHR-ih-kar-**DIE**-tis)	peri = surrounding card = heart itis = inflammation	inflammation of the fibrous sac surrounding the heart (the pericardium), usually due to infection
peripheral vascular disease	vascul = vessel ar = pertaining to	progressive disease in which the blood vessels of the legs become narrower, usually due to atherosclerosis
phlebitis (fluh-**BIE**-tis)	phleb = vein itis = inflammation	inflammation of a vein
Raynaud's phenomenon (ray-NOZE)	no word elements	vascular disorder in which the fingers and toes become cold, numb, and painful as a result of temporary constriction of blood vessels in the skin
rheumatic heart disease (roo-MAT-ick)	rheumat = watery flow ic = pertaining to	heart disease caused by rheumatic fever, in which persistent streptococcal infection causes inflammation and scarring of the valves, impairing their ability to open and close normally
secondary hypertension	hyper = excessive tension = blood pressure	type of hypertension in which blood pressure is elevated as a result of another condition, usually kidney disease
tachycardia (TACK-ee-**KAR**-dee-uh)	tachy = rapid cardi = heart a = condition	abnormally rapid heart rate, usually defined as 100 or more beats per minute
thrombophlebitis (THROM-boe-fluh-**BIE**-tis)	thrombo = clot phleb = vein itis = inflammation	inflammation of a vein complicated by the formation of a blood clot within the vein
thrombosis (throm-BOE-sis)	thromb = clot osis = condition	condition in which a stationary blood clot obstructs a blood vessel at the site of its formation
valvulitis (VAL-vyoo-**LIE**-tis)	valvul = valve itis = inflammation	inflammation of a valve, particularly one of the valves within the heart

Pathologic Conditions	Word Elements	Definition
varicose vein	varic = "twisted vein" ose = having qualities of	a superficial vein that has become enlarged and twisted, usually as a result of damage to a valve and subsequent pooling of blood in the vein
vasospasm (**VAY**-zoe-SPAZ-um)	vaso = vessel spasm = sudden contraction	sudden contraction of smooth muscle in a blood vessel wall, which can temporarily interrupt blood flow

Diagnostic Procedures	Word Elements	Definition
angiography (AN-jee-**OG**-ruh-fee)	angio = vessel graphy = recording	x-ray recording of the blood vessels after injection of a contrast agent
cardiac catheterization (KATH-eh-ter-ih-**ZAY**-shun)	cardi = heart ac = pertaining to catheter = "something inserted" ization = process	procedure in which a small tube is pushed through a blood vessel until it reaches the heart; used to withdraw a sample of blood directly from the heart and to evaluate the coronary arteries
echocardiography (EH-koe-kar-dee-**OG**-ruh-fee)	echo = returned sound cardio = heart graphy = recording	technique in which high-frequency sound waves are used to produce an image of the internal structures of the heart
electrocardiography (ih-LECK-troe-KAR-dee-**OG**-ruh-fee)	electro = electricity cardio = heart graphy = recording	technique in which electrodes placed on the surface of the body are used to record patterns of electrical activity in the heart; commonly referred to as ECG or EKG
pericardiocentesis (PEHR-ih-KAR-dee-oh-sen-**TEE**-sis)	peri = surrounding cardio = heart centesis = puncture	procedure in which a hollow needle is inserted through the chest wall into the fibrous sac surrounding the heart (the pericardium) to withdraw fluid for diagnostic purposes or to relieve pressure on the heart
sphygmomanometry (SFIG-moe-meh-**NOM**-eh-tree)	sphygmo = pulse mano = "thin" metry = measurement	measurement of blood pressure using a blood pressure cuff (a sphygmomanometer)
stress test	no word elements	use of a treadmill or other exercise equipment to measure a patient's cardiovascular response to exertion; changes in the ECG during exercise can provide evidence of various types of heart disease; also called an exercise tolerance test or ETT
venography (veh-NOG-ruh-fee)	veno = vein graphy = recording	technique in which x-rays are used to visualize the veins following injection of a contrast agent

Diagnostic Procedures	Word Elements	Definition
ventriculography (ven-TRICK-kyoo-**LOG**-ruh-fee)	ventriculo = ventricle graphy = recording	x-ray recording of a heart ventricle following injection of a contrast agent

Therapeutic Procedures	Word Elements	Definition
balloon angioplasty (**AN**-jee-oh-PLASS-tee)	angio = vessel plasty = surgical repair	procedure in which a deflated balloon is pushed through a blood vessel to a site of obstruction and is inflated to restore the vessel to its normal size; alternatively, the inflated balloon may be used to pull an embolus through the blood vessel for removal from the body; also called percutaneous transluminal coronary angioplasty, or PTCA
cardioversion (KAR-dee-oh-**VER**-zhun)	cardio = heart version = turning	application of an electrical shock to the chest to restore a normal rhythm to the heart beat; also referred to as defibrillation
coronary artery bypass graft	coron = heart; crown ary = pertaining to	procedure in which a vein taken from the leg or other part of the body is grafted onto the heart to circumvent an obstruction in a coronary artery; also referred to as CABG ("cabbage")
phlebotomy (fluh-BOT-uh-me)	phlebo = vein tomy = surgical incision	surgical opening of a vein (e.g., to draw blood or remove a blood clot)
valvotomy (val-VOT-uh-me)	valvo = valve tomy = surgical incision	surgical incision into a valve, usually to increase the size of the opening
valvuloplasty (**VAL**-vyoo-loe-PLASS-tee)	valvulo = valve plasty = surgical repair	surgical repair or replacement of a valve; if a balloon is used to open the defective valve, the procedure is called balloon valvuloplasty
venipuncture (**VEH**-nee-PUNK-chur)	veni = vein puncture = puncture	procedure in which a vein (usually in the forearm) is punctured with a needle, usually to withdraw blood for diagnostic purposes

Review Exercises

5. **Match** the following terms with their definitions.

_____ mitral stenosis

_____ balloon angioplasty

_____ arteriosclerosis

_____ atherosclerosis

_____ fibrillation

_____ echocardio-graphy

_____ sphygmo-manometry

_____ murmur

a. narrowing of the opening between the left atrium and left ventricle

b. measurement of blood pressure

c. irregular, quivering contractions of the ventricles

d. procedure in which a deflated balloon is pushed through a blood vessel to a site of obstruction

e. condition in which fatty deposits obstruct the flow of blood through a vessel

f. use of high-frequency sound waves to produce an image of structures within the heart

g. hardening of the arteries, usually occurring as a result of normal aging processes

h. abnormal blowing sound heard between beats of the heart in patients with damaged valves

6. **Break Down and Define** the word elements within each of the following terms, and then define the term itself.

   Example: hyper / tension   _excessive / blood pressure_   _elevated blood pressure_

a. electrocardiography

   _____

b. vasospasm

   _____

c. valvuloplasty

   _____

d. endocarditis

   _____

e. arrhythmia

   _____

f. venipuncture

   _____

g. phlebitis

   _____

h. angiography

_____

i. angiospasm

_____

j. atheroma

_____

k. embolism

_____

l. thrombophlebitis

_____

m. thrombosis

_____

n. venography

_____

o. phlebotomy

_____

p. ventriculography

_____

7. **Word Building and Spelling**. Spell out the medical term for each of the following definitions using the slashes provided to separate the word elements.

slow heart condition	*brady / cardi / a*

a. hardening of the arteries   _____ / _____

b. low blood pressure   _____ / _____

c. surgical incision into a valve   _____ / _____

d. any disease of the heart muscle   _____ / _____ / _____

e. narrowing of the aorta   _____ / _____

f. inflammation of a valve   _____ / _____

g. puncture of the fibrous sac surrounding the heart _____ / _____ / _____

h. surgical repair of a blood vessel   _____ / _____

i. excessive blood pressure   _____ / _____

8. *Circle* the choices that will make each statement true.

   a. *Brady*cardia is a condition characterized by a (fast/slow) heart rate, while *tachy*cardia is a condition characterized by a (fast/slow) heart rate.

   b. Inflammation of the heart muscle is (pericarditis/myocarditis), while inflammation of the fibrous sac surrounding the heart is (pericarditis/myocarditis).

   c. (Coarctation/Infarction) is an area of tissue death due to oxygen deprivation, while (coarctation/infarction) is the narrowing of a blood vessel due to a congenital malformation.

   d. (Cardiac arrest/Myocardial infarction) is the cessation of heart function, while (cardiac arrest/myocardial infarction) is the death of tissue in part of the heart due to impaired delivery of oxygen.

9. *Fill in the Blank.* Write in words to make the following sentences true.

   a. Elevated blood pressure of unknown cause is called _____ hypertension.

   b. Sustained, dangerously elevated blood pressure leading to vascular damage is called _____ _____ hypertension.

   c. Blood pressure which is elevated as a result of another condition is called _____ _____ hypertension.

   d. Palpitation is an unusually strong or rapid _____.

   e. Peripheral vascular disease is a progressive disease in which the blood vessels of the legs become _____, usually due to atherosclerosis.

   f. The vascular disorder in which the fingers and toes become cold, numb, and painful as a result of constriction of blood vessels in the skin is called _____.

   g. A superficial vein that has become enlarged and twisted is called a _____ vein.

   h. _____ is a condition in which a flap of the mitral valve collapses into the left atrium during systole.

   i. Rheumatic heart disease is a type of heart disease caused by _____.

   j. A balloon-like sac formed in a weak part of an arterial wall is called an _____.

   k. The application of an electrical shock to the chest to restore a normal rhythm to the heart beat is called _____.

   l. Heart block is a disturbance in the transmission of _____ through the heart.

Case Study. Read the case notes below. For each boldfaced term, provide a brief definition and indicate whether the term is spelled correctly; if it is misspelled, provide the correct spelling.

Example:
> **miocardial infraction:** *death of heart tissue due to impaired oxygen delivery*
>
> *Spelled correctly?* ☐ Yes ☑ No *myocardial infarction*

Patient presented as a 63-year-old diabetic female with shortness of breath, edema, chest pain, and elevated blood pressure. Patient reported that her doctor had found no evidence of **miocardial infraction** during a recent **stress test**. Patient was admitted for evaluation and treatment. Echocardiogram showed significant **left ventriculer hypertriphy**. **Cardiac cathaterization** revealed blockage at several sites in the coronary arteries. Preliminary diagnosis is **conjestive heart failure** secondary to longstanding **coronary artery disease** and hypertension. Treatment plan: meds for **angina pecteris,** hypertension, and edema; **coronary artery bypass graft** immediately following medical stabilization of patient.

a. stress test: _____

_____

Spelled correctly? ☐ Yes ☐ No _____

b. left ventriculer hypertriphy: _____

Spelled correctly? ☐ Yes ☐ No _____

c. cardiac cathaterization: _____

_____

Spelled correctly? ☐ Yes ☐ No _____

d. conjestive heart failure: _____

_____

Spelled correctly? ☐ Yes ☐ No _____

e. coronary artery disease: _____

_____

Spelled correctly? ☐ Yes ☐ No _____

f. angina pecteris: _____

_____

Spelled correctly? ☐ Yes ☐ No _____

g. coronary artery bypass graft: _____

_____

Spelled correctly? ☐ Yes ☐ No _____

Listen to the section on your audiotape cassette that corresponds to this chapter and write the terms below. Be careful to spell each term correctly.

1. _____   22. _____

2. _____   23. _____

3. _____   24. _____

4. _____   25. _____

5. _____   26. _____

6. _____   27. _____

7. _____   28. _____

8. _____   29. _____

9. _____   30. _____

10. _____   31. _____

11. _____   32. _____

12. _____   33. _____

13. _____   34. _____

14. _____   35. _____

15. _____   36. _____

16. _____   37. _____

17. _____   38. _____

18. _____   39. _____

19. _____   40. _____

20. _____   41. _____

21. _____   42. _____

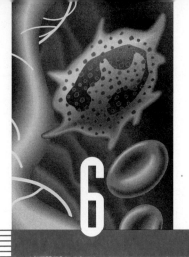

6

The Blood

Upon completing this chapter, you should be able to:

- Describe the blood and explain its primary components and functions
- Recognize, build, pronounce, and spell words that pertain to the blood
- Describe diseases, diagnostic tests, and therapeutic procedures that pertain to the blood

Overview   Blood is the bodily fluid in which nutrients, wastes, hormones, and other substances are transported throughout the body. As you learned in the preceding chapter, oxygen from the lungs and nutrients from the digestive tract are absorbed into the blood for transport to the tissues. At the same time, carbon dioxide and other waste products of cellular metabolism are absorbed from the tissues for transport to the organs of elimination. The blood also transports hormones from endocrine glands to their target organs. In addition, it contains cells and proteins that play a role in fighting infection and in blood clotting.

Word Elements

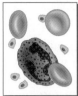

THE BLOOD – The following combining forms (CF) refer to the blood. Some are general terms, while others describe specific types of blood cells, blood-forming tissue, or blood constituents.

CF	Meaning	Example
bas/o	basic; alkaline	*baso*phil = type of blood cell that attracts alkaline dyes
eosin/o	red; dawn; rosy	*eosino*phil = type of blood cell that attracts red dyes
erythr/o	red	*erythro*cyte = red blood cell
granul/o	granules	*granulo*cyte = any granular blood cell
hem/o	blood	*hemo*lysis = the destruction of blood
hemat/o	blood	*hemato*logy = the study of blood
leuk/o	white	*leuko*cyte = white blood cell
lymph/o	lymph	*lympho*cyte = type of white blood cell
myel/o	bone marrow*	*myelo*suppression = suppression of the bone marrow
neutr/o	neutral	*neutro*phil = type of blood cell that attracts both acidic and alkaline dyes
sider/o	iron	*sidero*penia = iron deficiency

BLOOD PROCESSES – These combining forms describe processes in which the blood plays a key role. Normally beneficial, these processes can cause significant harm if they occur excessively.

CF	Meaning	Example
agglutin/o	clumping	*agglutin*ation = the process of clumping
coagul/o	clotting	*coagul*ation = the process of clotting
thromb/o	clot	*thrombo*lysis = the destruction or dissolution of a clot

SUFFIXES – The following suffixes pertain to the blood. They are commonly used to denote blood conditions or cell types.

Suffix	Meaning	Example
-emia	blood condition	an*emia* = blood condition characterized by red blood cell or iron deficiency
-phil	love; attraction	baso*phil* = type of blood cell that attracts alkaline dyes

*NOTE: Depending on the context, myel/o can also refer to the spinal cord (see Chapter 12).

Blood consists of cells suspended in a liquid medium called plasma. The functions of plasma and the various types of blood cells are described below.

Plasma

hem/o and hemat/o = blood

Plasma, the liquid portion of blood, consists of proteins, gases, nutrients, hormones, waste products, and other substances dissolved in water. As blood circulates throughout the body, it carries these substances to and from the tissues as needed. In addition, certain plasma proteins play an important role in maintaining the proper consistency of blood and in protecting the body from harm:

- **Albumin** (al-BYOO-min) is a protein that helps maintain the blood at the proper consistency.

globulin = protein

- **Globulins** (GLOB-yoo-linz) play a role in the immune system, helping to destroy foreign substances.

pro- = before
thromb/o = clot
-in = substance

- When activated, specific proteins called **fibrinogen** (fie-BRIN-oh-jin) and **prothrombin** (pro-THROM-bin) play an important role in blood clotting (see discussion of thrombocytes). When these clotting proteins are removed from plasma, the resulting fluid is called **serum**.

Blood Cells

myel/o = bone marrow
-poiesis = formation

All mature blood cells originate from immature cells called **stem cells** in the bone marrow. In a process called **hematopoiesis** (he-MAT-toe-poy-EE-sis), stem cells change in size and shape, becoming the various types of mature blood cells. The main classes of blood cells are erythrocytes, leukocytes, and thrombocytes.

erythr/o = red

The largest group of blood cells are **erythrocytes** (uh-RIH-throe-sites), commonly known as **red blood cells**. Their main functions are to carry oxygen from the lungs to the tissues, and to carry carbon dioxide from the tissues to the lungs. During maturation, the nuclei of erythrocytes are discarded, leaving them with a characteristic disk shape. This shape maximizes the surface area available for absorption of oxygen and carbon dioxide. In addition, erythrocytes produce an iron-containing protein called

-globin = protein

hemoglobin (**HE**-moe-GLOE-bin). Hemoglobin has a high affinity for oxygen, enabling erythrocytes to carry large amounts of oxygen through the blood. Hemoglobin also gives erythrocytes their red color.

leuk/o = white

Leukocytes (LOO-koe-sites), commonly known as **white blood cells**, are mainly responsible for protecting the body from bacteria and other potentially harmful foreign substances. There are five different types of leukocytes: three types of granulocytes and two types of agranulocytes.

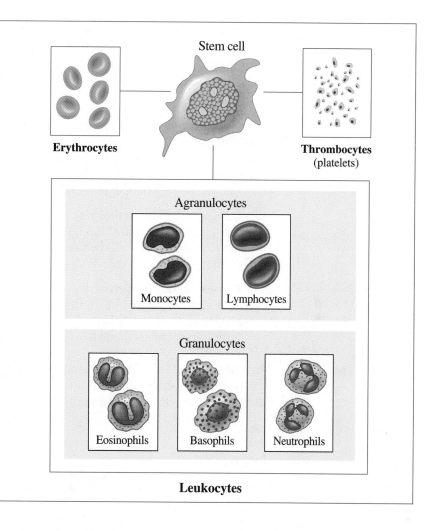

Figure 6-1:
Types of blood cells.

---

granul/o = granules

Granulocytes (GRAN-nyoo-loe-SITES) are characterized by the presence of visible particles (granules) in their cytoplasm and by their multi-lobed nuclei. Because of their oddly shaped nuclei, granulocytes are sometimes called **polymorphonuclear** (POL-ee-MOR-foe-**NOO**-klee-er) **leukocytes**, or **PMNs**. The three types of granulocytes are named for the types of dye they take up in laboratory tests.

poly- = many
morph/o = shape
nucle/o = nucleus

eosin/o = red; dawn;
rosy
-phil = love; attraction

- **Eosinophils** (EE-oh-**SIN**-oh-fills) take up a red acidic dye called eosin (EE-oh-sin); their main function is to detoxify foreign proteins, especially those causing allergic reactions.

bas/o = basic;
alkaline

- **Basophils** (BAY-zoe-fills) take up alkaline dyes; their main function is to release histamines (chemicals that initiate inflammation) and heparin (an anti-clotting chemical) at sites of injury.

neutr/o = neutral
phag/o = eat;
swallow

- **Neutrophils** (NOO-troe-fills) take up both acidic and alkaline dyes; they are phagocytic cells, responsible for ingesting and destroying bacteria and other foreign particles. Note that, although the term PMN technically refers to all three types of granulocytes, some physicians use the term to refer only to neutrophils.

Unlike granulocytes, **agranulocytes** (ay-**GRAN**-nyoo-loe-SITES) do not contain granules in their cytoplasm, nor do they have multi-lobed nuclei. Agranulocytes are characterized by the presence of a single large nucleus.

mono- = one
nucle/o = nucleus

As a result, they are sometimes called **mononuclear** (MON-oh-**NOO**-klee-er) **cells**. The two types of agranulocytes are monocytes and lymphocytes.

macro- = large

- Like neutrophils, **monocytes** (MON-oh-sites) are phagocytic cells that ingest and destroy foreign particles. In fact, many monocytes travel to the tissues and become larger phagocytic cells called **macrophages** (**MACK**-kroe-FAY-jez).

lymph/o = lymph

- **Lymphocytes** (LIM-foe-sites), on the other hand, mature in the lymph nodes and circulate in both the blood and lymphatic systems. They play an important role in the immune response, and will be discussed further in Chapters 7 and 8.

thromb/o = clot

Thrombocytes (THROM-boe-sites), commonly called **platelets** (PLATE-lets) because of their plate-like appearance, are actually cell fragments rather than complete cells. The main function of platelets is to initiate blood clotting at sites of vascular injury.

Coagulation

coagul/o = clotting

Blood clotting, also called **coagulation** (koe-AG-gyoo-**LAY**-shun), is a complex process involving several plasma proteins and clotting factors. The process is initiated when injured tissue and platelets release a protein called

thromb/o = clot
plast/o = formation
-in = substance

thromboplastin (THROM-boe-**PLASS**-tin). In the presence of calcium, thromboplastin causes the plasma protein prothrombin to turn into **thrombin**. Thrombin, in turn, causes the plasma protein fibrinogen to turn into **fibrin**. The tough threads of fibrin that result from this process become intertwined, forming a meshwork surrounding blood cells. This mass of fibrin and blood cells, called a **clot**, acts as a blockade, preventing further loss of blood from the injured area.

ABO Types

Based on the presence or absence of certain factors (specific of types antigens and antibodies), human blood is divided into four groups: Type A, Type B, Type AB, and Type O. Because the antibodies contained in Type

agglutin/o = clumping

A blood can cause Type B blood to **agglutinate** (uh-GLUE-tih-nate), and vice versa, donated blood must be typed before it can be **transfused** into a recipient. Only compatible blood should be given to a patient requiring a blood transfusion. Individuals with Type O blood are called "universal donors" because their blood can be given to anyone; conversely, individuals with Type AB blood are called "universal recipients" because they can receive blood from anyone.

Rh Factor

Blood contains many other factors in addition to the ABO antigens described above. Most of these substances are not clinically important and therefore are not generally typed. One, however, called the **Rh factor**, is important in pregnancy. When a pregnant woman delivers a baby, some of the baby's blood usually enters the mother's bloodstream. If the pregnant woman is Rh-negative (i.e., her blood does not contain Rh factor) and the fetus is Rh-positive (i.e., the fetus' blood contains Rh factor), the mother may develop antibodies against the Rh factor. If she then carries a second fetus with Rh-positive blood, her anti-Rh antibodies will attack the infant's blood, causing the baby to be born with a serious hemolytic blood disorder; to avoid complete destruction of the blood, the baby must receive a complete transfusion (i.e., all of the baby's blood must be removed and replaced with new blood).

-lytic = destroying

Review Exercises

1. **Match** the following suffixes and combining forms with their definitions.

_____	-emia	a. red
_____	-phil	b. red; dawn; rosy
_____	bas/o	c. white
_____	eosin/o	d. neutral
_____	erythr/o	e. basic; alkaline
_____	leuk/o	f. love; attraction
_____	neutr/o	g. blood condition
_____	myel/o	h. bone marrow

2. **Define** the following combining forms.

a. agglutin/o _____

b. coagul/o _____

c. thromb/o _____

d. granul/o _____

e. lymph/o _____

f. hem/o _____

g. hemat/o _____

h. sider/o _____

3. **Match** the following blood components with their descriptions.

_____ plasma

_____ erythrocytes

_____ leukocytes

_____ thrombocytes

a. hemoglobin-containing cells that transport oxygen and carbon dioxide through the blood

b. group of five cell types that help protect the body from infection and injury

c. liquid portion of blood that consists of water, proteins, gases, nutrients, and waste products

d. cell fragments that initiate blood clotting and prevent excessive bleeding at sites of injury

Terminology

The following are selected terms that pertain to pathology of the blood and to related diagnostic and therapeutic procedures. As you will see, most of the disorders listed result from a deficiency of particular types of blood cells or abnormalities in their function. Keeping this in mind will help you to understand other terms you may hear as well as the rationale behind the diagnosis and treatment of hematologic disorders.

Pathologic Conditions	Word Elements	Definition
anemia (uh-NEE-me-uh)	an = without; not emia = blood condition	condition characterized by a low red blood cell count or hemoglobin deficiency
aplastic anemia (ay-PLASS-tick)	a = without; not plast = formation ic = pertaining to	rare but serious form of anemia characterized by failure of the bone marrow to produce stem cells or by failure of stem cells to mature
blood dyscrasia (dis-KRAY-zee-uh)	dys = abnormal; difficult crasia = "temperament"	any abnormality of the blood

Pathologic Conditions	Word Elements	Definition
ecchymosis (ECK-kih-**MOE**-sis)	ec = out chym = to pour osis = condition	bruise (discoloration caused by leakage of blood under the skin following an injury); plural, ecchymoses
hemolytic anemia (HE-moe-**LIH**-tick)	hemo = blood lytic = destroying	form of anemia characterized by excessive destruction of red blood cells
hemophilia (HE-moe-**FEEL**-ee-uh)	hemo = blood phil = love; attraction ia = condition	hereditary disorder in which the lack of a clotting factor (Factor VIII) predisposes the patient to excessive bruising and bleeding
hemorrhage (HEH-mer-ehj)	hemo = blood rrhage = excessive flow	bleeding; usually refers to excessive or uncontrolled bleeding
iron-deficiency anemia	an = without; not emia = blood condition	most common form of anemia; caused by insufficient iron intake in the diet (iron is an essential component of hemoglobin)
leukemia (loo-**KEE**-me-uh)	leuk = white emia = blood condition	malignant disease of the bone marrow characterized by excessive production of leukocytes (white blood cells)
leukopenia (LOO-koe-**PEE**-nee-uh)	leuko = white penia = deficiency	leukocyte (white blood cell) deficiency
multiple myeloma (MY-ul-**LOE**-muh)	myel = bone marrow oma = tumor; growth	malignant disease arising from the bone marrow, usually involving plasma cells (a type of white blood cell that develops in the marrow)
pernicious anemia (per-**NIH**-shuss)	pernicious = "ruinous"	form of anemia characterized by deficient or abnormal maturation of red blood cells; caused by an inability to absorb vitamin B_{12}, which plays a role in hematopoiesis
polycythemia (POL-ee-sie-**THEE**-me-uh)	poly = many cyt = cell hem = blood ia = condition	condition in which increased production of blood cells without an increase in blood volume results in the formation of thick, sticky blood
purpura (PURR-purr-uh)	purpura = "purple"	condition in which small areas of bleeding under the skin and mucous membranes produce visible purplish or reddish-brown spots
sickle cell anemia	an = without; not emia = blood condition	hereditary form of anemia characterized by fragile, sickle-shaped red blood cells and a reduced oxygen-binding capacity in the hemoglobin; occurs almost exclusively in blacks

Pathologic Conditions	Word Elements	Definition
thalassemia (THAL-uh-**SEE**-me-uh)	thalass = "sea" emia = blood condition	inherited form of anemia characterized by impaired hemoglobin production; most commonly seen in individuals of Mediterranean, Southeast Asian, or Middle Eastern descent
thrombocytopenia (THROM-boe-SIE-toe-**PEE**-nee-uh)	thrombo = clot cyto = cell penia = deficiency	thrombocyte (platelet) deficiency

Diagnostic Procedures	Word Elements	Definition
bleeding time	no word elements	time required for a small puncture wound made in the earlobe or forearm to stop bleeding; used to evaluate the ability of blood to clot
bone marrow biopsy	bi = life opsy = view	use of a needle to extract bone marrow for examination and evaluation
complete blood count	no word elements	group of routine blood tests that measures the hemoglobin concentration and the numbers of red blood cells, white blood cells, and platelets in the blood; commonly referred to as a CBC
Coombs' test (KOOMZ)	no word elements	test used to detect the presence of antibodies directed toward red blood cells; often used to detect anti-Rh antibodies in infants of women with Rh-negative blood or to detect antibodies in the blood of patients with other hemolytic disorders
differential	differential = "to carry apart" or "separate"	routine test measuring each of the five types of white blood cells as a percentage of the total number of leukocytes in the blood; commonly referred to as a diff
erythrocyte sedimentation rate (SEH-dih-men-**TAY**-shun)	erythro = red cyte = cell sediment = "to settle" ation = process	test measuring the speed at which red blood cells settle to the bottom of a narrow tube; used in the diagnosis of inflammatory diseases, cancer, and other conditions that alter the consistency of blood; commonly called sed rate or ESR
finger prick	no word elements	pricking a finger and collecting blood using a capillary tube; used to obtain a blood sample when only a small volume is required; also called finger stick

Diagnostic Procedures	Word Elements	Definition
hematocrit (he-MAT-oh-krit)	hemato = blood crit = "to separate"	routine test used to measure the percentage of the total blood volume made up by red blood cells; along with other blood tests, used to diagnose various types of anemia; commonly called a crit
hemoglobin	hemo = blood globin = protein	routine test measuring the amount of hemoglobin in the blood; usually used in the diagnosis of anemia
partial thromboplastin time	thrombo = clot plast = formation in = substance	one of several tests used to evaluate the function of plasma clotting factors; often called PTT
prothrombin time	pro = before thromb = clot in = substance	one of several tests used to evaluate the function of plasma clotting factors; also called protime or PT
red blood count	no word elements	routine test measuring the number of red blood cells per cubic millimeter of blood
thrombin time	thromb = clot in = substance	one of several tests used to evaluate the function of plasma clotting factors
white blood count	no word elements	routine test measuring the number of white blood cells per cubic millimeter of blood; an increase is often a sign of infection

Therapeutic Procedures	Word Elements	Definition
blood transfusion	trans = through; across fusion = "pouring"	intravenous administration of blood, usually from a donor, into a patient; generally used to replace blood lost after injury, during surgery, or as a result of disease
bone marrow transplant	trans = through; across plant = plant	procedure in which a patient's diseased bone marrow is destroyed by irradiation and chemotherapy, then replaced with new bone marrow from a donor; used to treat aplastic anemia, leukemia, and certain cancers

Review Exercises

4. **Match** the following types of anemia with their descriptions.

_____ iron-deficiency

_____ hemolytic

_____ pernicious

_____ sickle cell

_____ aplastic

_____ thalassemia

a. characterized by failure of the bone marrow to produce stem cells or by failure of stem cells to mature

b. hereditary form characterized by fragile, abnormally-shaped red blood cells and a reduced oxygen-binding capacity; almost always seen in blacks

c. form characterized by deficient or abnormal red blood cell maturation due to an inability to absorb vitamin B_{12}

d. inherited form characterized by impaired hemoglobin production; most commonly found in individuals of Mediterranean descent

e. most common form; caused by insufficient iron intake in the diet

f. form characterized by excessive destruction of red blood cells

5. **Break Down and Define** the word elements within each of the following terms, and then define the term itself.

Example: hemo / lytic   _blood / destroying_   _pertaining to destruction of blood_

a. thrombocytopenia

_____

b. hemorrhage

_____

c. aplastic anemia

_____

d. hemolytic anemia

_____

e. erythrocyte

_____

f. hemophilia

_____

g. leukemia

_____

6. **Word Building and Spelling.** Spell out the medical term for each of the following definitions using the slashes provided to separate the word elements.

    stopping or controlling blood   *hemo / stasis*

a. deficiency of white cells   _____ / _____

b. blood protein   _____ / _____

c. condition characterized by many blood cells   _____ / _____ / _____

d. tumor arising from the bone marrow   _____ / _____

Case Study. Read the case notes below. For each boldfaced term, provide a brief definition and indicate whether the term is spelled correctly; if it is misspelled, provide the correct spelling.

Example:

perpera: *purple spots on the skin due to small areas of bleeding*

Spelled correctly?   ☐ Yes   ✔ No   *purpura*

Patient presented as a 27-year-old female complaining of dizziness and weakness. On examination, **perpera** and unexplained **eckymoses** were also noted, suggesting some type of **blood discrazia**. Ordered **complete blood count** and **differentiel**. Results of the lab tests were **hemoglobin** 7 mg/dl; **red blood count** 2,100/mm^3; **white blood count** 5,100/mm^3; platelet count 19,000/mm^3; differential 14% polymorphonuclear leukocytes, 81% lymphocytes, 4% monocytes, 1% eosinophils, 0% basophils. Suspected aplastic anemia. Ordered **bone marrow biopsy**. Examination of bone marrow revealed drastically reduced levels of all blood-forming elements. Diagnosis of aplastic anemia was confirmed. Treatment plan: **blood transfusions** until suitable bone marrow donor can be found, then **bone marrow tranplantation**.

a. eckymoses: _____

_____

Spelled correctly?   ☐ Yes   ☐ No _____

b. blood discrazia: _____

Spelled correctly?   ☐ Yes   ☐ No _____

c. complete blood count: _____

_____

Spelled correctly?   ☐ Yes   ☐ No _____

d. differentiel: _____

_____

Spelled correctly? ☐ Yes ☐ No _____

e. hemoglobin: _____

_____

Spelled correctly? ☐ Yes ☐ No _____

f. red blood count: _____

_____

Spelled correctly? ☐ Yes ☐ No _____

g. white blood count: _____

_____

Spelled correctly? ☐ Yes ☐ No _____

h. bone marow biopsy: _____

_____

Spelled correctly? ☐ Yes ☐ No _____

i. blood transfusions: _____

_____

Spelled correctly? ☐ Yes ☐ No _____

j. bone marrow tranplantation: _____

_____

Spelled correctly? ☐ Yes ☐ No _____

Listen to the section on your audiotape cassette that corresponds to this chapter and write the terms below. Be careful to spell each term correctly.

1. _____ 4. _____

2. _____ 5. _____

3. _____ 6. _____

7. _____

8. _____

9. _____

10. _____

11. _____

12. _____

13. _____

14. _____

15. _____

16. _____

17. _____

18. _____

19. _____

20. _____

21. _____

22. _____

23. _____

24. _____

25. _____

26. _____

27. _____

28. _____

29. _____

30. _____

31. _____

32. _____

33. _____

34. _____

35. _____

36. _____

37. _____

38. _____

39. _____

40. _____

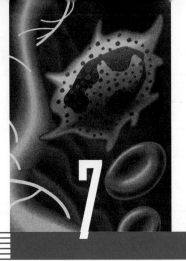

Lymphatic System

Upon completing this chapter, you should be able to:

- Describe the lymphatic system and explain the primary functions of its organs
- Recognize, build, pronounce, and spell words that pertain to the lymphatic system
- Describe diseases, diagnostic tests, and surgical procedures that pertain to the lymphatic system

Overview   The lymphatic system is related to the cardiovascular system in both structure and function. Like the cardiovascular system, the lymphatic system consists of a network of vessels and organs that transport fluid, cells, and other substances throughout the body. Its main functions are to drain fluid from the tissues and return it to the bloodstream, to transport proteins and other nutrients back and forth between the blood and tissues, to absorb fats from the digestive system and carry them to the bloodstream, and to produce lymphocytes and other immune cells that protect the body from injury and infection.

Word Elements

— The following combining forms (CF) pertain to the lymphatic system. They are used to denote the major lymphatic organs and structures.

CF	Meaning	Example
aden/o	gland	lymph*adeno*pathy = any disease of the lymph glands
adenoid/o	adenoids	*adenoid*itis = inflammation of the adenoids
angi/o	vessel	lymph*angio*graphy = x-ray of the lymph vessels
lymph/o	lymph	*lymph*oma = tumor of the lymph tissues
splen/o	spleen	*spleno*megaly = enlargement of the spleen
thym/o	thymus	*thym*itis = inflammation of the thymus
tonsill/o	tonsils	*tonsill*itis = inflammation of the tonsils

SUFFIX — The following suffix pertains to the lymphatic system. It describes where lymph, the fluid of the lymphatic system, originates.

Suffix	Meaning	Example
-stitial	to set; to be situated	inter*stitial* = situated in the spaces between the tissues

Anatomy and Physiology

The lymphatic system consists of lymph, lymph vessels, lymph nodes, and lymph organs (the spleen, thymus, and tonsils). These structures are described below.

Lymph

lymph/o = lymph

-stitial = to set; to be situated

Lymph (LIMF), the clear, watery fluid of the lymphatic system, actually originates from blood plasma. As blood circulates throughout the body, plasma seeps out of blood capillaries and into the spaces between the tissues. This fluid, called **interstitial** (IN-ter-**STIH**-shul) **fluid**, nourishes and bathes the tissues and collects cellular waste products, bacteria, and other debris. As fluid collects in the tissues, some of it drains into lymph vessels, where it is called lymph. Thus, lymph consists of water, nutrients, and debris from the tissues; it also contains lymphocytes and other immune cells manufactured in the lymph organs.

Lymph Vessels

angi/o = vessel

The lymphatic system contains an extensive network of **lymph vessels**, which are the vessels through which lymph is transported. These vessels originate in the tissues as capillaries that collect interstitial fluid; like blood capillaries, these tiny lymph vessels merge together, forming larger and larger vessels. Lymph vessels from the right chest and arm join together to form the **right lymphatic duct**; this duct drains lymph into the right subclavian vein of the cardiovascular system. Lymph vessels from all other parts of the body join together to form the **thoracic** (ther-RASS-ick) **duct**, which drains lymph into the left subclavian vein of the cardiovascular system.

thorac/o = chest

Lymph Nodes

aden/o = gland

Lymph nodes (also called lymph glands) are small masses of lymph tissue located at various places along the larger lymph vessels (see Figure 7-1). They tend to occur in clusters or chains; major groups are located in the

Figure 7-1:
Lymph vessels and lymph nodes.

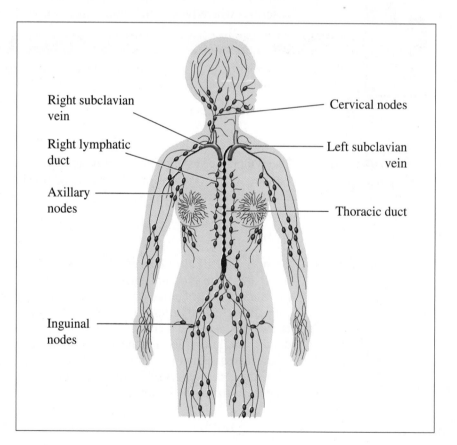

Right subclavian vein

Right lymphatic duct

Axillary nodes

Inguinal nodes

Cervical nodes

Left subclavian vein

Thoracic duct

Figure 7-2:
Organs of the
lymphatic system.

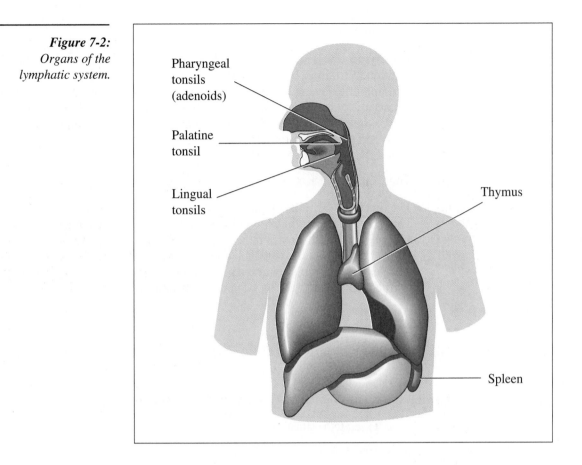

cervical (neck), axillary (armpit), and inguinal (groin) regions of the body. Lymph is filtered through these nodes as it passes through the lymph vessels. Thus, the main functions of the lymph nodes are to replenish lymph with lymphocytes, monocytes, and proteins. If too many bacteria accumulate in the lymph nodes, as during some types of bacterial infections, the lymph nodes can become swollen and tender.

The Spleen

splen/o = spleen

The **spleen** is an organ similar in structure and function to a lymph node, except that it is much larger. Like lymph nodes, the spleen filters lymph and manufactures lymphocytes and monocytes. It also destroys old red blood cells and stores new red blood cells for release into the bloodstream as needed. Unlike most other organs, the spleen is not essential to life; if the spleen is removed, other organs take over its functions.

The Thymus

thym/o = thymus

The **thymus** (THIE-muss) is a lymph gland located in between the lungs. In addition to filtering lymph, the thymus converts lymphocytes into specialized immune cells called T-cells in infants and young children, helping to protect them from disease. When children reach puberty, however, the thymus begins to wither away. In adults, the thymus is comprised mainly of fat and connective tissue.

The Tonsils

tonsill/o = tonsils
pharyng/o = pharynx
adenoid/o = adenoids
palat/o = palate
lingu/o = tongue

The **tonsils** (TON-sills) are masses of lymphatic tissue located in the throat. There are three sets: the **pharyngeal** (fer-RIN-jee-ul) **tonsils**, also called the adenoids (AD-dih-noydz); the **palatine** (PAL-uh-tine) **tonsils**; and the **lingual** (LING-gwul) **tonsils**. The adenoids and the palatine tonsils are those most commonly removed in children. All three sets of tonsils function to filter lymph and destroy bacteria entering the mouth and throat.

Review Exercises

1. ***Match*** the following suffix and combining forms with their definitions.

_____ thym/o	a.	to set; to be situated
_____ aden/o	b.	tonsils
_____ splen/o	c.	spleen
_____ adenoid/o	d.	thymus
_____ tonsill/o	e.	adenoids
_____ -stitial	f.	gland

2. ***Define*** the following combining form and compound combining forms.

a. lymph/o _____

b. lymphaden/o _____

c. lymphangi/o _____

3. **Match** the following lymphatic structures with their descriptions.

_____ tonsils

_____ thymus

_____ spleen

_____ lymph nodes

a. small masses scattered on the lymph vessels

b. destroy bacteria entering the mouth and throat

c. destroys old red blood cells and stores new red blood cells

d. thought to play an important role in immunity in young children but not in adults

Terminology

The following are selected terms that pertain to pathology of the lymphatic system and to associated diagnostic and surgical procedures. As you will see, most of the diseases listed result from inflammation, infection, obstruction, or cancer of lymphatic structures. Keeping this in mind will help you to understand other terms you may hear as well as the rationale behind treatment of lymphatic diseases.

Pathologic Conditions	Word Elements	Definition
adenoiditis (AD-dih-noyd-**EYE**-tis)	adenoid = adenoids itis = inflammation	inflammation of the adenoids, usually due to infection
asplenia (ay-SPLEE-nee-uh)	a = without; not splen = spleen ia = condition	absence of the spleen, either congenitally or as a result of surgical removal
elephantiasis (ELL-eh-fan-**TIE**-uh-sis)	elephant = elephant iasis = condition	condition involving massive swelling of the extremities due to chronic lymph vessel obstruction; usually caused by a parasitic worm infestation, but can be caused by other factors (e.g., cancer)
Hodgkin's disease (HODGE-kinz)	no word elements	malignant disease involving the lymph nodes and spleen; characterized by the presence of unique ("Reed-Sternberg") cells in the lymph nodes
lymphadenitis (LIM-fad-ih-**NIE**-tis)	lymph = lymph aden = gland itis = inflammation	inflammation of the lymph glands, usually due to infection
lymphadenopathy (LIM-fad-ih-**NOP**-uh-thee)	lymph = lymph adeno = gland pathy = disease	any disease of the lymph glands

Pathologic Conditions	Word Elements	Definition
lymphangioma (LIM-fan-jee-**OH**-muh)	lymph = lymph angi = vessel oma = tumor; growth	nodular tumor or swelling of the lymph vessels
lymphedema (LIM-feh-**DEE**-muh)	lymph = lymph edema = swelling	swelling of the tissues due to obstruction of the lymph vessels and accumulation of fluid
lymphoma (lim-FOE-muh)	lymph = lymph oma = tumor; growth	any malignant tumor of the lymph nodes or other lymph tissue
mononucleosis (MON-oh-NOO-klee-**OH**-sis)	mono = one nucle = nucleus osis = condition	acute infectious disease caused by Epstein-Barr virus characterized by enlarged, tender cervical nodes, sore throat, and fatigue
non-Hodgkin's lymphoma (non-HODGE-kinz lim-FOE-muh)	lymph = lymph oma = tumor; growth	any malignant disease of lymph tissue except for Hodgkin's disease; previously called lymphosarcoma
splenomegaly (SPLEH-noe-**MEG**-gull-lee)	spleno = spleen megaly = enlargement	abnormal enlargement of the spleen
tonsillitis (TON-sill-**LIE**-tis)	tonsill = tonsils itis = inflammation	inflammation of the tonsils, especially the palatine tonsils, usually due to infection

Diagnostic Procedure	Word Elements	Definition
lymphangiography (LIM-fan-jee-**OG**-ruh-fee)	lymph = lymph angio = vessel graphy = recording	x-ray recording of the lymph vessels after injection of a contrast agent

Surgical Procedures	Word Elements	Definition
adenoidectomy (AD-dih-noyd-**ECK**-tuh-me)	adenoid = adenoids ectomy = surgical removal	surgical removal of the adenoids
splenectomy (spleh-NECK-tuh-me)	splen = spleen ectomy = surgical removal	surgical removal of the spleen
tonsillectomy (TON-sill-**LECK**-tuh-me)	tonsill = tonsils	surgical removal of the tonsils, especially the palatine tonsils

Review Exercises

4. ***Match*** the following terms with their definitions.

_____ mononucleosis

_____ Hodgkin's disease

_____ non-Hodgkin's lymphoma

_____ lymphadenopathy

_____ elephantiasis

a. malignant disease of the lymph nodes and spleen with Reed-Sternberg cells present

b. any disease of the lymph glands

c. any malignant disease of lymph tissue except Hodgkin's disease

d. infection characterized by enlarged, tender cervical nodes, sore throat, and fever

e. massive swelling of the extremities due to chronic lymph vessel obstruction

5. ***Break Down and Define*** the word elements within each of the following terms, and then define the term itself.

    Example: thym / itis   *thymus / inflammation*   *inflammation of the thymus*

a. adenoidectomy

_____

b. asplenia

_____

c. lymphangiography

_____

d. lymphoma

_____

e. lymphadenoma

_____

f. lymphangioma

_____

g. lymphedema

_____

h. tonsillitis

_____

6. **Choose and Construct.** Choose the appropriate word elements from the list provided to construct terms for the following.

lymph/o	angi/o	-ectomy	-tomy
aden/o	-plasty	-graphy	

    surgical repair of lymph tissue   *lympho / plasty*

a. x-ray (recording) of lymph tissue   _____ / _____

b. x-ray (recording) of the lymph glands   _____ / _____ / _____

c. x-ray (recording) of the lymph vessels   _____ / _____ / _____

d. surgical incision in a lymph gland   _____ / _____ / _____

e. surgical incision in a lymph vessel   _____ / _____ / _____

f. surgical repair of a lymph vessel   _____ / _____ / _____

g. surgical removal of a lymph gland   _____ / _____ / _____

7. **Word Building and Spelling.** Spell out the medical term for each of the following definitions using the slashes provided to separate the word elements.

    inflammation of the tonsils   *tonsill / itis*

a. surgical removal of the tonsils   _____ / _____

b. enlargement of the spleen   _____ / _____

c. inflammation of the lymph glands   _____ / _____ / _____

d. inflammation of the adenoids   _____ / _____

e. surgical removal of the spleen   _____ / _____

f. any disease of the lymph   _____ / _____

g. any disease of the lymph glands   _____ / _____ / _____

Case Study. Read the case notes below. For each boldfaced term, provide a brief definition and indicate whether the term is spelled correctly; if it is misspelled, provide the correct spelling.

Example:

limfoma: *malignant tumor of the lymph tissues*

Spelled correctly? ☐ Yes ☑ No *lymphoma*

Patient presented as a 51-year-old female referred by her primary care physician with a preliminary diagnosis of **limfoma**. On questioning, she said that she'd had flu-like symptoms for three months accompanied by increasing fatigue, night sweats, and restless legs. She'd lost 25 pounds without explanation, but still felt abdominal pain and pressure. On examination, patient exhibited extensive **lymphadenapathy**, with multiple sites of enlarged, tender lymph nodes. The spleen was grossly enlarged; **splenomegaly** was probably the cause of her abdominal pain and pressure. Lymph node biopsies were positive, showing evidence of advanced, high grade, rapidly progressing **non-Hodgekin's lymphoma**. **Lymphangeography** also showed evidence of widespread lymphatic involvement. Treatment plan: chemotherapy plus radiation, **splinectomy** if warranted.

a. lymphadenapathy: _____

Spelled correctly? ☐ Yes ☐ No _____

b. splenomegaly: _____

Spelled correctly? ☐ Yes ☐ No _____

c. non-Hodgekin's lymphoma: _____

_____

Spelled correctly? ☐ Yes ☐ No _____

d. lymphangeography: _____

_____

Spelled correctly? ☐ Yes ☐ No _____

e. splinectomy: _____

Spelled correctly? ☐ Yes ☐ No _____

Listen to the section on your audiotape cassette that corresponds to this chapter and write the terms below. Be careful to spell each term correctly.

1. _____   3. _____

2. _____   4. _____

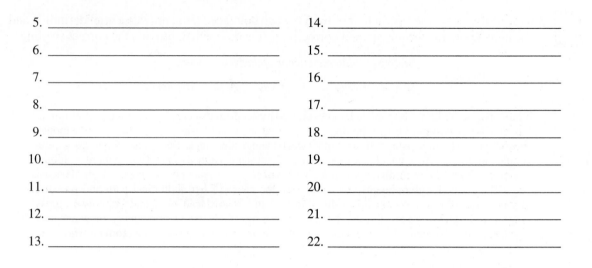

5. _____

6. _____

7. _____

8. _____

9. _____

10. _____

11. _____

12. _____

13. _____

14. _____

15. _____

16. _____

17. _____

18. _____

19. _____

20. _____

21. _____

22. _____

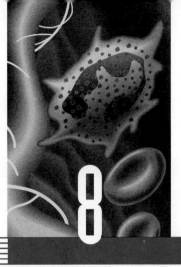

8

Immune System

Upon completing this chapter, you should be able to:

- Describe the immune system and explain the primary functions of its components
- Recognize, build, pronounce, and spell words that pertain to the immune system
- Describe diseases, diagnostic tests, and therapeutic procedures that pertain to the immune system

Overview   The immune system is responsible for defending the body against bacteria, viruses, and other foreign substances that enter the body. To do so, it must first recognize a substance as foreign ("non-self"), then take steps to remove the offending substance by inactivating or destroying it. This is achieved through defensive reactions called **immune responses**. Thus, unlike other body systems, the immune system encompasses reactions rather than organs. In effect, the immune system functions as a coordinator, activating and directing cells and proteins that the blood and lymphatic systems produce to protect the body from harm.

Word Elements

THE IMMUNE SYSTEM – The following combining forms (CF) pertain to the immune system. They are used to describe anything related to the immune system and to the process of engulfing foreign matter.

CF	Meaning	Example
immun/o	immune; protected	*immuno*logy = study of the immune system
phag/o	eat; swallow	*phago*cyte = cell that engulfs foreign matter

SUFFIX – The following suffix pertains to the immune system. It describes a protective immune process that can be dangerous if too extreme.

Suffix	Meaning	Example
-phylaxis	protection	ana*phylaxis* = type of protective reaction so extreme as to be life-threatening

Anatomy and Physiology

immun/o = immune; protected

Most bacteria, viruses, and other "non-self" substances that enter the body are destroyed by cells that react to any type of foreign substance. This general defensive reaction is called the **non-specific immune response**. If non-self substances enter the body in numbers too large for the non-specific immune response to handle, the immune system mobilizes to mount more intensive reactions directed specifically at the offending substance. These reactions, called **specific immune responses**, are carried out by lymphocytes. The various types of immune responses, as well as the types of protection they confer, are described below.

The Non-Specific Immune Response

phag/o = eat; swallow

The **non-specific immune response** occurs when bacteria, viruses, or any other type of foreign substance enters the body. The reaction is carried out by scavenger cells called **phagocytes** (FAG-go-sites) that engulf and digest any foreign substances they encounter. In some cases, a group of blood proteins known as **complement** assist phagocytes in destroying their targets. The two main types of phagocytes are **neutrophils** (NOO-troe-fills), which circulate in the blood, and **macrophages** (MACK-kroe-FAY-jez), which reside mainly in the tissues. In addition to digesting foreign particles, neutrophils and other white blood cells release proteins that attract more immune cells to the site of injury or infection and that cause local heat and inflammation.

The Humoral Immune Response

humor = fluid

The **humoral immune response** is a specific immune response that specialized lymphocytes called **B-cells** carry out in the blood and other body fluids. Each B-cell or group of B-cells reacts only to one specific type of foreign substance or **antigen** (AN-tih-jen). When a B-cell encounters the specific type of antigen that it can destroy, it becomes activated and turns into a **plasma cell**. This plasma cell then produces proteins called **antibodies** (**AN**-tih-**BOD**-eez) or **immunoglobulins** (IM-yoo-no-**GLOB**-yoo-linz) that react with and neutralize the antigen. In some cases, complement helps the antibodies destroy the antigen.

globulin = protein

The Cell-Mediated Immune Response

The **cell-mediated immune response** is a specific immune response that other specialized lymphocytes called **T-cells** carry out. Like B-cells, each T-cell or group of T-cells can react to only one type of antigen. When a T-cell encounters an antigen it recognizes, it multiplies very rapidly, creating a large number of activated T-cells capable of ingesting the antigen. In some cases, macrophages help T-cells clear away the antigen. Unlike B-cells, which mainly react to bacteria and viruses present in the blood or interstitial fluid, T-cells also react to cancer cells, infected tissue cells, and foreign tissues (e.g., transplanted organs).

Figure 8-1:
Immune responses that
can be triggered by a
foreign substance.

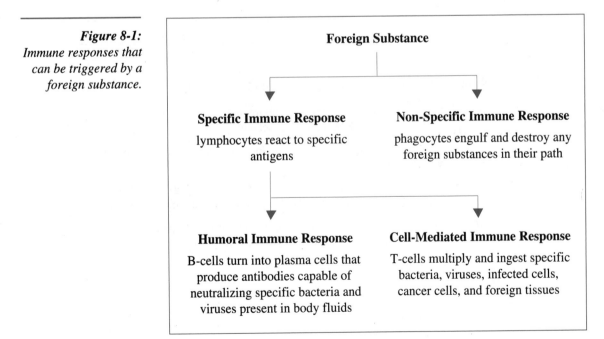

Types of Immunity

In some cases, a specific immune response can result in long-term immunity to a particular invader. This is why we contract some diseases only once in spite of repeat exposures. The body can acquire immunity in several ways. **Natural immunity** occurs when the body mounts an immune response on its own, while **artificially acquired immunity** results when vaccines (drugs that contain weakened or killed pathogens) are given to stimulate an immune response. Similarly, **active immunity** occurs when the body's own lymphocytes and antibodies are involved in the immune response, while **passive immunity** occurs when lymphocytes or antibodies are introduced to the body from other sources (e.g., from breast milk or from an immunoglobulin injection).

Review Exercises

1. **Define** the following word elements and terms.

   a. immun/o _____

   b. immunoglobulin _____

   c. phag/o _____

   d. phagocyte _____

   e. -phylaxis _____

2. **Match** the following types of immune responses with their descriptions.

   _____ specific

   _____ non-specific

   _____ humoral

   _____ cell-mediated

   a. immune response involving the production of antibodies (immunoglobulins) that react with and neutralize specific antigens

   b. immune response involving the destruction of specific antigens by activated T-cells

   c. general immune response involving the ingestion of all types of antigens by phagocytes (neutrophils and macrophages)

   d. any immune response involving the destruction of specific antigens by lymphocytes or their products

Terminology

The following are selected terms that pertain to pathology of the immune system and to related diagnostic and therapeutic procedures. As you will see, most of the diseases listed result from excessive or inadequate functioning of the immune system. Keeping this in mind will help you to understand other terms you may hear as well as the rationale behind treatment of immune system disorders.

Pathologic Conditions	Word Elements	Definition
acquired immune deficiency syndrome (AIDS)	syn = together drome = "running"	transmissible infection caused by human immunodeficiency virus (HIV); characterized by extreme immunodeficiency and the development of serious opportunistic infections and/or certain rare cancers
anaphylaxis (AN-uh-full-**LACK**-sis)	ana = backward phylaxis = protection	extreme allergic reaction characterized by a rapid drop in blood pressure, breathing difficulties, hives, and abdominal cramps
autoimmune disease (AW-toe-ih-**MYOON**)	auto = self immune = immune	any of several diseases caused by the failure of the body to distinguish between "self" and "nonself;" symptoms result from immune responses being directed against the individual's own tissues; examples include diabetes and psoriasis
HIV-positive	no word elements	state characterized by the presence of human immunodeficiency virus (HIV) or antibodies to HIV in the blood; generally used to refer to individuals who are infected with HIV but have not yet developed symptoms of AIDS
hypersensitivity (HI-per-sen-sih-**TIH**-vih-tee)	hyper = excessive sensitivity = state of being sensitive	condition in which the immune system produces an exaggerated response to a foreign substance, resulting in symptoms such as runny nose, swelling, and rash; commonly called allergy
immunodeficiency (IM-yoo-no-dee-**FIH**-shin-see)	immuno = immune deficiency = state of being deficient	state in which the immune system is unable to respond adequately, increasing susceptibility to infection; the deficiency can be caused by drugs or disease
opportunistic infection	no word elements	infection caused by pathogens that would not usually cause disease in healthy people; occurs mainly in patients whose resistance is low due to some type of immunodeficiency

Diagnostic Procedures	Word Elements	Definition
ELISA (uh-LIE-zuh)	no word elements	test used to screen blood for the presence of antibodies to HIV (or to other disease-causing substances)
skin tests	no word elements	tests used to evaluate the body's reaction to foreign substances by applying small amounts to the unbroken skin (patch tests) or lightly scratched skin (scratch tests), or by injecting small doses under the skin (intradermal skin tests)
Western blot	no word elements	test used to detect the presence of viral DNA in the blood; used to detect HIV and other viruses

Therapeutic Procedures	Word Elements	Definition
immunization (IM-yoo-nih-**ZAY**-shun)	immun = immune ization = process	process of inducing immunity to a particular infectious disease; may involve the administration of blood containing antibodies that provide short-term immunity (passive immunization) or the administration of weakened or killed microorganisms to induce an immune response (vaccination)
immunosuppression (IM-yoo-no-suh-**PREH**-shun)	immuno = immune suppression = suppression	use of drugs or surgery to suppress a patient's immune responses; used to prevent organ rejection after transplantation or to slow the progress of autoimmune diseases
immunotherapy (IM-yoo-no-**THER**-uh-pee)	immuno = immune therapy = treatment	treatment for allergy involving exposure to gradually increasing doses of the substance (allergen) to which the patient is allergic
vaccination (VACK-sih-**NAY**-shun)	vaccin = vaccine ation = process	administration of weakened or killed microorganisms to induce an immune response against the organism in order to induce immunity to an infectious disease

Review Exercises

3. *Match* the following terms with their definitions.

_____ vaccination

_____ immunotherapy

_____ anaphylaxis

_____ immunization

_____ skin tests

a. general term referring to any process in which immunity to a particular infectious disease is induced

b. specific type of immunization involving the administration of weakened or killed microorganisms

c. treatment for allergy involving exposure to increasing doses of an allergen

d. extreme allergic reaction characterized by a rapid drop in blood pressure and breathing difficulties

e. tests used to evaluate the body's reaction to foreign substances by applying or injecting small amounts on or into the skin

4. *Break Down and Define* the word elements within each of the following terms, and then define the term itself.

   Example: vaccin / ation   *vaccine / process*   *process of vaccinating*

a. immunosuppression

_____

b. autoimmune

_____

c. anaphylaxis

_____

d. immunoglobulin

_____

e. phagocyte

_____

f. phagocytosis

_____

g. immunogenic

_____

h. immunocompromised

_____

5. **Word Building and Spelling.** Spell out the medical term for each of the following definitions using the slashes provided to separate the word elements.

having immune responses to oneself   *auto / immune*

a. process of vaccinating   _____/_____

b. immune therapy   _____/_____

c. excessive sensitivity   _____/_____

d. suppression of immune responses   _____/_____

e. study of the immune system   _____/_____

f. study of the immune system and blood   _____/_____/_____

g. process of immunizing   _____/_____

Case Study. Read the case notes below. For each boldfaced term, provide a brief definition and indicate whether the term is spelled correctly; if it is misspelled, provide the correct spelling.

Example: **hiv-positive:** *state of having HIV or antibodies to HIV in the blood*

      Spelled correctly?   ☐ Yes   ☑ No   *HIV-positive*

Patient presented as a 28-year-old healthy female. Although she had no sign or symptom of disease, she was concerned that she might be **hiv-positive** because her boyfriend had just been diagnosed with **acquired immune deficiency sindrome.** She explained that her boyfriend was an intravenous drug user. He had gone through months of fever, diarrhea, night sweats, and weight loss, but had not sought treatment until finally he was hospitalized with severe pneumonia. Tests revealed that the pneumonia was an **oportunistic infection** resulting from severe **immunodeficiency**. She said that she and her boyfriend had had unprotected sex for nearly two years, which is why she wants to be tested. An initial **ELIZA** test was positive for HIV. A **Western blot** confirmed this result. Patient was referred to an ID specialist for prophylactic treatment for AIDS and to a social worker for counselling.

a. acquired immune deficiency sindrome: _____

_____

    Spelled correctly?   ☐ Yes   ☐ No _____

b. oportunistic infection: _____

_____

    Spelled correctly?   ☐ Yes   ☐ No _____

c. immunodeficiency: _____

_____

Spelled correctly? ☐ Yes ☐ No _____

d. ELIZA: _____

_____

Spelled correctly? ☐ Yes ☐ No _____

e. Western blot: _____

_____

Spelled correctly? ☐ Yes ☐ No _____

Listen to the section on your audiotape cassette that corresponds to this chapter and write the terms below. Be careful to spell each term correctly.

1. _____   12. _____

2. _____   13. _____

3. _____   14. _____

4. _____   15. _____

5. _____   16. _____

6. _____   17. _____

7. _____   18. _____

8. _____   19. _____

9. _____   20. _____

10. _____   21. _____

11. _____   22. _____

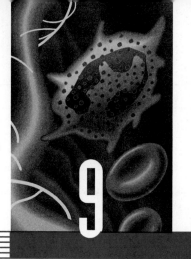

Respiratory System

Upon completing this chapter, you should be able to:

- Describe the respiratory system and explain the primary functions of its organs
- Recognize, build, pronounce, and spell words that pertain to the respiratory system
- Describe diseases, diagnostic tests, and surgical procedures that pertain to the respiratory system

Overview

The respiratory system is responsible for the exchange of gases between the body and the air, a process called **respiration**. Respiration consists of both external and internal processes. In external respiration, oxygen is inhaled into the lungs and absorbed into the bloodstream, while carbon dioxide passes from the blood into the lungs and is exhaled. In internal respiration, oxygen in the bloodstream passes into individual tissue cells, where it is used for energy; in exchange, carbon dioxide created as a waste product in the cells passes into the bloodstream for removal from the body.

Word Elements

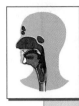

UPPER RESPIRATORY TRACT – By convention, the respiratory system is divided into the upper and lower respiratory tracts. The following combining forms (CF) pertain to the structures of the upper respiratory tract.

CF	Meaning	Example
laryng/o	larynx	*laryngo*plasty = surgical repair of the larynx
nas/o	nose	*nas*al = pertaining to the nose
or/o	mouth	*oro*pharynx = portion of the pharynx behind the mouth
pharyng/o	pharynx	*pharyng*itis = inflammation of the pharynx
rhin/o	nose	*rhino*plasty = plastic surgery of the nose
sin/o	sinus; sinus cavity	*sino*graphy = x-ray recording of the sinuses

LOWER RESPIRATORY TRACT – These combining forms pertain to the lower respiratory tract, including its major structures and the body cavity in which it is found.

CF	Meaning	Example
alveol/o	alveolus	*alveol*ar = pertaining to an alveolus
bronch/o	bronchus	*bronch*itis = inflammation of the bronchi
bronchiol/o	bronchiole	*bronchiol*ectasis = dilation of the bronchioles
lob/o	lobe (of the lung)	*lob*ar = pertaining to a lobe (of a lung)
pleur/o	pleura	*pleur*itis = inflammation of the pleura
pneum/o	lung; air	*pneumo*lith = a stone in the lungs
pneumon/o	lung; air	*pneumon*ia = lung condition (infection)
pulmon/o	lungs	*pulmon*ary = pertaining to the lungs
thorac/o	chest (thorax)	*thorac*ic = pertaining to the chest
trache/o	trachea	*tracheo*tomy = surgical incision into the trachea

RESPIRATION – These combining forms refer to respiration or breathing, the process by which oxygen is transported from the air to the tissues.

CF	Meaning	Example
ox/o	oxygen	hyp*ox*emia = reduced oxygen level in the blood
respir/o	breathing	*respir*ation = process of breathing
spir/o	breathing	*spiro*metry = measurement of breathing

SUFFIXES – The following suffixes pertain to the respiratory system. They are used to denote gas levels and processes related to respiration.

Suffix	Meaning	Example
-capnia	carbon dioxide	hyper*capnia* = excessive carbon dioxide in the blood
-ectasis	expansion; dilation	bronchi*ectasis* = dilation of the bronchi
-oxia	oxygen	hyp*oxia* = condition of reduced oxygen levels
-pnea	breathing	dys*pnea* = difficult or painful breathing

Anatomy and Physiology

The respiratory system consists of a series of tubes or airways that transport air into and out of the lungs. By convention, the respiratory system is divided into the upper respiratory tract (consisting of the nose, pharynx, and larynx) and the lower respiratory tract (consisting of the trachea, bronchi, and lungs). These structures are described below.

The Nose

nas/o and rhin/o = nose

septum = dividing wall
sin/o = sinus; sinus cavity

Air enters and leaves the body through the **nose**. The external portion of the nose is composed of cartilage and bone covered with skin. The entrance to the nose is known as the **nostrils** or **nares**. The internal portion of the nose is divided into left and right chambers by a dividing wall called the **septum**; air passing through these chambers also passes through the **sinuses**, which are hollow areas or cavities within the nasal cartilage. The internal nose and sinuses are lined by mucous membranes, which help to warm and filter air as it enters the respiratory system. Hairlike projections on the mucous membranes, called **cilia** (SILL-ee-uh), sweep dirt and foreign material towards the throat for elimination.

The Pharynx

pharyng/o = pharynx

or/o = mouth
laryng/o = larynx
hypo- = under

The **pharynx** (FEHR-inks), also known as the throat, is the airway that connects the mouth and nose to the larynx (voice box). Although the pharynx is a single organ, it is commonly divided into three sections: the **nasopharynx** (NAY-zoe-**FEHR**-inks), the upper portion located behind the nose; the **oropharynx** (OR-oh-**FEHR**-inks), the middle portion located behind the mouth; and the **laryngopharynx** (luh-RIN-go-**FEHR**-inks), also known as the **hypopharynx** (HI-poe-**FEHR**-inks), the lower portion located just behind the larynx.

Since the pharynx serves as a common passageway for both air from the nose and food from the mouth, there must be a mechanism to prevent food from accidentally entering the respiratory tract. During the act of swallowing, a

Figure 9-1:
*The upper
respiratory tract.*

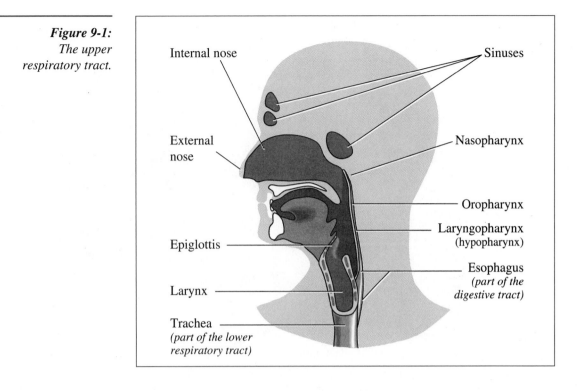

small flap of cartilage called the **epiglottis** (EH-pih-**GLOT**-iss) covers the opening of the larynx so that food cannot enter the larynx and lower airways while passing through the pharynx.

The Larynx

Also known as the voice box, the **larynx** (LEHR-inks) contains the structures which make vocal sounds possible (i.e., the vocal cords and supporting tissue). It is connected to the trachea.

The Trachea

trache/o = trachea   Air passing through the larynx enters the **trachea** (TRAY-kee-uh), which is the airway commonly known as the windpipe. The trachea extends into the chest and serves as a passageway for air to the bronchi. It lies in front of the esophagus, which is the tube through which food passes on its way to the stomach.

Figure 9-2: *The lower respiratory tract.*

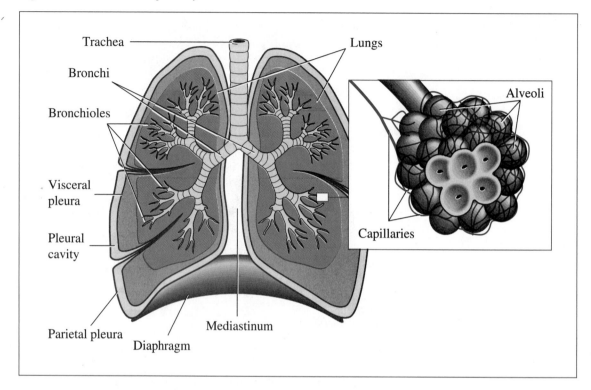

The Bronchi

bronch/o = bronchus
bronchiol/o = bronchiole
alveol/o = alveolus

The trachea branches into two tubes called **bronchi** (BRONG-kie). Each bronchus enters a lung, then subdivides into progressively smaller branches. The smallest branches of the bronchi are known as **bronchioles** (BRONG-kee-oles), which terminate at the **alveoli** (al-VEE-oh-lie), also known as air sacs.

The Lungs

*pneum/o, pneumon/o,
and pulmon/o = lungs*
lob/o = lobe

ox/o and -oxia = oxygen

-capnia = carbon dioxide

hem/o = blood
-globin = protein

The **lungs** are two cone-shaped, spongy organs consisting of alveoli, blood vessels, elastic tissue, and nerves. Each of the two lungs consists of smaller divisions called **lobes**; as shown in Figure 9-2, the left lung has two lobes, while the right lung is divided into three lobes. In the lungs, alveoli are surrounded by a network of tiny blood vessels called capillaries; oxygen from the lungs passes into these capillaries for distribution to tissue cells, while carbon dioxide from the blood passes into the lungs for removal from the body by exhalation. Once absorbed into blood cells, oxygen becomes attached to hemoglobin and is released to tissue cells as needed. Thus, the primary function of the lungs is to bring air into close contact with blood, which allows gas exchange to occur.

pleur/o = pleura

thorac/o = chest

The lungs are surrounded by a membrane called the **visceral pleura** (VIH-sir-ul PLOOR-uh). The space that the lungs occupy within the chest is called the **thoracic** (ther-RASS-ick) **cavity**, which is lined by a membrane called the **parietal** (per-RYE-eh-tul) **pleura**. The parietal and visceral pleurae lie very close to each other; the small space between these membranes, called the **pleural space**, is filled with a fluid that prevents friction when the two membranes slide against each other during respiration. In the central portion of the thoracic cavity (in the area between the lungs) is a space called the **mediastinum** (ME-dee-uh-STY-num), which contains the heart. A group of muscles called the **diaphragm** (DIE-uh-fram) separates the lower portion of the thoracic cavity from the abdomen.

Breathing

respir/o, spir/o, and -pnea = breathing

phren/o = diaphragm

Air is moved in and out of the lungs by a cyclic process called **ventilation**, also referred to as breathing (or respiration). Each ventilation cycle consists of an inhalation and an exhalation separated by a period of rest. The cycle begins when the **phrenic** (FREN-ick) nerve stimulates the diaphragm. This stimulation causes the diaphragm to drop and flatten, enlarging the chest cavity. As the chest cavity enlarges, air pressure within the chest cavity decreases, causing air to be pulled into the lungs. When the diaphragm returns to its raised state, shrinking the chest cavity, air is forced out of the lungs. Breathing is normally regulated unconsciously by the respiratory center in the brain.

Review Exercises

1. ***Match*** the following word elements with their definitions.

    _____ -capnia   a. oxygen

    _____ -ectasis   b. carbon dioxide

    _____ -oxia   c. breathing

    _____ -pnea   d. expansion; dilation

    _____ pulmon/o   e. lungs

2. ***Define*** the following combining forms.

    a. pleur/o   _____

    b. pneumon/o   _____

    c. ox/o   _____

d. trache/o _____

e. rhin/o _____

f. respir/o _____

g. alveol/o _____

h. bronchiol/o _____

i. lob/o _____

j. or/o _____

k. bronch/o _____

3. *Match* the following combining forms with their definitions.

_____ nas/o   a. larynx

_____ pharyng/o   b. pharynx

_____ spir/o   c. lung; air

_____ pneum/o   d. sinus; sinus cavity

_____ laryng/o   e. chest

_____ thorac/o   f. breathing

_____ sin/o   g. nose

4. *Match* the following respiratory terms with their common forms.

_____ trachea   a. "voice box"

_____ alveoli   b. "windpipe"

_____ larynx   c. "throat"

_____ ventilation   d. "air sacs"

_____ pharynx   e. "breathing"

Terminology

The following are selected terms that pertain to pathology of the respiratory system and to related diagnostic and surgical procedures. As you will see, most of the disorders listed result from inflammation or obstruction of the airways, abnormal fluid accumulation, or abnormal inflation of the lungs. Keeping this in mind will help you to understand other terms you may hear as well as the rationale behind treatment of respiratory disorders.

Pathologic Conditions	Word Elements	Definition
asthma (AZ-muh)	asthma = "panting"	respiratory condition characterized by obstruction of the bronchi, usually due to excessive mucus production or bronchial spasm
atelectasis (AT-ull-**LECK**-tuh-sis)	atel = incomplete ectasis = expansion	collapsed lung or incomplete expansion of a lung
bronchiectasis (BRONG-kee-**ECK**-tuh-sis)	bronchi = bronchus ectasis = expansion	abnormal condition of the lung characterized by irreversible dilation of the bronchi
bronchitis (brong-KIE-tis)	bronch = bronchus itis = inflammation	inflammation of the bronchi, usually due to infection
croup (CROOP)	no word elements	acute respiratory syndrome in children and infants characterized by obstruction of the larynx and a barking cough
cystic fibrosis (SIS-tick fie-BROE-sis)	cyst = cyst ic = pertaining to fibr = fiber osis = condition	genetic disease of the exocrine glands that results in excessive mucus production, leading to obstruction of the airways and recurrent respiratory infections
diphtheria (dif-THEER-ee-uh)	no word elements	serious acute bacterial infection characterized by sore throat and fever
dyspnea (DISP-nee-uh)	dys = difficult; painful pnea = breathing	difficult or painful breathing
emphysema (EM-fih-**SEE**-muh)	emphys = "to inflate" ema = condition	chronic lung disease characterized by the enlargement and destruction of alveoli
empyema (EM-pie-**EE**-muh)	em = in py = pus ema = condition	collection of pus in the pleural space
epistaxis (EH-pih-**STACK**-sis)	epi = above staxis = hemorrhage	hemorrhage from the nose (nosebleed)
hypoxemia (HI-pock-**SEE**-me-uh)	hyp = under; reduced ox = oxygen emia = blood condition	reduced level of oxygen in the blood; usually a sign of respiratory impairment
hypoxia (hi-POCK-see-uh)	hyp = under; reduced ox = oxygen ia = condition	reduced level of oxygen in the tissues; usually a sign of respiratory impairment
laryngitis (LEHR-in-**JIE**-tis)	laryng = larynx itis = inflammation	inflammation of the larynx, usually due to infection

Pathologic Conditions	Word Elements	Definition
pertussis (per-TUH-sis)	per = through tussis = cough	bacterial infection of the respiratory tract that mainly affects children; characterized by an explosive cough; also called whooping cough
pharyngitis (FEHR-in-**JIE**-tis)	pharyng = pharynx itis = inflammation	inflammation of the pharynx, usually due to infection
pleural effusion (PLOOR-ul eh-FYOO-zhun)	pleur = pleura al = pertaining to	accumulation of fluid in the pleural space
pleuritis (ploor-RYE-tis)	pleur = pleura itis = inflammation	inflammation of the pleura; previously called pleurisy
pneumoconiosis (NOO-moe-KOE-nee-**OH**-sis)	pneumo = lung; air conio = dust sis = condition	lung disease caused by inhalation of dust or other particles; also called black lung
pneumonia (noo-MOE-nyuh)	pneumon = lung; air ia = condition	inflammation of one or both lungs, usually due to infection
pneumothorax (NOO-moe-**THOR**-acks)	pneumo = lung; air thorax = chest	accumulation of air in the pleural space
rales (RAWLS)	rales = "rattles"	crackling sounds heard when using a stethoscope to listen to a patient's breathing; often a sign of pneumonia
rhinitis (rye-NIE-tis)	rhin = nose itis = inflammation	inflammation of the mucous membranes of the nose
rhonchi (RONG-kie)	rhonchi = "snores"	loud coarse sounds heard when using a stethoscope to listen to a patient's breathing; sign of obstructed airways
stridor (STRY-dor)	stridor = "a harsh sound"	high-pitched sound heard usually during inspiration caused by obstruction of the larynx or a bronchus
tuberculosis (too-BER-kyoo-**LOE**-sis)	tubercul = "small swelling" osis = condition	infectious disease caused by *Mycobacterium tuberculosis;* often affects the lungs
wheeze	no word elements	whistling sound heard usually during expiration; caused by narrowing of an airway

Diagnostic Procedures	Word Elements	Definition
arterial blood gases	arteri = artery al = pertaining to	group of tests measuring the oxygen and carbon dioxide concentrations in an arterial blood sample
bronchoscopy (brong-KOS-kuh-pee)	broncho = bronchus scopy = visual examination	visual examination of the bronchi using a bronchoscope
laryngoscopy (LEHR-rin-GOS-kuh-pee)	laryngo = larynx scopy = visual examination	visual examination of the larynx using a laryngoscope
pulmonary function tests	pulmon = lungs ary = pertaining to	tests (e.g., measurement of lung volume) used to evaluate lung function
spirometry (sper-ROM-eh-tree)	spiro = breathing metry = measurement	measurement of the breathing capacity of the lungs
sputum culture (SPEW-tum)	no word elements	test used to identify any bacteria present in a sample of coughed-up mucus (sputum)
thoracentesis (THOR-uh-sen-TEE-sis)	thora = chest centesis = puncture	use of a needle to puncture the chest wall to collect fluid from the pleural cavity for diagnostic tests

Surgical Procedures	Word Elements	Definition
laryngectomy (LEHR-rin-JECK-tuh-me)	laryng = larynx ectomy = surgical removal	surgical removal of the larynx
laryngoplasty (luh-RIN-go-PLASS-tee)	laryngo = larynx plasty = surgical repair	surgical repair of the larynx
lobectomy (loe-BECK-tuh-me)	lob = lobe (of the lung) ectomy = surgical removal	surgical removal of a lobe of a lung
rhinoplasty (RYE-no-PLASS-tee)	rhino = nose plasty = surgical repair	plastic surgery of the nose
tracheostomy (TRAY-kee-OS-tuh-me)	tracheo = trachea stomy = surgical opening	cutting of an opening through the neck into the trachea and insertion of a tube to facilitate air passage or to remove secretions
tracheotomy (TRAY-kee-OT-uh-me)	tracheo = trachea tomy = surgical incision	surgical incision through the neck into the trachea to gain access to an airway below a blockage

Review Exercises

5. **Match** the following terms with their definitions.

_____ pertussis

_____ empyema

_____ emphysema

_____ pneumoconiosis

_____ epistaxis

_____ stridor

a. collection of pus in the pleural space

b. black lung

c. high-pitched sound heard during inspiration

d. chronic lung disease characterized by the enlargement and destruction of alveoli

e. whooping cough

f. nosebleed

6. **Define** the following terms.

a. croup _____

b. diphtheria _____

c. pneumothorax _____

d. tuberculosis _____

e. rhonchi _____

7. **Break Down and Define** the word elements within each of the following terms, and then define the term itself.

Example: pleur / algia   *lung / painful*   *painful lungs*

a. tracheotomy

_____

b. spirometry

_____

c. lobectomy

_____

d. hypoxia

_____

e. hypoxemia

_____

f. pneumonia

_____

g. dyspnea

_____

h. pharyngitis

_____

i. rhinoplasty

_____

j. atelectasis

_____

k. pulmonology

_____

l. bronchitis

_____

m. rhinitis

_____

n. laryngoscopy

_____

o. pulmonary

_____

p. pneumonitis

_____

q. endotracheal

_____

r. bronchiectasis

_____

8. ***Choose and Construct.*** Choose the appropriate word elements from the list provided to construct terms for the following.

a-	tachy-	-capnia	-ectomy
dys-	laryng/o	-centesis	-plasty
hyper-	pneumon/o	-ectasis	-pnea

   excessive breathing   *hyper /pnea*

a. surgical repair of the larynx   _____ / _____

b. expansion of the lungs   _____ / _____

c. puncture of a lung   _____ / _____

d. fast breathing   _____ / _____

e. difficult breathing   _____ / _____

f. not breathing   _____ / _____

g. surgical removal of a lung   _____ / _____

h. excessive carbon dioxide   _____ / _____

9. ***Word Building and Spelling.*** Spell out the medical term for each of the following definitions using the slashes provided to separate the word elements.

    inflammation of the pharynx   *pharyng / itis*

a. surgical removal of the larynx   _____ / _____

b. visual examination of the bronchi _____ / _____

c. surgical opening in the trachea   _____ / _____

d. chest puncture   _____ / _____

e. inflammation of the larynx   _____ / _____

f. inflammation of the pleura   _____ / _____

g. inflammation of the trachea   _____ / _____

h. pertaining to the bronchioles   _____ / _____

Case Study. Read the case notes below. For each boldfaced term, provide a brief definition and indicate whether the term is spelled correctly; if it is misspelled, provide the correct spelling.

Example:

pnumonia: *inflammation of one or both lungs, usually due to infection*

Spelled correctly?   ☐ Yes ☑ No *pneumonia*

Patient presented as a 46-year-old male with signs of **pnumonia**. He appeared acutely ill, with fever, chills, cough, blue-tinged lips, and severe dyspnea. Fine **wheezes** could be heard on expiration, which he said was not unusual since he suffered from **azthma**. He said that his azthma was generally well controlled, but that **pulmonary function tests** usually show reduced lung capacity. Using a stethoscope, **rawls** could clearly be heard. A chest x-ray confirmed the diagnosis of pneumonia and also revealed a **plural effusion.** Ordered a **sputum culture** to determine the causative pathogen and **arterial blood gases** to assess the extent of respiratory impairment. Patient was admitted to the hospital for treatment. Treatment plan: intravenous antibiotics beginning immediately, to be adjusted pending results of sputum culture.

a. wheezes: _____

_____

Spelled correctly? ☐ Yes ☐ No _____

b. azthma: _____

_____

Spelled correctly? ☐ Yes ☐ No _____

c. pulmonary function tests: _____

_____

Spelled correctly? ☐ Yes ☐ No _____

d. rawls: _____

_____

Spelled correctly? ☐ Yes ☐ No _____

e. plural effusion: _____

_____

Spelled correctly? ☐ Yes ☐ No _____

f. sputum culture: _____

_____

Spelled correctly? ☐ Yes ☐ No _____

g. arterial blood gases: _____

_____

Spelled correctly? ☐ Yes ☐ No _____

Listen to the section on your audiotape cassette that corresponds to this chapter and write the terms below. Be careful to spell each term correctly.

1. _____ 4. _____

2. _____ 5. _____

3. _____ 6. _____

7. _____

8. _____

9. _____

10. _____

11. _____

12. _____

13. _____

14. _____

15. _____

16. _____

17. _____

18. _____

19. _____

20. _____

21. _____

22. _____

23. _____

24. _____

25. _____

26. _____

27. _____

28. _____

29. _____

30. _____

31. _____

32. _____

33. _____

34. _____

35. _____

36. _____

37. _____

38. _____

39. _____

40. _____

41. _____

42. _____

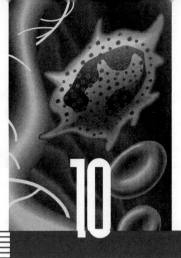

Digestive System

Upon completing this chapter, you should be able to:

- Describe the digestive system and explain the primary functions of its organs
- Recognize, build, pronounce, and spell words that pertain to the digestive system
- Describe diseases, diagnostic tests, and surgical procedures that pertain to the digestive system

Overview   The digestive system, also called the gastrointestinal or alimentary tract, contains the organs involved in the ingestion and processing of food. The digestive system plays a role in four major functions: ingestion, the entry of food into the body; digestion, the physical and chemical breakdown of food into nutrients that can be used by the body's cells; absorption, the passage of these nutrients from the gastrointestinal tract into the bloodstream; and elimination, the excretion of solid waste materials that cannot be absorbed into the blood.

Word Elements

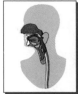

INGESTION – The digestive system includes structures involved in ingestion, digestion, and accessory digestive activities. The following combining forms (CF) pertain to ingestion and swallowing.

CF	Meaning	Example
aliment/o	food; nutrient	*aliment*ation = process of giving or taking nourishment
bucc/o	cheek	*bucc*al = pertaining to the cheek
esophag/o	esophagus	*esophag*eal = pertaining to the esophagus
gingiv/o	gum	*gingiv*itis = inflammation of the gums
or/o	mouth	*or*al = pertaining to the mouth
palat/o	palate	*palato*plasty = surgical repair of the palate
pharyng/o	pharynx	*pharyng*itis = inflammation of the pharynx
sial/o	saliva	*sialo*rrhea = excessive secretion of saliva
stomat/o	mouth	*stomat*itis = inflammation of the mouth

MAIN DIGESTIVE ORGANS – These combining forms refer to the main digestive organs. These structures act to digest food and excrete waste.

CF	Meaning	Example
an/o	anus	*an*al = pertaining to the anus
cec/o	cecum	*cec*al = pertaining to the cecum
col/o	colon; large intestine	*col*itis = inflammation of the colon
duoden/o	duodenum	*duodeno*scopy = visual examination of the duodenum
enter/o	small intestine	*enter*itis = inflammation of the small intestine
fec/o	feces	*fec*al = pertaining to the feces
gastr/o	stomach	*gastro*cele = hernial protrusion of the stomach
ile/o	ileum	*ile*ectomy = surgical removal of the ileum
jejun/o	jejunum	*jejun*itis = inflammation of the jejunum
proct/o	anus; rectum	*procto*logy = study of the anus/rectum
pylor/o	pylorus; pyloric sphincter	*pylor*algia = pain in the area of the pylorus
rect/o	rectum	*rect*al = pertaining to the rectum
sigmoid/o	sigmoid colon	*sigmoido*tomy = surgical incision into the sigmoid colon

ACCESSORY DIGESTIVE ORGANS — These combining forms refer to the accessory digestive organs. Most of these organs secrete substances that aid in digestion. One, the peritoneum, lines the digestive organs.

CF	Meaning	Example
append/o	appendix	*append*ectomy = surgical removal of the appendix
bil/i	bile; gall	*bili*ary = pertaining to the bile or gallbladder
chol/e	bile; gall	*chole*lith = a gallstone
choledoch/o	common bile duct	*choledocho*stomy = surgical creation of an opening into the common bile duct
hepat/o	liver	*hepato*toxic = poisonous to the liver
pancreat/o	pancreas	*pancreat*itis = inflammation of the pancreas
peritone/o	peritoneum	*peritone*al = pertaining to the peritoneum

SUFFIXES — The following suffixes pertain to the digestive system. They are used to refer to digestive processes and properties.

Suffix	Meaning	Example
-emesis	vomiting	hyper*emesis* = excessive vomiting
-orexia	appetite	an*orexia* = lack of appetite
-pepsia	digestion	dys*pepsia* = indigestion

Anatomy and Physiology

Anatomically, the digestive system consists of a 30-foot long, mucous membrane-lined tube beginning at the mouth, where food enters the body, and ending at the anus, where solid waste is excreted; the organs forming this tube include the mouth, pharynx, esophagus, stomach, small intestine, and large intestine. The digestive system also contains so-called "accessory organs," including the liver, gallbladder, and pancreas; although food does not pass through these organs, they aid in the processing of food and nutrients. The organs of the digestive system are illustrated in Figure 10-1 and described in the paragraphs below.

Structures of the Mouth

or/o and stomat/o = mouth
aliment/o = food; nutrient
bucc/o = cheek

The **mouth**, also called the **oral cavity** or **buccal** (BUCK-ul) **cavity**, is the opening through which food enters the body. The **lips** form the opening to the mouth, while the **cheeks** or **bucca** (BUCK-uh) form the borders of the oral cavity. The structures within the oral cavity, including the teeth, tongue, and palate, are involved in the chewing (mastication) and swallowing (deglutition) of food. They also play a role in speech.

Figure 10-1: *Organs of the digestive system.*

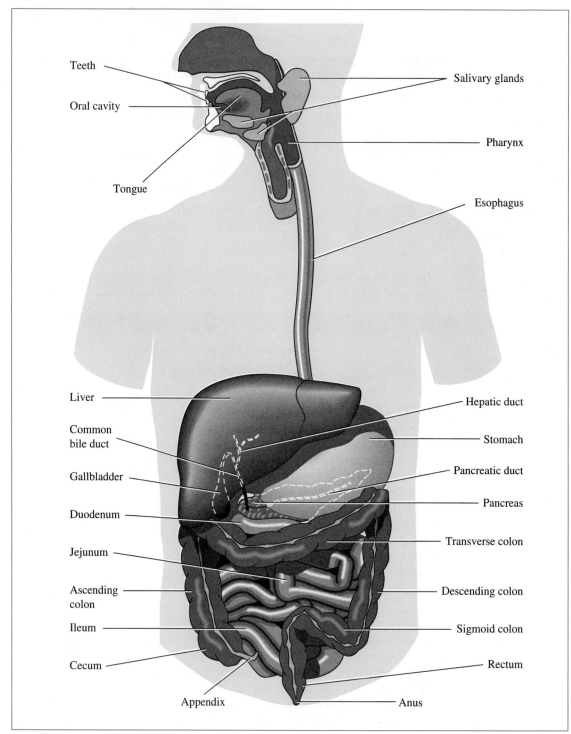

The **teeth** are used to cut, tear, and crush food into smaller pieces. Types of teeth include incisors and cuspids (in the front of the mouth) and molars (in the back of the mouth). Each tooth consists of a mass of nerves and blood vessels, called pulp, surrounded by a hard bone-like substance called cementum (see-MEN-tum) and a white, smooth substance called enamel (uh-NAM-ul). The teeth are embedded in pink fleshy tissue called **gums** or **gingivae** (jin-JIE-vee). Together, the gums and other structures that support the teeth are known as the **periodontium** (PEHR-ee-oh-**DON**-chum).

gingiv/o = gums

The **tongue** is the muscular organ that extends across the floor of the mouth. It is used to manipulate food in the mouth during chewing and swallowing. On the top surface of the tongue are bumps called **taste buds** or **papillae** (puh-PILL-ee) that sense flavors, such as bitter, sweet, salty, and sour.

palat/o = palate

The **palate** (PAL-ut) forms the roof of the mouth. It is divided into two parts: the hard palate (the front half) and the soft palate (the back half). The cone-shaped projection hanging from the back of the soft palate is called the **uvula** (YOO-vyoo-luh). During swallowing, the soft palate and uvula move upward to prevent food from entering the nasal cavity; the uvula also helps to guide the food into the pharynx.

Figure 10-2: Structures of the mouth.

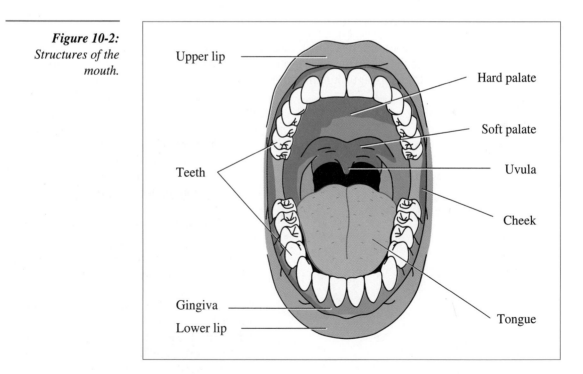

Upper lip

Hard palate

Soft palate

Teeth

Uvula

Cheek

Gingiva

Tongue

Lower lip

sialaden/o = salivary gland

sial/o = saliva

Located around the oral cavity are three pairs of **salivary** (SAL-ih-VEHR-ee) **glands** (shown in Figure 10-1), which produce **saliva** (suh-LIE-vuh). Saliva contains fluid and enzymes that help dissolve and digest food in the mouth.

The Pharynx

pharyng/o = pharynx

The **pharynx** (FEHR-inks), or throat, is a muscular tube that serves as a passageway for food from the mouth to the esophagus and as a passageway for air from the nose to the larynx (voice box). The latter function is described in *Chapter 9: Respiratory System.*

The Esophagus

esophag/o = esophagus

The **esophagus** (eh-SOF-uh-gus) is a long muscular tube extending from the pharynx to the stomach. Food is pushed toward the stomach by rhythmic, wavelike contractions of muscles in the walls of the esophagus; this process, called **peristalsis** (PEHR-ih-**STALL**-sis), is also how food is moved through the stomach and intestines.

The Stomach

gastr/o = stomach

The **stomach**, a pouch-like organ located in the upper part of the abdominal cavity, connects the esophagus with the small intestine. Entry of food from the esophagus into the stomach is controlled by a ring of muscles known as the **cardiac sphincter** (SFINK-ter). Food that passes through the cardiac sphincter enters the upper portion of the stomach, known as the **fundus** (FUN-duss). Peristaltic motion causes the food to descend through the central section of the stomach, called the **body**, to the lower section, called the **antrum** (antrum = "cave-like"), and finally to the lower end of the stomach, known as the **pylorus** (pie-LORE-us). A second ring of muscles, called the **pyloric sphincter**, controls the passage of food from the stomach to the small intestine.

When the stomach is empty, the mucous membranes lining its walls are highly folded; buried within these folds, or **rugae** (ROO-jee), are numerous digestive glands. As the stomach fills, the rugae unfold, exposing the digestive glands and stimulating them to secrete digestive enzymes and hydrochloric acid.

Figure 10-3: *The stomach.*

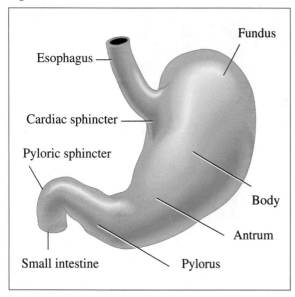

chym/o = to pour

These substances help transform food present in the stomach into a semi-fluid substance called **chyme** (KIME). The pyloric sphincter allows food to pass into the small intestine only after it has been transformed into chyme.

The Small Intestine

enter/o = small intestine

The **small intestine**, also known as the **small bowel**, is a coiled, 20-foot-long tube that winds from the pyloric sphincter of the stomach to the beginning of the large intestine, filling much of the abdominal cavity. By convention, the small intestine is divided into three sections: the **duodenum** (DOO-oh-**DEE**-num), a 10-inch section that receives chyme from the stomach; the **jejunum** (juh-JOO-num), an 8-foot long central section; and the **ileum** (ILL-lee-um), a 12-foot long section that ends at the large intestine.

duoden/o = duodenum

jejun/o = jejunum
ile/o = ileum

In the small intestine, digestion of food (chyme) is completed with the aid of enzymes secreted by glands in the small intestine and secretions from the accessory organs (the liver, gallbladder, and pancreas). As digestion is completed, nutrients are absorbed into the bloodstream and lymphatic system through tiny fingerlike projections, called **villi** (VILL-eye), that line the small intestine. Materials that cannot be absorbed pass from the small intestine to the large intestine.

The Large Intestine

col/o = colon; large intestine

The **large intestine**, also known as the **large bowel**, is a 5-foot long tube extending from the small intestine to the end of the gastrointestinal tract. By convention, the large intestine is divided into three sections: the cecum, the colon, and the rectum.

cec/o = cecum

The **cecum** (SEE-kum) is a pouch-like structure connected to the small intestine by the **ileocecal** (ILL-ee-oh-**SEE**-kul) **valve**, which controls the passage of fluid waste from the small intestine into the large intestine. Hanging off of the cecum is the **appendix**, a small organ with no apparent function; if it becomes infected and inflamed, however, the appendix can cause considerable pain and must be surgically removed.

append/o = appendix

The **colon** (KOE-lun), which comprises the main length of the large intestine, is itself divided into four sections: the **ascending colon**, extending from the cecum to the upper abdominal area; the **transverse colon**, extending from one side of the abdomen to the other; the **descending colon**, extending from the upper to the lower abdominal area; and the **sigmoid** (SIG-moyd) **colon**, the S-shaped end of the colon that leads into the rectum. As fluid waste from the small intestine passes through the various sections of the colon, water is reabsorbed into the body; as a result, the previously fluid waste turns into a solid material known as **feces** (FEE-seez) or **stool**.

sigmoid/o = sigmoid colon

fec/o = feces

rect/o = rectum *an/o = anus*	The **rectum** (RECK-tum) serves as a reservoir for feces; it leads to the **anus** (AY-nuss), the external opening through which feces are excreted.

Accessory Digestive Organs

hepat/o = liver	The **liver** is a large glandular organ located in the upper right portion of the abdominal cavity. The liver manufactures blood proteins, destroys old red blood cells, removes poisons from the blood, stores and releases glycogen (the stored form of glucose) as needed by the body, and manufactures bile.
bil/i and chol/e = *bile; gall*	**Bile** is a thick, yellowish-brown fluid that aids in the digestion of fats. Bile manufactured in the liver passes through the hepatic (heh-PAT-ick) duct to the cystic (SIS-tick) duct and into the gallbladder.
cholecyst/o = gallbladder	The **gallbladder**, a pear-shaped sac located behind the lower portion of the liver, concentrates and stores the bile it receives from the liver. When the stomach and duodenum are full, the gallbladder contracts, forcing bile to
choledoch/o = *common bile duct*	pass through the cystic duct to the **common bile duct** and into the duodenum. In the duodenum, bile aids in digestion.
pancreat/o = pancreas	The **pancreas** (PAN-kree-us), an elongated organ located just behind the stomach, produces digestive juices containing enzymes that aid in the digestion of proteins, starches, and fats. These digestive juices pass into the duodenum via the pancreatic duct. The pancreas also secretes insulin and glucagon, two hormones that help regulate carbohydrate metabolism and blood glucose levels.
peritone/o = peritoneum	Note that the abdominal cavity and all of its organs, including the organs of the digestive system, are lined by a membrane called the **peritoneum** (PEHR-ih-tuh-**NEE**-um). The portion of the peritoneum that surrounds the abdominal organs is called the **visceral** (VIH-sir-ul) **peritoneum**, while the portion that lines the abdominal wall is referred to as the **parietal** (per-RYE-uh-tul) **peritoneum**.

Review Exercises

1. *Spell* the combining forms that have the following meanings.

    a. colon; large intestine _____

    b. duodenum   _____

    c. small intestine _____

    d. ileum   _____

    e. jejunum   _____

f. pancreas _____

g. pharynx _____

h. pylorus _____

i. rectum _____

2. **Match** the following word elements with their definitions.

_____ -emesis   a. appetite

_____ -pepsia   b. food; nutrient

_____ -orexia   c. saliva

_____ bil/i   d. digestion

_____ sial/o   e. bile; gall

_____ aliment/o   f. feces

_____ fec/o   g. vomiting

3. **Match** the following combining forms with their definitions.

_____ bucc/o   a. mouth

_____ or/o   b. cheek

_____ proct/o   c. anus; rectum

_____ hepat/o   d. gum

_____ gingiv/o   e. liver

_____ sigmoid/o   f. palate

_____ palat/o   g. stomach

_____ gastr/o   h. peritoneum

_____ esophag/o   i. esophagus

_____ peritone/o   j. sigmoid colon

4. **Define** the following combining forms and compound combining forms.

a. chol/e _____

b. cholecyst/o _____

c. choledoch/o _____

d. cholangi/o _____

e. sialaden/o   _____

f. an/o   _____

g. cec/o   _____

h. append/o   _____

i. stomat/o   _____

5. **Match** the following digestive structures with their functions.

_____ stomach	a. serves as an entry for food and contains the structures responsible for chewing and swallowing
_____ large intestine	b. transforms food into chyme with the aid of digestive enzymes and hydrochloric acid
_____ small intestine	c. completes digestion of food and serves as the main site of absorption of nutrients into the blood
_____ rectum	d. transforms fluid waste into feces
_____ oral cavity	e. stores feces and leads to the opening (the anus) through which feces are excreted

Terminology

The following are selected terms that pertain to pathology of the digestive system and to related diagnostic and surgical procedures. As you will see, most of the symptoms and disorders listed result from inflammation, ulceration, or obstruction of the digestive organs. Keeping this in mind will help you to understand other terms you may hear as well as the rationale behind treatment of digestive disorders.

Pathologic Conditions	Word Elements	Definition
anorexia (AN-ner-**RECK**-see-uh)	an = without; not orexia = appetite	lack of appetite
appendicitis (uh-PEN-dih-**SIE**-tis)	appendic = appendix itis = inflammation	inflammation of the appendix, usually due to obstruction or infection
cholelithiasis (KOE-lee-lih-**THIE**-uh-sis)	chole = bile; gall lith = stone iasis = condition	condition characterized by the presence or formation of stones in the gallbladder
cirrhosis (sir-ROE-sis)	cirrh = yellow osis = condition	chronic liver disease characterized by the destruction of liver cells; eventually leads to impaired liver function and jaundice

Pathologic Conditions	Word Elements	Definition
colitis (koe-LIE-tis)	col = colon; large intestine itis = inflammation	inflammation of the colon or large intestine, usually due to infection
constipation (KON-stih-**PAY**-shun)	constip = "to press together" ation = process	difficult or infrequent elimination of hard, dry feces
Crohn's disease (KROHNZ)	no word elements	type of chronic inflammatory bowel disease that usually affects the ileum
diarrhea (DIE-er-**REE**-uh)	dia = through rrhea = discharge	elimination of unusually loose, watery stools, often with increased frequency
diverticulosis (DIE-ver-TIH-kyoo-**LOE**-sis)	diverticul = "things that turn aside" osis = condition	condition characterized by the presence of diverticula (abnormal outpouchings of the intestinal wall); if the diverticula are inflamed, the condition is called diverticulitis
dyspepsia (dis-PEP-see-uh)	dys = difficult; painful pepsia = digestion	indigestion
emesis (EH-muh-sis)	emesis = vomiting	vomiting
enteritis (EN-ter-**EYE**-tis)	enter = small intestine itis = inflammation	inflammation of the small intestine, usually due to irritation or infection
gastritis (gas-TRY-tis)	gastr = stomach itis = inflammation	inflammation of the stomach, usually due to irritation, infection, or stress
gastroenteritis (GAS-troe-EN-ter-**EYE**-tis)	gastro = stomach enter = small intestine itis = inflammation	inflammation of the stomach and small intestine, usually due to irritation or infection
hematemesis (HEH-muh-**TEE**-muh-sis)	hemat = blood emesis = vomiting	vomiting blood
hematochezia (HE-muh-toe-**KEE**-zee-uh)	hemato = blood chezia = "to go into the stools"	excretion of stools containing red blood; bloody stools
hemorrhoids (HEH-mer-roydz)	hemorrhoid = "vein liable to bleed"	swollen veins in the lining of the anus, often causing rectal bleeding and pain
hepatitis (HEH-puh-**TIE**-tis)	hepat = liver itis = inflammation	inflammation of the liver, usually caused by viral infection; the infection is generally transmitted through blood products or sexual contact

Pathologic Conditions	Word Elements	Definition
hepatomegaly (heh-PAT-oh-**MEH**-gull-lee)	hepato = liver megaly = enlargement	enlargement of the liver
hiatal hernia (hi-AY-tul HER-nee-uh)	hiat = opening al = pertaining to hernia = rupture	condition characterized by the protrusion of the upper part of the stomach through the diaphragm
ileitis (ILL-ee-**EYE**-tis)	ile = ileum itis = inflammation	inflammation of the ileum
inguinal hernia (ING-wuh-nul HER-nee-uh)	inguin = groin al = pertaining to hernia = rupture	condition characterized by the protrusion of a portion of an intestine through the lower abdominal wall (in the groin area)
irritable bowel syndrome	no word elements	combination of lower abdominal pain, diarrhea, and constipation occurring in the absence of known disease; thought to be associated with stress; also called spastic colon
jaundice (JAWN-diss)	jaundice = "yellowed"	yellow discoloration of the skin due to abnormally high levels of bilirubin (a pigment) in the blood; usually a sign of liver dysfunction or obstruction of the bile ducts
nausea (NAW-zee-uh)	nausea = "seasickness"	unpleasant sensation in the stomach, usually with a feeling of the need to vomit
pancreatitis (PAN-kree-uh-**TIE**-tis)	pancreat = pancreas itis = inflammation	inflammation of the pancreas, often resulting in damage to the tissue by digestive enzymes
peptic ulcer (PEP-tick ULL-sir)	pept = digestion ic = pertaining to	an open sore or lesion on the mucous membrane lining the stomach or intestine; usually found in the highly acidic regions of the duodenum or stomach
peritonitis (PEHR-ih-tuh-**NIE**-tis)	periton = peritoneum itis = inflammation	inflammation of the peritoneum, usually due to infection
pyrosis (pie-ROE-sis)	pyr = fever; fire osis = condition	a burning sensation in the chest, often caused by backflow of stomach acid into the esophagus; commonly called heartburn
stomatitis (STOE-muh-**TIE**-tis)	stomat = mouth itis = inflammation	inflammation of the mouth, especially the mucosal linings of the mouth

Diagnostic Procedures	Word Elements	Definition
barium enema (BEHR-ee-um EN-uh-muh)	no word elements	x-ray of the rectum and colon following administration of barium sulfate (a substance that x-rays cannot penetrate) into the rectum; also called a "lower GI"
barium swallow (BEHR-ee-um)	no word elements	x-ray of the esophagus, stomach, and small intestine following oral administration of barium sulfate; also called an "upper GI series"
cholangiography (koe-LAN-jee-**OG**-ruh-fee)	chol = bile; gall angio = vessel graphy = recording	x-ray recording of the bile ducts; if a contrast agent is injected into the blood first, the procedure is called intravenous cholangiography; if a contrast agent is injected through the skin directly into the liver, the procedure is called percutaneous transhepatic cholangiography (PER-kyoo-**TAY**-nee-us TRANZ-heh-**PAT**-ick KOE-lan-jee-**OG**-ruh-fee), or PTC
cholecystography (KOE-luh-sih-**STOG**-ruh-fee)	chole = bile; gall cysto = bladder graphy = recording	x-ray recording of the gallbladder, usually following oral administration of a contrast agent that accumulates in the gallbladder
gastrointestinal endoscopy (en-DOS-kuh-pee)	endo = inside scopy = visual examination	visual examination of one or more digestive system organs using an endoscope; depending on the organ(s) examined, the procedure may be called esophagoscopy, gastroscopy, colonoscopy, sigmoidoscopy, proctoscopy, anoscopy, etc.
liver function tests	no word elements	tests involving measurement of the levels of certain enzymes (ALT, AST, and ALK) and bilirubin in the blood; elevated levels are suggestive of impaired liver function or liver damage
liver scan	no word elements	injection of radioactive material capable of penetrating liver cells, followed by use of a special scanner to record the radiation emitted from the cells
stool guaiac (GWIE-ack)	no word elements	addition of a substance called guaiac to a stool sample to detect the presence of blood in the feces; occasionally called Hemoccult (the tradename of a modified guaiac test)

Surgical Procedures	Word Elements	Definition
appendectomy (AP-pen-**DECK**-tuh-me)	append = appendix ectomy = surgical removal	surgical removal of the appendix
cholecystectomy (KOE-luh-sis-**TECK**-tuh-me)	chole = bile; gall cyst = bladder ectomy = surgical removal	surgical removal of the gallbladder; if the procedure is performed through a tube placed into the abdomen, it is called laparoscopic cholecystectomy
choledocholithotomy (KOE-luh-DOE-koe-lih-**THOT**-uh-me)	choledocho = common bile duct litho = stone tomy = surgical incision	surgical incision into the common bile duct to remove gallstones
colectomy (koe-**LECK**-tuh-me)	col = colon; large intestine ectomy = surgical removal	surgical removal of all or part of the colon, often to treat patients with chronic colitis or Crohn's disease
colostomy (koe-**LOSS**-tuh-me)	colo = colon; large intestine stomy = surgical opening	surgical creation of an opening between the colon and the surface of the abdomen, usually to allow elimination of the feces into a bag attached to the skin
hemorrhoidectomy (HEH-muh-royd-**ECK**-tuh-me)	hemorrhoid = "vein liable to bleed" ectomy = surgical removal	surgical removal of one or more hemorrhoids
ileostomy (ILL-ee-**OS**-tuh-me)	ileo = ileum stomy = surgical opening	surgical creation of an opening between the ileum and the surface of the abdomen to allow feces to be discharged into a bag attached to the skin; often a permanent means of elimination following a colectomy

Review Exercises

6. **Define** the following terms.

a. diarrhea _____

b. diverticulosis _____

c. hiatal hernia _____

d. irritable bowel syndrome _____

e. peptic ulcer _____

f. pyrosis _____

g. barium swallow _____

7. **Match** the following terms with their definitions.

_____ appendicitis

_____ hematochezia

_____ emesis

_____ stool guaiac

_____ barium enema

_____ constipation

_____ Crohn's disease

a. vomiting

b. x-ray of the rectum and colon following administration of barium into the rectum

c. bloody stools

d. type of chronic inflammatory bowel disease usually affecting the ileum

e. inflammation of the appendix

f. test used to detect the presence of blood in the feces

g. difficult or infrequent elimination of hard, dry feces

8. **Break Down and Define** the word elements within each of the following terms, and then define the term itself.

     Example: appendic / itis   *appendix / inflammation*   *inflammation of the appendix*

a. cholelithiasis

_____

b. hepatomegaly

_____

c. gastroenteritis

_____

d. stomatitis

_____

e. sigmoidoscopy

_____

f. esophagoscopy

_____

g. ileostomy

_____

h. hematemesis

_____

i. gastritis

_____

j. ileitis

_____

k. colostomy

_____

l. pancreatitis

_____

m. choledocholithotomy

_____

n. anorexia

_____

o. gastrointestinal

_____

p. endoscopy

_____

9. ***Choose and Construct.*** Choose the appropriate word elements from the list provided to construct terms for the following.

angi/o	cyst/o	jejun/o	-itis
chol/e	enter/o	-ectomy	-stomy
col/o	gastr/o	-graphy	

surgical opening into the jejunum　　　　　　　　*jejuno / stomy*

a. inflammation of the colon

_____ / _____

b. x-ray (recording) of the bile ducts

_____ / _____ / _____

c. surgical removal of the colon

_____ / _____

d. surgical removal of the gallbladder

_____ / _____ / _____

e. inflammation of the stomach and colon

_____ / _____ / _____

f. surgical opening between the small intestine and colon

_____ / _____ / _____

g. surgical opening between the stomach and jejunum

_____ / _____ / _____

h. surgical opening between the stomach and small intestine

_____ / _____ / _____

10. **Word Building and Spelling**. Spell out the medical term for each of the following definitions using the slashes provided to separate the word elements.

enlargement of the liver	*hepato / megaly*

a. surgical removal of the appendix   _____ / _____

b. difficult or painful digestion   _____ / _____

c. inflammation of the liver   _____ / _____

d. x-ray (recording) of the gallbladder   _____ / _____ / _____

e. inflammation of the small intestine   _____ / _____

f. surgical removal of hemorrhoids   _____ / _____

g. surgical opening into the ileum   _____ / _____

h. inflammation of the peritoneum   _____ / _____

Case Study. Read the case notes below. For each boldfaced term, provide a brief definition and indicate whether the term is spelled correctly; if it is misspelled, provide the correct spelling.

Example: **anerexia:** *lack of appetite*

              Spelled correctly? ☐ Yes ☑ No *anorexia*

Patient presented as a 54-year-old male complaining of fatigue, weakness, **anerexia, nausea**, swelling in the legs and abdomen, itching, and yellowing of the skin. The symptoms, especially the **jaundis**, were highly suggestive of liver disease. With the exception of **hemoroids** and previous surgery for an **iguanal hernia**, patient's history appeared unremarkable. On questioning, however, patient acknowledged longstanding alcoholism. Suspect **serosis**. Ordered **liver function tests** and a **liver scan**. Results consistent with serosis. Treatment plan: medications to alleviate symptoms, enrollment in alcohol treatment program, low protein diet.

a. nausea: _____

_____

Spelled correctly? ☐ Yes ☐ No _____

b. jaundis: _____

_____

Spelled correctly? ☐ Yes ☐ No _____

c. hemoroids: _____

_____

Spelled correctly? ☐ Yes ☐ No _____

d. iguanal hernia: _____

_____

Spelled correctly? ☐ Yes ☐ No _____

e. serosis: _____

_____

Spelled correctly? ☐ Yes ☐ No _____

f. liver function tests: _____

_____

Spelled correctly? ☐ Yes ☐ No _____

g. liver scan: _____

_____

Spelled correctly? ☐ Yes ☐ No _____

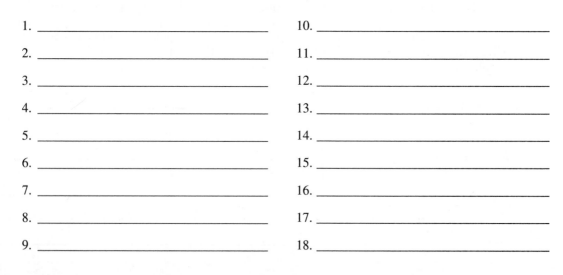

Listen to the section on your audiotape cassette that corresponds to this chapter and write the terms below. Be careful to spell each term correctly.

1. _____   10. _____

2. _____   11. _____

3. _____   12. _____

4. _____   13. _____

5. _____   14. _____

6. _____   15. _____

7. _____   16. _____

8. _____   17. _____

9. _____   18. _____

19. _____

20. _____

21. _____

22. _____

23. _____

24. _____

25. _____

26. _____

27. _____

28. _____

29. _____

30. _____

31. _____

32. _____

33. _____

34. _____

35. _____

36. _____

37. _____

38. _____

39. _____

40. _____

41. _____

42. _____

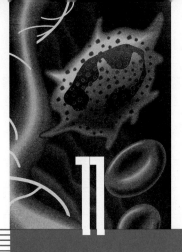

Urinary System

Upon completing this chapter, you should be able to:

- Describe the urinary system and explain the primary functions of its organs
- Recognize, build, pronounce, and spell words that pertain to the urinary system
- Describe diseases, diagnostic tests, and therapeutic procedures that pertain to the urinary system

Overview   The main function of the urinary system is to selectively remove cellular waste products, excess electrolytes, and other potentially harmful substances from the blood. The urinary system accomplishes this task by extracting these substances from the blood during the process of creating urine. The primary component of urine is urea, a waste product resulting from cellular metabolism of protein. The urinary system also regulates the balance of electrolytes (sodium, potassium, and calcium) in the blood, the amount of water in the blood and tissues, and the acidity of the blood.

Word Elements

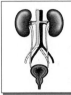

URINARY STRUCTURES — The following combining forms (CF) refer to the major organs of the urinary system, including the structures that make up the kidneys (the organs that filter blood and produce urine).

CF	Meaning	Example
cyst/o	urinary bladder	*cyst*itis = inflammation of the urinary bladder
glomerul/o	glomerulus	*glomerulo*sclerosis = hardening of the glomeruli
nephr/o	kidney	*nephr*ectomy = surgical removal of a kidney
pyel/o	renal pelvis	*pyelo*nephritis = inflammation of the body and pelvis of the kidney
ren/o	kidney	*ren*al = pertaining to the kidney
ureter/o	ureter	*uretero*stenosis = narrowing of a ureter
urethr/o	urethra	*urethr*itis = inflammation of the urethra
vesic/o	urinary bladder	*vesico*cele = hernial protrusion of the urinary bladder

URINE — These combining forms refer to urine, as well as to constituents of urine that can be evidence of disease.

CF	Meaning	Example
albumin/o	albumin	*albumin*uria = excessive albumin in the urine
keton/o	ketones	*keton*uria = excessive ketones in the urine
ur/o	urine; urea	*ur*emia = excessive urea in the blood

SUFFIX — The following suffix pertains to the urinary system. It is used to denote urinary conditions.

Suffix	Meaning	Example
-uria	urine condition	py*uria* = presence of pus in the urine

Anatomy and Physiology

The urinary system consists of the kidneys, ureters, bladder, and urethra. These structures are illustrated in Figure 11-1 and described in the following paragraphs.

Figure 11-1: The urinary system.

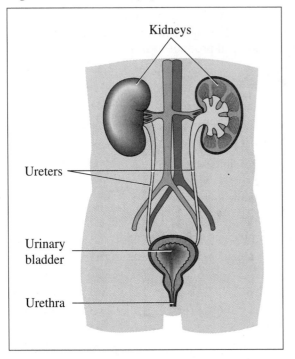

Kidneys

Ureters

Urinary
bladder

Urethra

*ren/o = kidney
(generally refers to
structure)*

*nephr/o = kidneys
(generally refers to
function)*

The Kidneys

The **kidneys** (KID-neez) are the primary functional organs of the urinary system, responsible for filtering urea and other waste products from the blood. In the process of filtering blood, the kidneys also help maintain the proper balance of water and electrolytes in the body by secreting some substances into the urine and retaining others. In addition, the kidneys secrete **renin** (REE-nin or REH-nin), an enzyme involved in the control of blood pressure, and **erythropoietin** (eh-RITH-roe-**POY**-uh-tin), a hormone that regulates the production of red blood cells. The kidneys also activate **Vitamin D**, which stimulates calcium absorption from the intestines.

Structurally, each kidney is comprised of an outer layer, called the **renal cortex** (REE-nul KOR-tecks), and an inner region, called the **renal medulla** (meh-DULL-uh). Blood enters the kidney through a blood vessel called the **renal artery**. Inside the kidney, the renal artery branches into smaller and smaller arteries, eventually leading to microscopic filtering units called **nephrons** (NEH-fronz), where the blood is filtered and urine is formed. Filtered blood is transported out of the kidney via the **renal vein**, while the forming urine left behind is carried to a central collecting area in the kidney called the **renal pelvis** (PEL-vis).

Nephrons, the microscopic filtering units of the kidney, are complex structures designed to efficiently filter urea and other waste materials from the blood. There are about a million nephrons in each kidney. Structurally, each nephron consists of two components: a **renal corpuscle** (KOR-pus-sul) and a **renal tubule** (TOOB-yule).

The renal corpuscle is the site of blood filtration in the nephron; it consists of a **glomerulus** (gluh-MEHR-yoo-lus), which is a cluster of capillaries originating from the renal artery, and a **Bowman's** (BOE-menz) **capsule**, a cup-like structure that encases the glomerulus (see Figure 11-3). As blood passes through the glomerulus, water, electrolytes, sugar, amino acids, and waste products of protein metabolism (urea, creatinine, and uric acid) are absorbed into the Bowman's capsule. In healthy individuals, proteins, blood cells, and other large substances cannot pass through the walls of the glomerulus, so they remain in the blood and return to the systemic circulation via the renal vein. The waste-containing fluid absorbed into the Bowman's capsule is called **glomerular** (gluh-MEHR-yoo-ler) **filtrate**.

Figure 11-2:
The kidney.

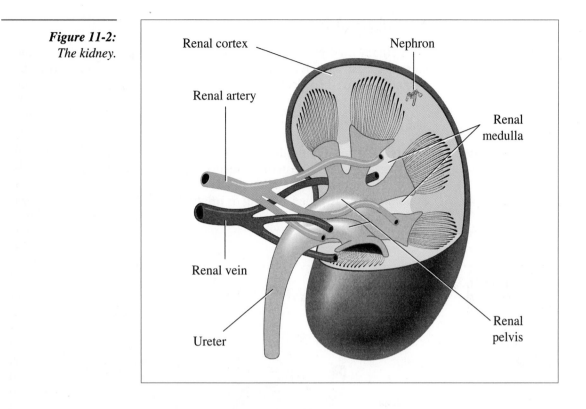

This glomerular filtrate flows from the Bowman's capsule into the renal tubule, a long, twisted, tubular structure consisting of four sections: the **proximal** (PROX-ih-mul) **tubule**, the **loop of Henle** (HEN-lee), the **distal** (DIS-tul) **tubule**, and the **collecting duct**. As the glomerular filtrate flows through these four sections of the renal tubule, substances that the body needs (e.g., water, salts, and sugar) re-enter the bloodstream through the **peritubular** (PEHR-ih-**TOOB**-yoo-ler) **capillaries** surrounding the renal tubule; this process is called **reabsorption**. At the same time, specialized cells of the collecting duct transfer additional waste products from the peritubular capillaries into the duct, a process called **secretion**. The resulting fluid, now called urine, flows from the renal tubule of the nephron to the renal pelvis.

The Ureters

ureter/o = ureters

Each renal pelvis (one from each kidney) narrows to form a **ureter** (YER-ruh-ter), a muscular tube lined with mucous membranes. When the muscles of the ureters contract, urine is pushed away from the kidneys and into the urinary bladder.

The Urinary Bladder

cyst/o and vesic/o =
urinary bladder

The **urinary bladder**, usually referred to simply as the bladder, is a hollow, muscular sac in the pelvic cavity. It serves as a temporary reservoir for urine, expanding as urine collects and contracting when urine is excreted.

The Urethra

urethr/o = urethra

The **urethra** (yer-EE-thruh) is a tube extending from the urinary bladder to the external opening, the **urinary meatus** (me-AY-tus). The urethra serves as the passageway for excretion of urine from the bladder. The process of excreting urine is called **voiding** or **micturition** (MICK-tyer-**RIH**-shun). In men, the urethra also serves as a passageway for semen during ejaculation (see Chapter 14).

Figure 11-3:
The nephron.

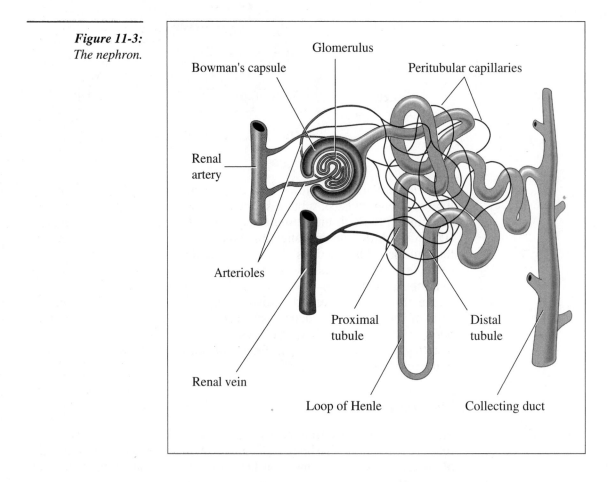

Review Exercises

1. **Match** the following combining forms with their definitions.

_____	nephr/o	a.	urinary bladder
_____	ureter/o	b.	glomerulus
_____	vesic/o	c.	ureter
_____	pyel/o	d.	renal pelvis
_____	glomerul/o	e.	kidney
_____	ur/o	f.	urine; urea

2. **Define** the following suffix and combining forms.

a. keton/o _____

b. -uria _____

c. urethr/o _____

d. ren/o _____

e. cyst/o _____

f. albumin/o _____

3. **Match** the following structures with their descriptions.

_____	nephrons	a.	the microscopic filtering units of the kidney
_____	renal tubule	b.	a cluster of capillaries in the nephron through which blood is filtered
_____	glomerulus		
_____	renal pelvis	c.	the cup-like structure in the nephron that collects glomerular filtrate
_____	ureters	d.	the long twisted tube in the nephron through which glomerular filtrate passes
_____	Bowman's capsule		
_____	peritubular capillaries	e.	tiny blood vessels that reabsorb water and nutrients from the renal tubule
		f.	the central collecting area for urine in the kidney
_____	urinary bladder	g.	muscular tubes that convey urine from the kidneys to the bladder
		h.	the muscular sac that serves as a reservoir for urine until it is excreted

Terminology

The following are selected terms that pertain to pathology of the urinary system and to related diagnostic and therapeutic procedures. As you will see, most of the disorders listed result from inflammation, tissue damage, or abnormalities in blood filtration or urination. Keeping this in mind will help you to understand other terms you may hear as well as the rationale behind treatment of urinary disorders.

Pathologic Conditions	Word Elements	Definition
anuria (an-NYER-ree-uh)	an = without; not uria = urine condition	absence of urine formation (reduced or no urination)
cystitis (sis-TIE-tis)	cyst = urinary bladder itis = inflammation	inflammation of the urinary bladder, usually due to infection
cystocele (SIS-toe-seel)	cysto = urinary bladder cele = hernia; swelling	protrusion of the urinary bladder through the wall of the vagina
cystolith (SIS-toe-lith)	cysto = urinary bladder lith = stone	bladder stone, usually caused by crystallization of waste products in the urine
diuresis (DIE-yer-**EE**-sis)	diure = "to urinate" sis = condition	increased excretion of urine; in some cases, an early sign of diabetes
dysuria (dis-YER-ee-uh)	dys = painful; difficult uria = urine condition	painful or difficult urination
end-stage renal disease	ren = kidney al = pertaining to	any type of kidney disease that has advanced to the point that the kidneys can no longer adequately filter the blood; also called ESRD
enuresis (EN-yer-**EE**-sis)	en = in; surrounded by ur = urine; urea esis = condition	urinary incontinence, including bedwetting (nocturnal urinary incontinence)
glomerulonephritis (gluh-MEHR-yoo-loe-neh-**FRY**-tis)	glomerulo = glomerulus nephr = kidney itis = inflammation	inflammation of the glomeruli of the kidney
hydronephrosis (HI-droe-neh-**FROE**-sis)	hydro = water nephr = kidney osis = condition	excessive accumulation of urine in the renal pelvis due to obstruction of a ureter
nephritis (neh-**FRY**-tis)	nephr = kidney itis = inflammation	inflammation of a kidney, usually due to infection

Pathologic Conditions	Word Elements	Definition
nephrolithiasis (NEH-froe-lih-**THIE**-uh-sis)	nephro = kidney lith = stone iasis = condition	disorder characterized by the presence of stones in the kidney
nephroma (neh-**FROE**-muh)	nephr = kidney oma = tumor; growth	tumor arising from kidney tissue
nephropathy (neh-**FROP**-uh-thee)	nephro = kidney pathy = disease	any type of kidney disease or damage
nephrosclerosis (NEH-froe-sklur-**OH**-sis)	nephro = kidney sclerosis = hardening	disorder characterized by hardening of kidney tissue
nephrosis (neh-**FROE**-sis)	nephr = kidney osis = condition	disorder of the kidney characterized by excessive protein loss in the urine
nocturia (nock-**TYER**-ee-uh)	noct = night uria = urine condition	excessive urination at night
oliguria (OL-ih-**GYER**-ee-uh)	olig = scanty; few uria = urine condition	scanty production of urine
polyuria (POL-ee-**YER**-ee-uh)	poly = many uria = urine condition	excretion of an unusually large amount of urine; in some cases, a sign of diabetes
pyelonephritis (PIE-ull-loe-neh-**FRY**-tis)	pyelo = renal pelvis nephr = kidney itis = inflammation	inflammation of the body and pelvis of the kidney, usually due to infection
renal colic (REE-nul KOL-ick)	ren = kidney al = pertaining to	painful contractions of a ureter, usually due to obstruction by (or passing of) a kidney stone
uremia (yer-**EE**-me-uh)	ur = urine; urea emia = blood condition	elevated level of urea or other protein waste products in the blood
ureterostenosis (yer-**REE**-ter-oh-sten-**NO**-sis)	uretero = ureter stenosis = narrowing	narrowing of one or both ureters
urethritis (YER-ee-**THRIE**-tis)	urethr = urethra itis = inflammation	inflammation of the urethra, usually due to infection
urinary retention	no word elements	inability to expel urine

Diagnostic Procedures	Word Elements	Definition
blood urea nitrogen	no word elements	laboratory test that measures the amount of urea in the blood; since the kidneys normally filter urea from the blood, a high result is suggestive of impaired kidney function
catheterization (KATH-eh-ter-ih-**ZAY**-shun)	catheter = "something inserted" ization = process	insertion of a catheter (tube) through the urethra and into the bladder to withdraw urine
cystography (sis-TOG-ruh-fee)	cysto = urinary bladder graphy = recording	x-ray recording of the bladder following administration of a contrast agent via a urinary catheter
intravenous pyelography (PIE-ull-**LOG**-ruh-fee)	pyelo = renal pelvis graphy = recording	x-ray recording of the kidneys, ureters, bladder, and urethra following intravenous injection of a contrast agent; commonly called IVP
retrograde pyelography (REH-troe-grade PIE-ull-**LOG**-ruh-fee)	retro = backward grade = step pyelo = renal pelvis graphy = recording	x-ray recording of the urinary collecting system following the introduction of a contrast agent into the ureters via a cystoscope
urinalysis (YER-ih-**NAL**-ih-sis)	urin = urine alysis = analysis	physical, microscopic, or chemical examination of urine
voiding cystourethrography (SIS-toe-yer-ee-**THROG**-ruh-fee)	cysto = urinary bladder urethro = urethra graphy = recording	x-ray recording of the bladder and urethra while the patient is expelling urine; a contrast agent is administered prior to the procedure

Urinalysis Results	Word Elements	Definition
albuminuria (al-BYOO-min-**NYER**-ee-uh)	albumin = albumin uria = urine condition	presence of abnormally high levels of albumin in the urine; proteinuria; a sign of abnormal kidney function
bacteriuria (back-TEER-ee-**YER**-ee-uh)	bacteri = bacteria uria = urine condition	presence of bacteria in the urine; a sign of urinary tract infection
glycosuria (GLIE-koe-**SYER**-ee-uh)	glycos = sugar uria = urine condition	presence of abnormally high levels of sugar in the urine; often a sign of diabetes
hematuria (HE-muh-**TYER**-ee-uh)	hemat = blood uria = urine condition	presence of blood in the urine; a sign of damage to or infection of one or more urinary structures
ketonuria (KEE-tone-**NYER**-ee-uh)	keton = ketones uria = urine condition	presence of abnormally high levels of ketones in the urine; usually a sign of excessive fasting (starvation) or diabetes

Urinalysis Results	Word Elements	Definition
proteinuria (PRO-teen-**NYER**-ee-uh)	protein = protein uria = urine condition	presence of abnormally high levels of protein (usually albumin) in the urine; a sign of abnormal kidney function
pyuria (pie-YER-ee-uh)	py = pus uria = urine condition	presence of pus in the urine; a sign of urinary tract infection

Therapeutic Procedures	Word Elements	Definition
cystectomy (sis-TECK-tuh-me)	cyst = urinary bladder ectomy = surgical removal	surgical removal of the bladder
cystoplasty (**SIS**-toe-PLASS-tee)	cysto = urinary bladder plasty = surgical repair	surgical repair of the bladder, often to remove a cystocele
hemodialysis (HE-moe-die-**AL**-lih-sis)	hemo = blood dia = through lysis = dissolution	purification of the blood by pumping it through a mechanical filtration device; used to treat patients with severely impaired kidney function
lithotripsy (**LIH**-thoe-TRIP-see)	litho = stone tripsy = crushing	crushing of a stone (in the bladder or urethra)
nephrectomy (neh-FRECK-tuh-me)	nephr = kidney ectomy = surgical removal	surgical removal of a kidney
peritoneal dialysis (PEHR-ih-tuh-**NEE**-ul die-AL-lih-sis)	peritone = peritoneum al = pertaining to dia = through lysis = dissolution	removal of toxic substances from the body by draining waste products through a tube inserted into the peritoneal (abdominal) cavity; used to treat patients with severely impaired kidney function
pyeloplasty (**PIE**-ull-loe-PLASS-tee)	pyelo = renal pelvis plasty = surgical repair	surgical repair of the renal pelvis
renal biopsy	bi = life opsy = view	surgical extraction of kidney tissue for microscopic examination
renal transplantation	trans = through; across plant = plant ation = process	surgical implantation of a kidney from a compatible donor into a recipient; used to treat end-stage renal disease
ureteroplasty (yer-**REE**-ter-oh-PLASS-tee)	uretero = ureter plasty = surgical repair	surgical repair of a ureter
urethroplasty (yer-**EE**-throe-PLASS-tee)	urethro = urethra plasty = surgical repair	surgical repair of the urethra

Review Exercises

4. **Match** the following terms with their definitions.

_____	diuresis	a.	presence of pus in the urine
_____	urinary retention	b.	inability to expel urine
_____	enuresis	c.	kidney disorder involving excessive protein loss in the urine
_____	cystocele	d.	painful contractions of a ureter due to the presence of a kidney stone
_____	renal colic	e.	urinary incontinence
_____	hydronephrosis	f.	increased excretion of urine
_____	nephrosis	g.	surgical removal of kidney tissue for examination
_____	hemodialysis	h.	insertion of a tube into the bladder to withdraw urine
_____	renal biopsy	i.	protrusion of the urinary bladder through the wall of the vagina
_____	pyuria	j.	excessive collection of urine in the renal pelvis
_____	catheterization	k.	purification of the blood using a mechanical filtration device

5. **Break Down and Define** the word elements within each of the following terms, and then define the term itself.

Example: urethr / itis *urethra / inflammation* *inflammation of the urethra*

a. anuria

_____

b. nephrectomy

_____

c. dysuria

_____

d. oliguria

_____

e. lithotripsy

_____

f. ureterostenosis

_____

g. hematuria

_____

h. uremia

_____

i. urethroplasty

_____

j. bacteriuria

_____

k. ketonuria

_____

l. pyeloplasty

_____

m. nephrolithiasis

_____

n. nephrosclerosis

_____

o. cystoplasty

_____

p. polyuria

_____

6. ***Choose and Construct.*** Choose the appropriate word elements from the list provided to construct terms for the following.

albumin/o	nephr/o	-ectomy	-oma
cyst/o	urethr/o	-graphy	-pathy
glycos/o		-itis	-uria

surgical removal of a kidney   *nephr / ectomy*

a. x-ray (recording) of the urinary bladder   _____ / _____

b. x-ray (recording) of the urinary bladder and urethra   _____ / _____ / _____

c. surgical removal of the urinary bladder   _____ / _____

d. (excessive) albumin in the urine   _____ / _____

e. (excessive) sugar in the urine   _____ / _____

f. inflammation of the kidney   _____ / _____

g. tumor of the kidney   _____ / _____

h. any disease of the kidney   _____ / _____

7. ***Word Building and Spelling.*** Spell out the medical term for each of the following definitions using the slashes provided to separate the word elements.

     bacteria in the urine   *bacteri / uria*

a. inflammation of the urinary bladder   _____ / _____

b. x-ray (recording) of the renal pelvis   _____ / _____

c. bladder stone   _____ / _____

d. inflammation of the renal pelvis and whole kidney   _____ / _____ / _____

e. inflammation of the glomeruli of the kidney   _____ / _____ / _____

f. night urination   _____ / _____

g. inflammation of the urethra   _____ / _____

h. surgical repair of a ureter   _____ / _____

Case Study. Read the case notes below. For each boldfaced term, provide a brief definition and indicate whether the term is spelled correctly; if it is misspelled, provide the correct spelling.

Example: **glumerulonephritis:** *inflammation of the glomeruli of the kidney*

            Spelled correctly?   ☐ Yes   ☑ No   *glomerulonephritis*

Patient presented as an ill 52-year-old with chronic **glumerulonephritis**. Patient was diagnosed four years ago when a **uranalysis** revealed **proteenuria** and **hematuria**, a physical examination revealed high blood pressure, and a **renal biopsy** confirmed kidney damage consistent with glomerulonephritis. Over the years, patient's kidney function has steadily decreased, with **blood uria nitrogen** levels steadily rising. For the last six months, patient has been undergoing **periteoneal dialysis** due to kidney failure. Patient was diagnosed with **end-stage renal disease** and referred to me for evaluation as a candidate for **renal transplantation**. Following a complete work-up, placed patient's name on waiting list for a donor organ. Treatment plan: continue dialysis, monitor for complications until donor organ can be found.

a. uranalysis: _____

_____

Spelled correctly? ☐ Yes ☐ No _____

b. proteenuria: _____

_____

Spelled correctly? ☐ Yes ☐ No _____

c. hematuria: _____

_____

Spelled correctly? ☐ Yes ☐ No _____

d. renal biopsy: _____

_____

Spelled correctly? ☐ Yes ☐ No _____

e. blood uria nitrogen: _____

_____

Spelled correctly? ☐ Yes ☐ No _____

f. periteoneal dialysis: _____

_____

Spelled correctly? ☐ Yes ☐ No _____

g. end-stage renal disease: _____

_____

Spelled correctly? ☐ Yes ☐ No _____

h. renal transplantation: _____

_____

Spelled correctly? ☐ Yes ☐ No _____

Listen to the section on your audiotape cassette that corresponds to this chapter and write the terms below. Be careful to spell each term correctly.

1. _____
2. _____
3. _____
4. _____
5. _____
6. _____
7. _____
8. _____
9. _____
10. _____
11. _____
12. _____
13. _____
14. _____
15. _____
16. _____
17. _____
18. _____
19. _____
20. _____

21. _____
22. _____
23. _____
24. _____
25. _____
26. _____
27. _____
28. _____
29. _____
30. _____
31. _____
32. _____
33. _____
34. _____
35. _____
36. _____
37. _____
38. _____
39. _____
40. _____

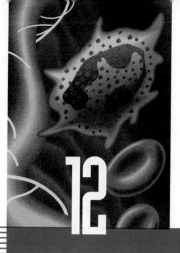

12

Nervous System

Upon completing this chapter, you should be able to:

- Describe the nervous system and explain the primary functions of its two major divisions
- Recognize, build, pronounce, and spell words that pertain to the nervous system
- Describe diseases, diagnostic tests, and surgical procedures that pertain to the nervous system

Overview   The nervous system functions as the body's master control center, coordinating all of the body's conscious and unconscious responses to environmental stimuli. As such, the nervous system includes some components that are responsible for detecting and interpreting changes in the environment, and others that enable the body to generate an appropriate response. The nervous system is also responsible for discriminatory functions, such as thinking and feeling.

Word Elements

STRUCTURES OF NERVES – Neurons, or nerve cells, are the main building blocks of nervous tissue. The following combining forms (CF) refer to the structures that make up neurons and connections between neurons.

CF	Meaning	Example
ax/o	axon	*axo*dendritic = pertaining to an axon-dendrite synapse
dendr/o	dendrite	*dendr*itic = pertaining to a dendrite
myelin/o	myelin	*myelino*pathy = any disease of the myelin
neur/o	nerve; nerve tissue	*neur*algia = pain along the path of a nerve
neuron/o	neuron	*neuron*al = pertaining to a neuron
synapt/o	synapse	pre*synapt*ic = situated or occurring before a synapse

THE CENTRAL NERVOUS SYSTEM – These combining forms pertain to the central nervous system. They refer to the structures of the brain and spinal cord, and the structures that support and protect the brain and spinal cord.

CF	Meaning	Example
cerebell/o	cerebellum	*cerebell*itis = inflammation of the cerebellum
cerebr/o	cerebrum	*cerebr*al = pertaining to the cerebrum
cortic/o	cortex	*cortic*al = pertaining to the cortex
encephal/o	brain	*encephal*itis = inflammation of the brain
gli/o	glia	*gli*oma = tumor of the glia
hypo-thalam/o	hypothalamus	*hypothalamo*tomy = surgical creation of incisions in the hypothalamus
medull/o	medulla	*medull*ary = pertaining to the medulla
mening/e	membranes; meninges	*mening*itis = inflammation of the meninges
mes-encephal/o	midbrain	*mesencephalo*tomy = surgical creation of incisions in the midbrain
myel/o	spinal cord*	*myelo*graphy = x-ray recording of the spinal cord
pont/o	pons	*ponto*bulbia = presence of cavities in the pons
thalam/o	thalamus	*thalam*ectomy = surgical removal of part of the thalamus
thec/o	sheath; covering	intra*thec*al = pertaining to inside a sheath
ventricul/o	ventricle	*ventriculo*graphy = x-ray recording of the ventricles

*NOTE: Depending on the context, myel/o can also refer to the bone marrow (see Chapters 6 and 16).

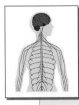

THE PERIPHERAL NERVOUS SYSTEM — These combining forms pertain to the peripheral nervous system, which consists of all of the neurons and nervous structures outside of the brain and spinal cord.

CF	Meaning	Example
ganglion/o	ganglion	*ganglion*ated = provided with ganglia
para-sympath/o	parasympathetic nervous system	*parasympatho*mimetic = having effects similar to those of the parasympathetic nervous system
sympath/o	sympathetic nervous system	*sympatho*mimetic = having effects similar to those of the sympathetic nervous system

SUFFIXES — The following suffixes pertain to the nervous system. They are used to denote processes and symptoms mediated by nervous mechanisms.

SUFFIX

Suffix	Meaning	Example
-algesia	sensitivity to pain	an*algesia* = insensitivity to pain
-algia	pain	neur*algia* = pain along the path of a nerve
-asthenia	weakness	my*asthenia* = muscle weakness
-esthesia	feeling; sensation	an*esthesia* = without feeling or sensation
-lepsy	seizure	epi*lepsy* = a type of seizure disorder
-mentia	thinking	de*mentia* = loss of the ability to think clearly
-mnesia	memory	a*mnesia* = without memory
-paresis	partial paralysis	hemi*paresis* = partial paralysis of half of the body
-plegia	paralysis	quadri*plegia* = paralysis of the arms and legs
-somnia	sleep	in*somnia* = inability to sleep

Anatomy and Physiology

Anatomically, the nervous system can be separated into two major divisions: the central nervous system, consisting of the brain and spinal cord, and the peripheral nervous system, consisting of the bundles of nerve cells that relay information between the central nervous system and other organs. Both systems, and the structures that comprise them, are described below.

STRUCTURAL ELEMENTS OF THE NERVOUS SYSTEM

The Neuron

neuron/o = neuron

The functional and structural subunit of the nervous system is the **neuron** (NOOR-on), or individual nerve cell. Neurons are specialized cells capable of conducting an electrical impulse from one location to another. The

Figure 12-1: *The neuron and neurotransmission.*

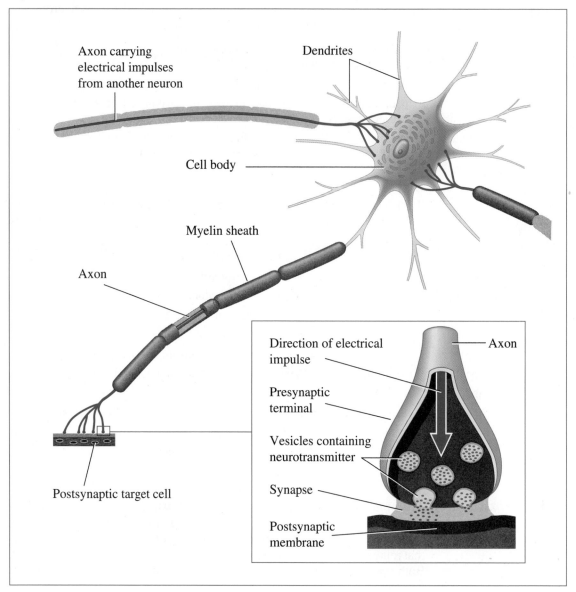

complicated circuits that make up the nervous system are actually networks of interconnected neurons.

The general structure common to most neurons is illustrated in Figure 12-1. Most neurons have a bipolar structure in which signals are received at one end and are transmitted from the other. At its receptive end, the neuron

dendr/o = dendrite   consists of numerous highly branched projections, called **dendrites** (DENdrites), that extend out from the round or elongated neuronal **cell body**. The dendrites are the sites at which the majority of inputs from other nerve cells are received. Signals received by the dendrites are conveyed to the cell body, where they are integrated to produce a single output. The integrated signal is carried away from the cell body by the **axon** (ACKS-on), a single projection which extends to the neuron's target cell or tissue.

ax/o = axon

Axons vary a great deal in length; although some are less than a millionth of an inch long, others extend all the way from a cell body in the brain to muscles in the toes. Depending on its size, an axon may be surrounded by a fatty coating called a **myelin** (MY-ull-lin) **sheath** that insulates the axon and increases the efficiency of impulse conduction. Due to their fatty coating, myelinated (**MY**-ull-lin-**AY**-ted) axons take on a whitish appearance. Because of this, groups of myelinated axons constitute the "white matter" of the brain and spinal cord, while groups of dendrites and nerve cell bodies are referred to as the "gray matter."

myelin/o = myelin

Individual neurons communicate with one another in a process called **neurotransmission** (NOOR-oh-tranz-**MIH**-shun). This process occurs at a narrow gap between two cells called a **synapse** (SIN-aps). In the **presynaptic** (PRE-sin-**AP**-tick) neuron, specialized chemicals known as **neurotransmitters** (NOOR-oh-**TRANZ**-mih-terz) are stored in tiny sacs called **vesicles** (VEH-sih-kulls). When an electrical signal reaches the terminal of the presynaptic axon, these vesicles release a neurotransmitter into the synapse. Specialized proteins known as **receptors** (ree-SEP-torz) on the surface of the **postsynaptic** (POST-sin-**AP**-tick) cell detect the presence of the neurotransmitter and generate an electrical signal of their own. In this way, the signal is passed from the presynaptic cell to the postsynaptic cell.

neur/o = nerve; nerve tissue
synapt/o = synapse
presynaptic = before the synapse

postsynaptic = after the synapse

The Nerves

In contrast with neurons, which are individual cells, **nerves** are bundles of axons following a common pathway. Whereas a single neuron can be compared with a wire conducting an electrical impulse, a nerve is more like a cable carrying thousands of individual wires. Unlike individual axons, which can be seen only with the help of a microscope, most nerves are visible to the naked eye.

In the periphery (i.e., outside the brain and spinal cord), nerve bundles are surrounded by a thin, external membrane called the **neurolemma** (NOOR-uh-**LEH**-muh). The neurolemma is thought to play a role in determining whether a damaged neuron will regenerate, since regeneration can occur in the periphery but not in the central nervous system.

-lemma = "rind; husk"

-ferent = carry
afferent = carry
toward
efferent = carry away

Depending on the direction in which they transmit information, neurons and nerves are classified as **afferent** (AF-fehr-unt) or **efferent** (EE-fehr-unt). Because they transmit impulses from the sensory organs *to* the central nervous system, sensory neurons and nerves are afferent. Likewise, because they carry information *away* from the central nervous system toward muscles and organs in the periphery, motor neurons and nerves are efferent. Nerves that carry both afferent and efferent fibers are referred to as **mixed nerves**.

THE CENTRAL NERVOUS SYSTEM

By definition, the **central nervous system** (CNS) consists of the brain, spinal cord, and related supporting tissues. Each of these structures is described below.

The Brain

The brain is one of the most complicated organs in the body. Although little is known about the mechanisms by which the brain regulates and coordinates all of the body's voluntary and involuntary activities, it is clear that primary control over various functional activities is localized to different areas of the brain.

cerebr/o = cerebrum

The largest functional division of the brain is the **cerebrum** (sir-EE-brum), a highly convoluted mass of tissue that accounts for nearly half of the brain's total volume and weight. The cerebrum is divided into two halves, or **hemispheres**, which are connected by a bundle of fibers known as the **corpus callosum** (KOR-puz kul-LOE-sum). Each hemisphere is further divided into four subunits, or lobes, named for the cranial bones that overlie them: the **frontal** (FRUN-tul) lobe, the **parietal** (per-RYE-eh-tul) lobe, the **occipital** (ock-SIH-pih-tul) lobe, and the **temporal** (TEM-purr-ul) lobe. Architecturally, the cerebrum consists of an outer layer of cell bodies and dendrites, called the **cerebral cortex** (sir-EE-brul KOR-tecks), over an intricate network of fibers that connect various regions of the cortex with one another and with other neural tissues. Different areas of the cerebral cortex are responsible for most "higher" functions, including speech, vision, motor control, associative reasoning, and memory.

cortic/o = cortex

thalam/o = thalamus

hypothalam/o = hypothalamus

Just below the cerebrum is a large collection of neurons called the **thalamus** (THAL-luh-muss), which acts as a processing center for sensory and motor impulses passing into and out of the cerebral cortex. The **hypothalamus** (HI-poe-**THAL**-luh-muss), located just below the thalamus, coordinates more primitive aspects of behavior, including appetite, sleep, sexual desire,

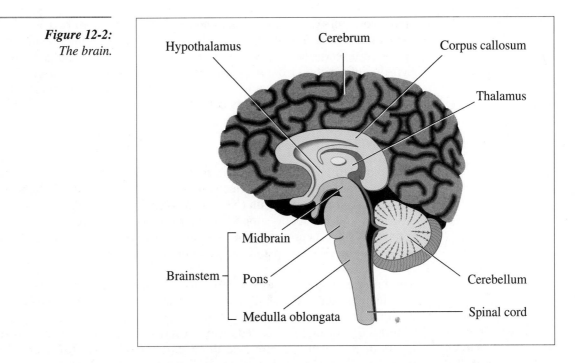

Figure 12-2:
The brain.

Hypothalamus

Cerebrum

Corpus callosum

Thalamus

Brainstem — Midbrain

Pons

Medulla oblongata

Cerebellum

Spinal cord

and emotions such as fear and pleasure. By regulating the release of hormones from the nearby pituitary gland, the hypothalamus also acts to coordinate the responses of the nervous and endocrine systems.

mesencephal/o = midbrain
pont/o = pons
medull/o = medulla

Even more rudimentary processes are regulated by the **brainstem**, which consists of the **midbrain**, the **pons**, and the **medulla oblongata** (meh-DULL-luh OB-long-**GOT**-tuh). Small collections of neurons in the brainstem regulate involuntary processes such as respiration, heart rate, and blood pressure. In addition, the brainstem is the site where motor neurons cross from one side of the body to the other, so that the right half of the brain controls movement involving the left side of the body and vice versa.

cerebell/o = cerebellum

Attached to the brainstem is the **cerebellum** (SEHR-uh-**BELL**-um), which plays a role in equilibrium, posture, and muscular coordination.

The Spinal Cord

myel/o = spinal cord

The **spinal cord** is a cylindrical column of nervous tissue which is surrounded and protected by the vertebrae. Continuous with the medulla oblongata, the spinal cord extends approximately two-thirds of the way down the vertebral column, to about the small of the back. It consists of a central core of cell bodies and dendrites, surrounded by numerous defined pathways, or **tracts,** through which millions of axons travel up and down the spinal column. These fibers enter and leave the spinal cord by way of 31 pairs of nerves positioned along the length of the cord. Functionally, the spinal cord serves as a relay station between the brain and the periphery. Sensory information from the periphery passes to the brain via **ascending tracts** in the spinal cord, while motor influences pass from the brain to the periphery via **descending tracts** in the spinal cord.

Supporting Structures

gli/o = glia

In addition to neurons, the central nervous system also contains a huge number of supporting cells collectively referred to as **glia** (GLEE-uh) or, less commonly, as **neuroglia** (NOOR-oh-**GLEE**-uh). Glial cells provide structural and metabolic support to neurons; they also mount defensive responses when neuronal tissue is injured or infected. Unlike neurons, however, glia do not transmit electrical impulses.

mening/e = meninges
dura mater = "tough or strong mother"
arachnoid = "spiderlike"
pia mater = "tender mother"

The brain and spinal cord are protected mainly by the bony structures surrounding them: the skull and the vertebral column, respectively. In addition, however, the brain and spinal cord are surrounded by three layers of protective membranes called the **meninges** (muh-NIN-jeez). The three layers of the meninges are: the **dura mater** (DURE-uh MOT-er), the outermost layer, named for its tough, fibrous appearance; the **arachnoid** (uh-RACK-noyd), the middle layer, named for its spider-web appearance; and the **pia mater** (PEE-uh MOT-er), the innermost layer, named for its role in nurturing as well as protecting the underlying tissue. The space between the dura mater and the arachnoid is referred to as the **subdural space**; similarly, the space between the arachnoid and the pia mater is called the **subarachnoid space**. Injections directly into the subarachnoid space (e.g.,

thec/o = sheath; covering

to administer chemotherapeutic drugs) are referred to as **intrathecal** (IN-truh-**THEE**-kull) injections.

ventricul/o = ventricle

The brain and spinal cord are bathed by **cerebrospinal** (sir-EE-broe-**SPY**-null) **fluid**, or **CSF**, a liquid similar in composition to the plasma or lymph. The CSF circulates through the brain and spinal cord in a series of interconnected canals called **ventricles** (VEN-trih-kulls). The CSF also bathes the meninges, keeping them moist. In addition to supplying nutrients, the CSF serves a protective function, acting as a shock absorber when there is a shift in the position of the head or vertebral column.

THE PERIPHERAL NERVOUS SYSTEM

Anatomically, the **peripheral nervous system (PNS)** is defined to include all of the nervous tissue found outside of the skull and vertebral column. Functionally, it consists of two subsystems: the somatic nervous system and the autonomic nervous system.

Figure 12-3:
Divisions of the peripheral nervous system.

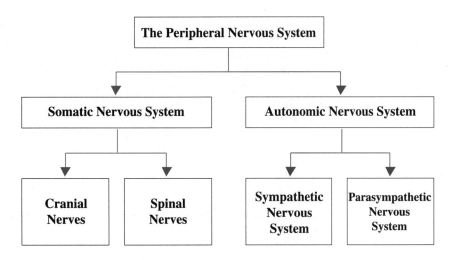

The **somatic** (so-MAT-tick) **nervous system** is responsible for the relay of sensory information from the periphery to the central nervous system and for the execution of voluntary activities involving the peripheral musculature. It consists of 12 pairs of **cranial nerves** that emerge from the brainstem and 31 pairs of **spinal nerves** that emerge from the spinal cord. Neurons of the somatic nervous system extend uninterrupted from the brain or spinal cord to their peripheral targets.

crani/o = skull

The **autonomic** (AW-toe-**NOM**-ick) **nervous system** is responsible for coordinating the organs and systems involved in involuntary activities such as respiration, cardiovascular function, and digestion. Unlike somatic fibers, autonomic neurons form one synapse before reaching their targets in the periphery. These synapses occur within **ganglia** (GANG-glee-uh), which are collections of neurons located outside the central nervous system. The autonomic nervous system responds to environmental stimuli by increasing or decreasing the rate and intensity of physiologic processes. To accomplish this, the autonomic nervous system is further divided into two subdivisions; the **sympathetic** (SIM-puh-**THEH**-tick) and **parasympathetic** (PEHR-uh-SIM-puh-**THEH**-tick) nervous systems.

ganglion/o = ganglia
sing. = ganglion
sympath/o = sympathetic nervous system
parasympath/o = parasympathetic nervous system

In general, the sympathetic and parasympathetic nervous systems exert opposing actions. Activation of the sympathetic nervous system causes the rate and intensity of physiologic processes to increase, preparing the body for "fight or flight" responses. Conversely, activation of the parasympathetic nervous system decreases the rate and intensity of these processes, preparing the body to engage in restorative functions such as sleep, digestion, and excretion. At any given time, the actual rate and intensity of physiologic processes reflects the balance between sympathetic and parasympathetic influences on target organs. Because its actions are mediated in large part by the neurotransmitter **norepinephrine** (NOR-eh-pih-**NEH**-frin), also called **noradrenaline** (NOR-uh-**DREH**-null-lin), the sympathetic nervous system is sometimes referred to as the **adrenergic** (AD-reh-**NER**-jick) system. Similarly, because its actions are mediated by the neurotransmitter **acetylcholine** (uh-SEE-tul-**KOE**-leen), the parasympathetic nervous system is sometimes referred to as the **cholinergic** (KOE-lih-**NER**-jick) system.

Review Exercises

1. **Match** the following suffixes with their definitions.

_____	-asthenia	a. pain
_____	-esthesia	b. sensitivity to pain
_____	-algia	c. feeling; sensation
_____	-plegia	d. sleep
_____	-algesia	e. seizure
_____	-lepsy	f. weakness
_____	-somnia	g. paralysis

2. **Match** the following structures of the nervous system with the functions they perform.

_____	afferent fibers	a. central control of involuntary processes
_____	thalamus	b. increases the rate and intensity of physiologic processes
_____	sympathetic nervous system	c. coordinates nervous and endocrine responses
_____	cerebellum	d. "higher" functions such as speech and memory
_____	parasympathetic nervous system	e. decreases the rate and intensity of physiologic processes
_____	cerebrum	f. carry information toward the CNS
_____	hypothalamus	g. carry information away from the CNS
_____	efferent fibers	h. equilibrium, posture, and muscular coordination
_____	brainstem	i. processes sensory and motor inputs to the cerebral cortex

3. *Match* the following combining forms with their definitions.

_____ cerebell/o   a. thalamus

_____ cortic/o   b. sympathetic nervous system

_____ dendr/o   c. cerebellum

_____ mesencephal/o   d. dendrite

_____ thalam/o   e. spinal cord

_____ myelin/o   f. midbrain

_____ myel/o   g. cortex

_____ sympath/o   h. myelin

4. *Define* the following suffixes and combining forms.

a. -paresis _____

b. neur/o _____

c. hypothalam/o _____

d. encephal/o _____

e. synapt/o _____

f. ventricul/o _____

g. gli/o _____

h. thec/o _____

i. -mentia _____

j. -mnesia _____

5. *Spell* the combining forms that have the following meanings.

a. neuron _____

b. ganglion _____

c. axon _____

d. cerebrum _____

e. pons _____

f. medulla _____

g. meninges _____

h. parasympathetic _____
   nervous system

Terminology

The following are selected terms that pertain to pathology of the nervous system and to related diagnostic and surgical procedures. As you will see, most of the disorders listed result from structural changes in the nervous system that produce functional deficits reflecting the site of damage. Keeping this in mind will help you to understand other terms you may hear as well as the rationale behind treatment of nervous disorders.

Pathologic Conditions	Word Elements	Definition
akinesia (AY-kih-**NEE**-zyuh)	a = without kinesia = movement	inability to move due to a loss of voluntary muscle control
Alzheimer's disease (ALZ-hime-erz)	no word elements	degenerative disorder in which the progressive loss of brain cells leads to memory loss and other cognitive deficits
anesthesia (AN-ehz-**THEE**-zyuh)	an = without; not esthesia = feeling; sensation	insensitivity to pain, heat, or other stimuli
aphasia (uh-FAY-zyuh)	a = without phasia = speech	inability to produce or to understand spoken language
ataxia (ay-TACK-see-uh)	a = without taxia = muscular coordination	loss of muscular coordination characterized by difficulty in walking
Bell's palsy (BELZ PAWL-zee)	palsy = paralysis	reversible disorder characterized by facial numbness or paralysis, including loss of the blink reflex, due to dysfunction of the nerve that controls the facial muscles
cerebral palsy (sir-EE-brul PAWL-zee)	cerebr = cerebrum al = pertaining to palsy = paralysis	disorder in which damage to the brain at birth or during infancy leads to motor deficits, including paralysis or loss of muscular coordination
cerebrovascular accident (sir-EE-broe-**VAS**-kyoo-ler)	cerebro = cerebrum vascul = vessel ar = pertaining to	damage to brain tissue resulting from an interruption of the blood supply, usually due to the formation of a clot or rupture of a blood vessel; the resulting functional deficit depends on the area of the brain affected; also called stroke, apoplexy, or CVA
coma (KOE-muh)	coma = "a deep sleep"	deep unconsciousness, characterized by a complete or nearly complete loss of responsiveness to external stimuli

Pathologic Conditions	Word Elements	Definition
concussion (kun-KUH-shun)	concussion = "to shake violently"	transient loss of consciousness as a result of trauma to the head
dementia (dee-MEN-shuh)	de = without mentia = thinking	loss of the ability to think clearly, usually as a result of aging or disease
dyslexia (dis-LECK-see-uh)	dys = difficult lexia = word; phrase	difficulty in interpreting written language
encephalitis (en-SEF-ull-**LIE**-tis)	encephal = brain itis = inflammation	inflammation of the brain, usually due to infection
epilepsy (**EH**-pih-LEP-see)	epi = above lepsy = seizure	CNS disorder in which abnormal electrical activity in the brain produces symptoms ranging from a transient loss of consciousness to muscular twitches or seizures
glioma (glee-OH-muh)	gli = glia oma = tumor; growth	tumor arising from non-neuronal cells (glia) in the brain
grand mal (GRON MOL)	grand mal = "great evil"	type of seizure characterized by jerking motions in the limbs and a temporary loss of consciousness; also referred to as tonic-clonic seizures or convulsions
hemiparesis (HEM-ee-per-**REE**-sis)	hemi = half paresis = partial paralysis	muscular weakness affecting only the right or left side of the body (e.g., following a stroke)
hemiplegia (HEM-ee-**PLEE**-jyuh)	hemi = half plegia = paralysis	paralysis affecting only the right or left side of the body (e.g., following a stroke)
Huntington's chorea (kor-EE-uh)	chorea = "to dance"	hereditary degenerative disorder in which the progressive loss of brain cells leads to bizarre, involuntary, dance-like movements
lethargy (LEH-ther-jee)	lethargy = "drowsiness"	drowsiness or sluggishness; indifference to external stimuli
Lou Gehrig's disease (GEHR-igz)	no word elements	degenerative disorder in which the progressive loss of motor neurons in the spinal cord leads to muscular weakness and paralysis; also called ALS (amyotrophic lateral sclerosis)
meningitis (MEH-nin-**JIE**-tis)	mening = membrane itis = inflammation	inflammation of the membranes (meninges) surrounding the brain and/or spinal cord, usually due to infection

Pathologic Conditions	Word Elements	Definition
multiple sclerosis (sklur-OH-sis)	sclerosis = hardening	chronic, progressive disorder in which hardening of the myelin sheaths of motor neurons in the spinal cord produces weakness and other muscular symptoms
myasthenia gravis (MY-uh-**STHEE**-nee-uh GRAV-iss)	my = muscle asthenia = weakness gravis = "heavy"	chronic, progressive disorder in which a loss of neurotransmitter receptors produces increasingly severe muscular weakness
myelitis (MY-ull-**LIE**-tis)	myel = spinal cord itis = inflammation	inflammation of the spinal cord, often due to infection
narcolepsy (**NAR**-koe-LEP-see)	narco = sleep lepsy = seizure	disorder characterized by sudden, recurrent attacks in which the patient falls into a brief but deep sleep
neuralgia (noor-AL-jyuh)	neur = nerve; nerve tissue algia = pain	sharp pain that occurs along the path followed by a nerve
neuritis (noor-EYE-tis)	neur = nerve; nerve tissue itis = inflammation	inflammation of a nerve due to infection; also used to denote any type of nerve damage or disease
neuroblastoma (NOOR-oh-blass-**TOE**-muh)	neuro = nerve; nerve tissue blast = immature oma = tumor	tumor arising from immature nerve cells (neuroblasts); seen mainly in children
neuroma (noor-OH-muh)	neuro = nerve; nerve tissue oma = tumor	tumor arising from neuronal tissue
paraplegia (PEHR-ruh-**PLEE**-jyuh)	para = beside plegia = paralysis	paralysis of the lower portion of the body, including both legs
paresthesia (PEHR-rehs-**THEE**-zyuh)	par = beside esthesia = sensation	feeling of numbness or tingling; also referred to as a "pins and needles" sensation
Parkinson's disease	no word elements	degenerative disorder in which the progressive loss of brain cells leads to impairments in motor function, including tremor, muscular rigidity, and a slowing of movement
petit mal (PEH-tee MOL)	petit mal = "little evil"	type of seizure characterized by minor muscular twitches or a loss of contact with the environment lasting for less than 30 seconds; also called an absence seizure
poliomyelitis (POE-lee-oh-MY-ull-**LIE**-tis)	polio = gray matter myel = spinal cord itis = inflammation	disease in which the gray matter of the spinal cord is destroyed by a slow-acting virus, eventually leading to paralysis and muscular atrophy

Pathologic Conditions	Word Elements	Definition
quadriplegia (KWOD-rih-**PLEE**-jyuh)	quadri = four plegia = paralysis	paralysis of both arms and both legs; often, the trunk is also affected
sciatica (sie-**AT**-tih-kuh)	sciat = hip ic = pertaining to a = condition	sharp, "shooting" pain that follows the route of the sciatic nerve, which travels from the hip to the foot
seizure (SEE-zyur)	seizure = "to take possession of"	behavioral manifestation of abnormal electrical activity in the brain, usually involving impaired consciousness and/or involuntary motor activity
shingles (SHING-gulls)	shingles = "girdle"	chronic, intermittent viral disease in which painful blisters appear on the skin along the course of a peripheral nerve
somnambulism (som-**NAM**-byoo-LIH-zum)	somn = sleep ambul = walking ism = condition	sleepwalking; engaging in purposeful activity while asleep
stupor (STOO-per)	stupor = "numbness"	near unconsciousness, characterized by responsiveness only to vigorous stimulation
syncope (SIN-koe-pee)	syncop = "to cut off or cut short" e = condition	loss of consciousness occurring as a result of diminished blood flow to the brain
transient ischemic attack (iss-KEE-mick)	isch = "to hold back" emic = pertaining to a blood condition	temporary loss of function due to a transient decrease in the blood supply of an area of the brain; also called a TIA or mini-stroke
tremor (TREH-mer)	tremor = "to shake"	involuntary shaking or trembling in a muscle, usually involving the extremities

Diagnostic Procedures	Word Elements	Definition
carotid ultrasound (kehr-ROT-id)	ultra = beyond sound = sound	procedure in which high-frequency sound waves are used to generate an image of the carotid arteries that supply the brain with blood; used to identify blockages
cerebral angiography (sir-EE-brul AN-jee-**OG**-ruh-fee)	cerebr = cerebrum al = pertaining to angio = vessel graphy = recording	technique in which x-rays of the head are used to visualize the cerebral vasculature following injection of a contrast agent into the arteries

Diagnostic Procedures	Word Elements	Definition
computerized tomography (toe-MOG-ruh-fee)	tomo = section graphy = recording	procedure in which a series of cross-sectional x-rays are taken of the brain; a computer then generates an image of the brain based on variations in x-ray absorption
electroencephalography (ih-LECK-troe-en-SEF-full-**LOG**-ruh-fee)	electro = electricity encephalo = brain graphy = recording	technique in which electrodes on the scalp are used to record patterns of electrical activity within the brain; commonly referred to as EEG
lumbar puncture (LUM-bar)	lumb = loin; waist ar = pertaining to	procedure in which a hollow needle is inserted through the lower back into the subarachnoid space to withdraw CSF for diagnostic purposes or to relieve pressure within the brain or spinal cord; also called a spinal tap, spinal puncture, or LP
magnetic resonance imaging	magnet = magnet ic = pertaining to resonance = "to resound"	technique in which magnetic waves are used to produce a detailed image of structures within the brain; also referred to as MRI
myelography (MY-ull-**LOG**-ruh-fee)	myelo = spinal cord graphy = recording	technique in which x-rays are used to visualize the spinal cord following injection of a contrast agent into the spinal canal
positron emission tomography (POZ-ih-tron ee-MIH-shun toe-MOG-ruh-fee)	tomo = section graphy = recording	technique in which the distribution of radioactive glucose molecules is monitored to map activity in various parts of the brain; also referred to as PET scan

Surgical Procedures	Word Elements	Definition
laminectomy (LAM-mih-**NECK**-tuh-me)	lamin = layer ectomy = surgical removal	removal of a vertebra in order to gain access to a disk or to relieve pressure on the spinal cord
lobotomy (loe-BOT-uh-me)	lobo = lobe tomy = surgical incision	surgical incision into the frontal lobe of the brain to relieve pain or to alter behavior; no longer widely performed
neurotomy (noor-OT-uh-me)	neuro = nerve; nerve tissue tomy = surgical incision	surgical cutting of a nerve, usually to relieve severe pain
sympathectomy (SIM-puh-**THECK**-tuh-me)	sympath = sympathetic nervous system ectomy = surgical removal	surgical removal of a portion of the sympathetic nervous system
trephination (TREH-fih-**NAY**-shun)	trephin = "bore" ation = process	removal of a circular disk of bone using a specialized saw called a trephine (TREH-fine); performed to reveal brain tissue during neurosurgery or to relieve intracranial pressure

Review Exercises

6. **Match** the following terms with their definitions.

_____ trephination

_____ Parkinson's disease

_____ lumbar puncture

_____ poliomyelitis

_____ Alzheimer's disease

_____ sciatica

_____ dyslexia

    a. difficulty in interpreting written language

    b. degenerative disorder characterized by memory loss and other cognitive deficits

    c. sharp pain that follows the route of the sciatic nerve

    d. diagnostic procedure in which a needle is used to extract CSF from the spinal cord

    e. disorder in which the gray matter of the spinal cord is destroyed by a slow-acting virus

    f. degenerative disorder characterized by tremor, muscular rigidity, and a slowing of movements

    g. removal of a circular disk of bone using a special saw

7. **Define** the following terms.

a. Bell's palsy _____

b. cerebral palsy _____

c. Huntington's chorea _____

d. Lou Gehrig's disease _____

e. multiple sclerosis _____

f. shingles _____

8. **Break Down and Define** the word elements within each of the following terms, and then define the term itself.

    Example: a / mnesia   *without / memory*   *memory loss*

a. anesthesia

_____

b. electroencephalography

_____

c. meningitis

_____

d. dementia

_____

e. sympathectomy

_____

f. ataxia

_____

g. quadriplegia

_____

h. neuritis

_____

i. akinesia

_____

j. lobotomy

_____

k. myasthenia

_____

l. narcolepsy

_____

m. paraplegia

_____

n. paresthesia

_____

o. somnambulism

_____

p. laminectomy

_____

9. **_Word Building and Spelling_**. Spell out the medical term for each of the following definitions using the slashes provided to separate the word elements.

       inflammation of the meninges   _mening_ **/** _itis_

    a. x-ray (recording) of the spinal cord   _____ / _____

    b. tumor arising from a nerve   _____ / _____

    c. inflammation of the brain   _____ / _____

d. surgical incision in a nerve   _____ / _____

e. inflammation of the spinal cord   _____ / _____

f. nerve pain   _____ / _____

g. tumor of the glia   _____ / _____

h. tumor of immature nerve tissue   _____ / _____ / _____

Case Study. Read the case notes below. For each boldfaced term, provide a brief definition and indicate whether the term is spelled correctly; if it is misspelled, provide the correct spelling.

Example:

hemiperesis: *muscular weakness affecting the left or right side of the body*

Spelled correctly? ☐ Yes ☑ No *hemiparesis*

Patient presented to the emergency room as a confused, ill 63-year-old male. His wife explained that he had complained of sudden headache and weakness, then became dizzy, unsteady, confused, and had difficulty communicating. On examination, patient had difficulty responding to commands and had difficulty moving his right arm. **Hemiperesis**, but not **hemiplejia**, was also evident in patient's facial responses. Hearing and vision appeared to be normal, but **aphasia** made testing difficult. Blood pressure was elevated. On questioning, patient's wife indicated that he had no known history of **sincope**, **transient iskemic attack**, or other neurologic disease. He had a single **siezure** 20 years ago, but there was no recurrence and he was not diagnosed with **epilespy**. Patient has been on medication for hypertension for 15 years. Preliminary diagnosis: **cerebrovascular accident**. Treatment plan: admit patient to hospital for treatment; conduct **cerebral angiogrophy** and **magnetic resonance imaging** to assess sites and extent of damage.

a. hemiplejia: _____

_____

Spelled correctly? ☐ Yes ☐ No _____

b. aphasia: _____

_____

Spelled correctly? ☐ Yes ☐ No _____

c. sincope: _____

_____

Spelled correctly? ☐ Yes ☐ No _____

d. transient iskemic attack: _____

_____

Spelled correctly?   ☐ Yes   ☐ No _____

e. siezure: _____

_____

Spelled correctly?   ☐ Yes   ☐ No _____

f. epilespy: _____

_____

Spelled correctly?   ☐ Yes   ☐ No _____

g. cerebrovascular accident: _____

_____

Spelled correctly?   ☐ Yes   ☐ No _____

h. cerebral angiogrophy: _____

_____

Spelled correctly?   ☐ Yes   ☐ No _____

i. magnetic resonance imaging: _____

_____

Spelled correctly?   ☐ Yes   ☐ No _____

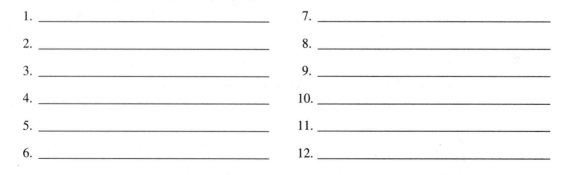

Listen to the section on your audiotape cassette that corresponds to this chapter and write the terms below. Be careful to spell each term correctly.

1. _____   7. _____

2. _____   8. _____

3. _____   9. _____

4. _____   10. _____

5. _____   11. _____

6. _____   12. _____

13. _____

14. _____

15. _____

16. _____

17. _____

18. _____

19. _____

20. _____

21. _____

22. _____

23. _____

24. _____

25. _____

26. _____

27. _____

28. _____

29. _____

30. _____

31. _____

32. _____

33. _____

34. _____

35. _____

36. _____

37. _____

38. _____

39. _____

40. _____

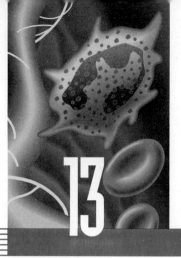

Endocrine System

Upon completing this chapter, you should be able to:

- Describe the endocrine system and explain the primary functions of its organs
- Recognize, build, pronounce, and spell words that pertain to the endocrine system
- Describe diseases, diagnostic tests, and therapeutic procedures that pertain to the endocrine system

Overview   The endocrine system is a network of glandular structures that function in close coordination with the nervous system. Like the nervous system, the endocrine system controls and integrates many bodily functions. Processes under direct endocrine control include growth, reproduction, cellular metabolism, and the regulation of blood levels of many important nutrients. In contrast with the rapid electrical responses of the nervous system, the endocrine system uses chemicals called hormones to generate responses that are more cyclical in nature, occurring over hours or days rather than seconds or minutes. Integration of nervous and endocrine influences on the body occurs in the hypothalamus, a structure of the central nervous system.

Word Elements

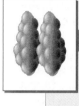

GENERAL TERMS – The following combining forms (CF) are used to construct general terms pertaining to the endocrine system. They refer to glands generally or to gland function (hormone secretion).

CF	Meaning	Example
aden/o	gland	*adeno*pathy = any gland disease
crin/o	secrete	*crin*ology = study of secretions
hormon/o	hormone	*hormon*al = pertaining to a hormone

ENDOCRINE GLANDS – These combining forms refer to the specific glands that make up the endocrine system. They form the foundation of many of the terms introduced in this chapter.

CF	Meaning	Example
adren/o	adrenal glands	*adreno*pathy = any disease of the adrenal glands
cortic/o	cortex	*cortico*tropic = acting upon the cortex
gonad/o	gonads	hyper*gonad*ism = overactivity of the gonads
hypophys/o	pituitary	*hypophys*eal = pertaining to the pituitary
medull/o	medulla	*medull*ectomy = surgical removal of the medulla
pancreat/o	pancreas	*pancreat*itis = inflammation of the pancreas
parathyroid/o	parathyroid glands	*parathyroid*oma = tumor of the parathyroid glands
pineal/o	pineal gland	*pineal*ism = condition of abnormal pineal activity
pituit/o	pituitary	*pituit*ectomy = surgical removal of the pituitary
thym/o	thymus	*thym*itis = inflammation of the thymus
thyr/o	thyroid	*thyro*megaly = enlargement of the thyroid
thyroid/o	thyroid	hyper*thyroid*ism = overactivity of the thyroid

SUFFIXES – The following suffixes pertain to the endocrine system. They are used to refer to effects of hormones or processes regulated by hormones.

Suffix	Meaning	Example
-trophic	nourishment; growth	hyper*trophic* = characterized by excessive growth
-tropic	turning; changing; acting upon	cortico*tropic* = acting upon the cortex

Anatomy and Physiology

aden/o = gland
endo- = inward

hormon/o = hormone

-trophic = nourish-
ment; growth
-tropic = changing;
acting upon

The endocrine system consists of a network of **glandular** (GLAN-dyoo-ler) structures distributed throughout the body. Unlike the **exocrine** (ECK-so-krin) **glands** that secrete chemical substances onto the surface of the body or into specific organs, the **endocrine** (EN-doe-krin) **glands** secrete chemical substances called **hormones** (HOR-moanz) directly into the bloodstream.

By definition, a hormone is a chemical substance that is synthesized by one organ or tissue and is carried in the blood to another tissue, called a **target organ**, where its actions are exerted. Because they travel in the blood, hormones reach all of the tissues in the body; only target organs, however, have receptors that recognize a particular hormone. These receptors, in turn, regulate the tissue's responsiveness to hormonal stimulation.

Hormones are generally secreted continuously. Endocrine regulation of target organs occurs via increases or decreases in the rate of hormonal secretion, which in turn stimulate or inhibit cellular processes. Hormones that regulate processes involving the growth or development of tissue are called **trophic** (TROE-fick) hormones; those that regulate the rate or intensity of particular metabolic reactions are referred to as **tropic** (TROE-pick) hormones.

The organs that make up the endocrine system are illustrated in Figure 13-1. Each of these structures, and the hormones they produce, are described below.

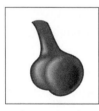

The Pituitary Gland

The **pituitary** (pih-**TOO**-ih-TEHR-ee) **gland** is a tiny, pea-shaped structure hanging from the base of the brain. It is attached to the hypothalamus by a bundle of nerve fibers and connective tissue called the **infundibular** (IN-fun-**DIH**-byoo-ler) **stalk**. Because it produces hormones that regulate the function of other endocrine structures, the pituitary gland is sometimes referred to as the "master gland" of the body.

pituit/o and
hypophys/o = pituitary

Structurally, the pituitary gland is divided into three lobes, each of which secretes different types of hormones.

The **anterior lobe** of the pituitary, also called the **adenohypophysis** (AD-deh-no-hi-**POF**-ih-sis), secretes six hormones:

- **somatotropin** (so-**MAT**-toe-TROE-pin), or **growth hormone**, which regulates the growth of bones and other tissues
- **thyroid-stimulating hormone**, or **TSH**, which regulates the activity of the thyroid gland (see below)

Figure 13-1: The endocrine system.

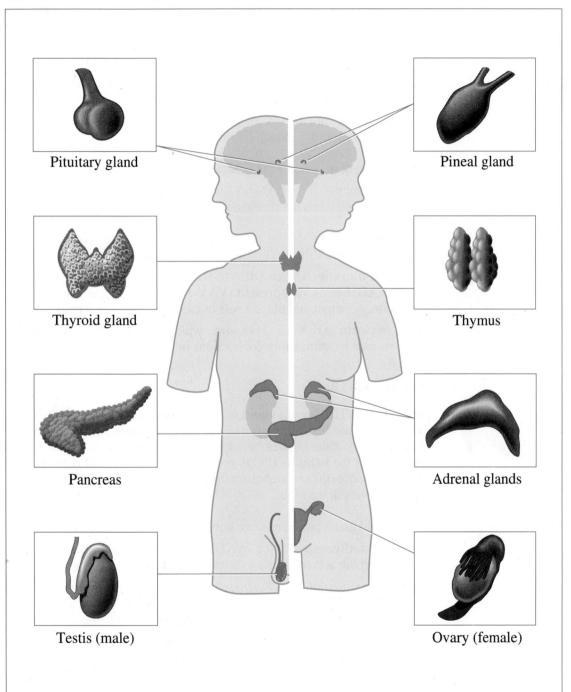

- **adrenocorticotropic** (uh-DREH-no-KOR-tih-koe-**TROE**-pick) **hormone**, or **ACTH**, which regulates the production of steroid hormones by the adrenal gland (see below)
- **follicle** (FOL-lih-kull)**-stimulating hormone**, or **FSH**, which stimulates egg production in the ovaries or sperm production in the testes
- **luteinizing** (**LOO**-tih-NIE-zing) **hormone**, or **LH**, which stimulates the production of sex hormones by the ovaries or testes
- **prolactin** (pro-LACK-tin), which stimulates the growth of breast tissue and milk production in females

The **intermediate lobe** of the pituitary produces a single hormone:

- **melanocyte** (mel-LAN-no-site)**-stimulating hormone**, or **MSH**, which regulates the pigmentation of the skin

The **posterior lobe** of the pituitary, also called the **neurohypophysis** (NOOR-oh-hi-**POF**-ih-sis) produces two hormones:

- **anti-diuretic** (AN-tee-DIE-yer-**REH**-tick) **hormone**, also referred to as **ADH** or as **vasopressin** (**VAY**-zoe-PREH-sin), which regulates urinary output and plays a role in blood pressure regulation
- **oxytocin** (OCK-see-**TOE**-sin), which induces labor in pregnant women by stimulating contractions in the uterus

The Thyroid Gland

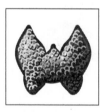

The **thyroid** (THIE-royd) **gland** is an H-shaped organ located in the front of the throat, just below the larynx (voicebox). It consists of two lobes, one on either side of the trachea (windpipe), connected by a narrow bridge of tissue called the **isthmus** (ISTH-muss). The thyroid gland regulates the overall state of cellular metabolism in the body and plays a role in regulating calcium levels in the blood.

thyr/o and thyroid/o = thyroid

The thyroid gland produces three hormones:

- **triiodothyronine** (TRY-eye-OH-doe-**THIE**-roe-neen), also called T_3, which acts to increase the rate of cellular metabolism
- **thyroxine** (thie-ROCK-sin), also called **tetraiodothyronine** (TEH-truh-eye-OH-doe-**THIE**-roe-neen) or T_4, which acts to increase the rate of cellular metabolism after being converted to T_3 in the tissues
- **calcitonin** (KAL-sih-**TOE**-nin), which acts in conjunction with parathyroid hormone (see below) to regulate calcium levels in the blood

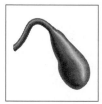

The Parathyroid Glands

The **parathyroid** (PEHR-ruh-**THIE**-royd) **glands** are two pairs of pea-shaped organs located on the undersides of the thyroid gland; in some individuals, a fifth gland or third pair of glands may be present.

The parathyroid glands produce a single hormone:

parathyroid/o =
parathyroid

- **parathyroid hormone**, or **PTH**, which acts in conjunction with calcitonin (see above) to regulate calcium and phosphate levels in the blood

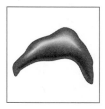

The Adrenal Glands

The **adrenal** (uh-DREE-nul) **glands** are a pair of triangular organs situated atop the kidneys; because of their location, they are sometimes alternatively referred to as the **suprarenal** (SOO-pruh-**REE**-null) **glands**. Structurally, the adrenal glands have two distinct divisions: an outer layer of cells known as the **adrenal cortex** and an inner core of cells known as the **adrenal medulla**.

adren/o = adrenal glands

cortic/o = cortex

The adrenal cortex produces three types of hormones:

- **cortisol** (KOR-tih-sol) and other **glucocorticoids** (gloo-koe-**KOR**-tih-koyds), which regulate the metabolism of complex molecules such as carbohydrates and proteins
- **aldosterone** (al-DOS-ter-ohn) and other **mineralocorticoids** (MIN-er-ul-oh-**KOR**-tih-koyds), which regulate water balance and mineral levels in the body
- **androgen** (AN-droe-jin) and other **androsterones** (AN-droe-**STEHR**-ohns), which serve as precursors for the sex hormones manufactured in the ovaries and testes (see below)

medull/o = medulla

The adrenal medulla produces three additional hormones:

- **epinephrine** (EH-pih-**NEH**-frin), also called **adrenaline** (uh-DREH-null-lin), which acts in conjunction with the sympathetic nervous system to stimulate "fight or flight" reactions in response to stress
- **norepinephrine** (NOR-eh-pih-**NEH**-frin), also called **noradrenaline** (NOR-uh-**DREH**-null-lin), which reduces the diameter of blood vessels in the periphery
- **dopamine** (DOE-puh-meen), which opposes the action of norepinephrine on the blood vessels and stimulates blood flow to the kidneys

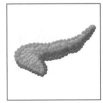

pancreat/o = pancreas

The Pancreas

The **pancreas** (PAN-kree-us) is an elongated organ located just below the stomach, in the back of the abdomen. The pancreas acts as both an exocrine and endocrine organ. In its exocrine role, it produces digestive juices that assist in the breakdown of proteins, starches, and fats within the small intestines. Its endocrine functions are mediated by **pancreatic islet** (PAN-kree-**AT**-ick EYE-let) **cells** located in the area of the pancreas known as the **isles of Langerhans** (LANG-ger-honz).

The pancreas produces two hormones:

- **insulin** (IN-sul-lin), which acts to clear sugar molecules from the blood by promoting their storage in the tissues as carbohydrates when blood glucose levels are high
- **glucagon** (GLOO-kuh-gon), which stimulates the release of sugar from storage sites in the liver when blood glucose levels are low

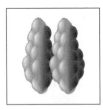

pineal/o = pineal gland

The Pineal Gland

The **pineal** (pie-NEE-ul) **gland** is a small, pine cone-shaped organ located deep within the brain, just behind the thalamus. In part because of its limited accessibility, the function of the pineal gland is less well understood than the function of other endocrine organs.

The pineal gland produces a single hormone:

- **melatonin** (MEL-luh-**TOE**-nin), which influences the maturation of sexual organs during puberty and may play a role in the regulation of circadian rhythms; circadian, literally meaning "about a day," refers to cyclical processes such as sleep and wakefulness that occur in regular patterns over the course of a day

The Thymus

The **thymus** (THIE-muss) is a butterfly-shaped organ located between the lungs in infants and young children; during puberty, the thymus begins to wither away, leaving adults with fat and connective tissue in its place.

The thymus produces a single hormone:

- **thymosin** (THIE-muh-sin), which plays a role in the development of the immune response in newborns

thym/o = thymus

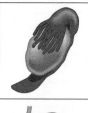

gonad/o = gonads

The Gonads

The **gonads** (GO-nadz) are the organs of the reproductive system that are responsible for producing sex hormones. In females, these organs are known as the **ovaries** (OH-ver-reez); in males, they are called the **testes** (TESS-teez).

The ovaries produce the two female sex hormones:

- **estradiol** (ESS-truh-**DIE**-ol), also called **estrogen** (ESS-troe-jin), which is responsible for the development of secondary sexual characteristics (e.g., breasts and pubic hair) and which plays a role in regulating cyclic changes in the lining of the uterus

- **progesterone** (pro-JESS-ter-ohn), which complements the action of estradiol in regulating cyclic changes in the lining of the uterus

The testes produce the male sex hormone:

- **testosterone** (tess-TOS-ter-ohn), which is responsible for the development of secondary sexual characteristics (e.g., beard and pubic hair) and which plays a role in regulating numerous metabolic and behavioral processes in males

Review Exercises

1. ***Match*** the following suffixes and combining forms with their definitions.

_____ thym/o	a.	nourishment; growth
_____ cortic/o	b.	turning; changing; acting upon
_____ -tropic	c.	medulla
_____ thyroid/o	d.	cortex
_____ hormon/o	e.	hormone
_____ -trophic	f.	pituitary
_____ medull/o	g.	thyroid
_____ pituit/o	h.	thymus

2. ***Define*** the following combining forms.

a. crin/o   _____

b. gonad/o   _____

c. thyr/o _____

d. pancreat/o _____

e. pineal/o _____

f. aden/o _____

g. adren/o _____

h. hypophys/o _____

i. parathyroid/o _____

3. **Match** the following endocrine structures with their descriptions.

_____ thymus

_____ parathyroid glands

_____ pineal gland

_____ pituitary gland

_____ adrenal glands

_____ gonads

_____ thyroid

_____ pancreas

a. tiny, pea-shaped structure hanging from the brain

b. two pairs of pea-shaped organs located on the underside of the thyroid gland

c. butterfly-shaped organ located between the lungs in infants and small children

d. triangular organs situated atop the kidneys

e. H-shaped organ located in the front of the throat

f. pine cone-shaped organ located deep in the brain

g. elongated organ located just below the stomach

h. female ovaries; male testes

4. **Match** the following endocrine structures with the hormones they produce.

_____ thymus

_____ parathyroid glands

_____ pituitary gland

_____ adrenal glands

_____ gonads

_____ thyroid

_____ pancreas

_____ pineal gland

a. aldosterone

b. melatonin

c. progesterone

d. insulin

e. parathyroid hormone

f. thyroxine

g. somatotropin

h. thymosin

Terminology

The following are selected terms that pertain to pathology of the endocrine system and to associated diagnostic and therapeutic procedures. As you will see, most of the diseases listed result from over- or underproduction of the various hormones. Keeping this in mind will help you to understand other terms you may hear as well as the rationale behind treatment of endocrine diseases.

Pathologic Conditions	Word Elements	Definition
acromegaly (ACK-kroe-**MEH**-gull-lee)	acro = extremities megaly = enlargement	enlargement of bones in the extremities and head due to overproduction of growth hormone (somatotropin) after puberty
Addison's disease (AD-dih-sunz)	no word elements	condition in which decreased production of glucocorticoids and mineralocorticoids by the adrenal glands leads to weakness, fatigue, weight loss, and increased pigmentation of the skin
aldosteronism, primary (al-**DOS**-ter-ohn-IZ-um)	aldosteron = aldosterone ism = condition	condition in which the blood contains high levels of aldosterone due to dysfunction of the adrenal gland
aldosteronism, secondary (al-**DOS**-ter-ohn-IZ-um)	aldosteron = aldosterone ism = condition	condition in which the blood contains high levels of aldosterone due to dysfunction of organs other than the adrenal gland (e.g., the pituitary gland)
Cushing's disease (KUH-shingz)	no word elements	disorder in which dysfunction of the anterior pituitary or adrenal glands leads to overproduction of glucocorticoids by the adrenal glands
diabetes insipidus (DIE-uh-**BEE**-teez in-SIH-pih-dus)	diabetes = "passing through" insipidus = "without taste"	disorder characterized by excessive thirst (polydipsia) and excessive urination (polyuria) due to inadequate production of anti-diuretic hormone
diabetes mellitus (DIE-uh-**BEE**-teez MEL-luh-tuss or mull-LIE-tuss)	diabetes = "passing through" mellitus = "honey-like; sweet"	disorder of carbohydrate metabolism in which decreased production of or responsiveness to insulin results in high levels of glucose in the blood
endemic goiter (en-DEH-mick GOY-ter)	en = in dem = people ic = pertaining to goiter = "throat"	enlargement of the thyroid (goiter) occurring as a result of a dietary iodine deficiency; rare, except in specific geographic areas
exophthalmos (ECK-sof-**THAL**-muss)	ex = out ophthalm = eye os = condition	protrusion of the eyeball; often a symptom of hyperthyroidism

Pathologic Conditions	Word Elements	Definition
gigantism (**JIE**-gan-TIH-zum)	gigant = giant ism = condition	excessive growth of the body or a part of the body resulting from overproduction of growth hormone (somatotropin)
Graves' disease	no word elements	hyperthyroidism characterized by goiter and exophthalmos; thought to be due to an autoimmune reaction to thyroid tissue
hyperglycemia (HI-per-glie-**SEE**-me-uh)	hyper = excessive glyc = sugar emia = blood condition	abnormally high levels of glucose in the blood
hypergonadism (HI-per-**GO**-nad-dih-zum)	hyper = excessive gonad = gonads ism = condition	overproduction of sex hormones by the ovaries or testes
hyperparathyroidism (HI-per-PEHR-ruh-**THIE**-royd-ih-zum)	hyper = excessive parathyroid = parathyroid ism = condition	overproduction of parathyroid hormone by the parathyroid gland, usually resulting in elevated calcium levels in the blood
hyperpituitarism (HI-per-pih-**TOO**-ih-tehr-ih-zum)	hyper = excessive pituitar = pituitary ism = condition	overactivity of the anterior pituitary gland
hyperthyroidism (HI-per-**THIE**-royd-ih-zum)	hyper = excessive thyroid = thyroid ism = condition	overactivity of the thyroid gland
hypogonadism (HI-poe-**GO**-nad-dih-zum)	hypo = under; reduced gonad = gonads ism = condition	underproduction of sex hormones by the ovaries or testes
hypoparathyroidism (HI-poe-PEHR-ruh-**THIE**-royd-ih-zum)	hypo = under; reduced parathyroid = parathyroid ism = condition	underproduction of parathyroid hormone by the parathyroid gland
hypothyroidism (HI-poe-**THIE**-royd-ih-zum)	hypo = under; reduced thyroid = thyroid ism = condition	underactivity of the thyroid gland
insulinoma (IN-sull-lin-**NO**-muh)	insulin = insulin oma = tumor; growth	tumor of the islets of Langerhans in the pancreas
ketoacidosis (KEE-toe-ass-ih-**DOE**-sis)	keto = ketones acid = acid osis = condition	acidification of the blood and urine due to improper metabolism of fats, seen mainly in patients with diabetes mellitus

Pathologic Conditions	Word Elements	Definition
myxedema (MICK-seh-**DEE**-muh)	myx = mucus edema = swelling	collections of mucus-like material in the subcutaneous tissue resulting in swelling, usually in the shins and face; a symptom of hypothyroidism
panhypopituitarism (PAN-hi-poe-pih-**TOO**-ih-tehr-ih-zum)	pan = all hypo = under; reduced pituitar = pituitary ism = condition	condition in which production of all pituitary hormones is reduced
pheochromocytoma (FEE-oh-KROE-moe-sie-**TOE**-muh)	pheo = dark; dusky chromo = color cyt = cell oma = tumor; growth	usually benign tumor of the adrenal medulla, characterized by increased production of epinephrine and norepinephrine
pituitarism (pih-TOO-ih-tehr-ih-zum)	pituitar = pituitary ism = condition	any disorder of the pituitary gland
pituitary dwarfism	no word elements	condition in which the bones remain small and underdeveloped due to congenital underproduction of growth hormone (somatotropin) by the anterior pituitary
syndrome of inappropriate ADH secretion	no word elements	condition in which overproduction of anti-diuretic hormone results in decreased sodium levels in the blood and weight gain; also called SIADH
thyroiditis (THIE-royd-**EYE**-tis)	thyroid = thyroid itis = inflammation	inflammation of the thyroid gland due to any of several causes
thyromegaly (THIE-roe-**MEH**-gull-lee)	thyro = thyroid megaly = enlargement	enlargement of the thyroid gland; also referred to as goiter
thyrotoxicosis (THIE-roe-TOCK-sih-**KOE**-sis)	thyro = thyroid toxic = poisonous osis = condition	general term for any toxic reaction resulting from overactivity of the thyroid gland (hyperthyroidism)

Diagnostic Procedures	Word Elements	Definition
glucose tolerance test	no word elements	procedure in which blood sugar levels are monitored in a patient who has ingested a known amount of glucose after a 12-hour fast; used to screen for diabetes mellitus
radioactive iodine uptake test	no word elements	procedure in which levels of radioactivity are measured in the thyroid following administration of a known quantity of radioactive iodine; used to monitor the ability of the thyroid to take up iodine from the blood; also called RAIU

Diagnostic Procedures	Word Elements	Definition
radioimmunoassay (RAY-dee-oh-IH-myoo-no-**ASS**-ay)	radio = radioactivity immuno = immune assay = test; measurement	technique that measures hormone levels in the blood by monitoring their ability to interfere with the binding of radioactive hormones to antibody molecules
thyroid-stimulating hormone (TSH) assay	no word elements	sensitive technique used to evaluate thyroid function by measuring thyroid-stimulating hormone levels in the blood
thyroxine (T_4) test (thie-ROCK-sin)	no word elements	technique that evaluates thyroid function by determining the amount of thyroxine present in a blood sample
triiodothyronine (T_3) uptake test (TRY-eye-OH-doe-**THIE**-roe-neen)	no word elements	technique that evaluates thyroid function by monitoring the amount of thyroid hormone bound to the protein present in a blood sample; also called a T_3 test

Therapeutic Procedures	Word Elements	Definition
adenectomy (AD-ih-**NECK**-tuh-me)	aden = gland ectomy = surgical removal	surgical removal of a gland
adrenalectomy (uh-DREE-null-**LECK**-tuh-me)	adrenal = adrenal glands ectomy = surgical removal	surgical removal of an adrenal gland
hormone replacement therapy	no word elements	oral administration or injection of synthetic hormones to patients with hormone deficiencies
hypophysectomy (HI-poe-fih-**ZECK**-tuh-me)	hypophys = pituitary ectomy = surgical removal	surgical removal of the pituitary gland
lobectomy (loe-BECK-tuh-me)	lob = lobe ectomy = surgical removal	surgical removal of a lobe of an organ; in the treatment of endocrine disorders, usually refers to the removal of one lobe of the thyroid gland
pinealectomy (pie-NEE-ull-**LECK**-tuh-me)	pineal = pineal gland ectomy = surgical removal	surgical removal of the pineal gland
thymectomy (thie-MECK-tuh-me)	thym = thymus ectomy = surgical removal	surgical removal of the thymus gland
thyroidectomy (THIE-royd-**ECK**-tuh-me)	thyroid = thyroid ectomy = surgical removal	surgical removal of the thyroid gland

Review Exercises

5. **Match** the following terms with their definitions.

_____ diabetes
  insipidus

_____ Cushing's
  disease

_____ glucose
  tolerance test

_____ radioimmuno-
  assay

_____ Addison's
  disease

_____ Graves'
  disease

_____ diabetes
  mellitus

_____ radioactive iodine
  uptake test

a. form of diabetes associated with decreased production of anti-diuretic hormone

b. form of diabetes associated with decreased production of or responsiveness to insulin

c. autoimmune disorder characterized by goiter, exophthalmos, and other signs of hyperthyroidism

d. diagnostic test that measures hormone levels in the blood

e. diagnostic test used to assess the function of the thyroid gland

f. condition characterized by decreased production of glucocorti-coids by the adrenal glands

g. condition characterized by increased production of glucocorti-coids by the adrenal glands

h. diagnostic test in which blood sugar levels are monitored in a patient who has ingested a known amount of glucose after fasting for 12 hours

6. **Define** the following terms.

a. endemic goiter _____

_____

b. insulinoma _____

_____

c. gigantism _____

_____

d. pheochromocytoma _____

_____

e. ketoacidosis _____

_____

7. **Break Down and Define** the word elements within each of the following terms, and then define the term itself.

　　　Example:　thyroid / itis　　　*thyroid / inflammation*　　　*inflammation of the thyroid*

a. adrenalectomy

　　　_____

b. thyromegaly

　　　_____

c. exophthalmos

　　　_____

d. hypergonadism

　　　_____

e. hyperglycemia

　　　_____

f. hypothyroidism

　　　_____

g. thyrotoxicosis

　　　_____

h. hypophysectomy

　　　_____

i. pituitarism

　　　_____

j. hyperpituitarism

　　　_____

k. panhypopituitarism

　　　_____

l. acromegaly

　　　_____

m. aldosteronism

　　　_____

n. hypogonadism

　　　_____

o. hypoparathyroidism

　　　_____

p. myxedema

　　　_____

8. **Word Building and Spelling.** Spell out the medical term for each of the following definitions using the slashes provided to separate the word elements.

any disease of a gland   *adeno / pathy*

a. surgical removal of the pineal gland   _____ / _____

b. inflammation of the thyroid gland   _____ / _____

c. excessive parathyroid condition   _____ / _____ / _____

d. surgical removal of the thymus   _____ / _____

e. surgical removal of a gland   _____ / _____

f. surgical removal of a lobe   _____ / _____

g. reduced sugar in the blood   _____ / _____ / _____

Case Study. Read the case notes below. For each boldfaced term, provide a brief definition and indicate whether the term is spelled correctly; if it is misspelled, provide the correct spelling.

Example: **mixedema:** *collections of mucus-like material in the skin, causing swelling*

Spelled correctly? ☐ Yes ☑ No *myxedema*

Patient presented as a 52-year-old female with vague complaints of numbness of the hands, unsteadiness, fatigue, dry skin, constipation, and a vague feeling of depression. Her physical appearance was striking: a dull facial expression; puffiness around the eyes consistent with **mixedema**; dry, coarse, thick skin; coarse, gray hair. Patient said that she had been diagnosed with **thyromegully** and **thyrotoxicosis** three years ago. She was treated with radioactive iodine, not **thyroydectomy**. She was monitored for **hypothyrodism** after RAI treatment, but did not exhibit clinically significant symptoms for one year. After that, she discontinued seeing her doctor. She could not pinpoint a time of onset for her current symptoms. Ordered a **thyroxin (T_4) test** and a **thyroid-stimulating hormone (TSH) assay**. T_4 was low, TSH was high. Diagnosis: Hypothyroidism. Treatment plan: **hormone replacement therapy** with thyroxine.

a. thyromegully: _____

_____

Spelled correctly? ☐ Yes ☐ No _____

b. thyrotoxicosis: _____

_____

Spelled correctly? ☐ Yes ☐ No _____

c. thyroydectomy: _____

_____

Spelled correctly?   ☐ Yes   ☐ No _____

d. hypothyrodism: _____

_____

Spelled correctly?   ☐ Yes   ☐ No _____

e. thyroxin (T_4) test: _____

_____

Spelled correctly?   ☐ Yes   ☐ No _____

f. thyroid-stimulating hormone (TSH) assay: _____

_____

Spelled correctly?   ☐ Yes   ☐ No _____

g. hormone replacement therapy: _____

_____

Spelled correctly?   ☐ Yes   ☐ No _____

Listen to the section on your audiotape cassette that corresponds to this chapter and write the terms below. Be careful to spell each term correctly.

1. _____   10. _____

2. _____   11. _____

3. _____   12. _____

4. _____   13. _____

5. _____   14. _____

6. _____   15. _____

7. _____   16. _____

8. _____   17. _____

9. _____   18. _____

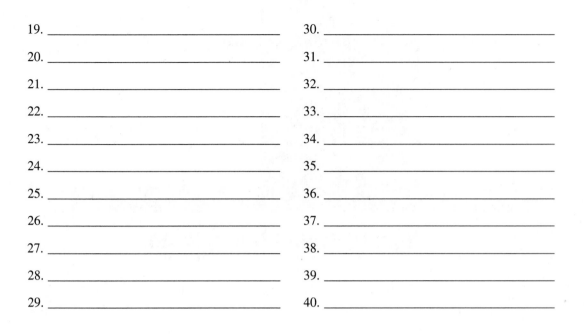

19. _____
20. _____
21. _____
22. _____
23. _____
24. _____
25. _____
26. _____
27. _____
28. _____
29. _____

30. _____
31. _____
32. _____
33. _____
34. _____
35. _____
36. _____
37. _____
38. _____
39. _____
40. _____

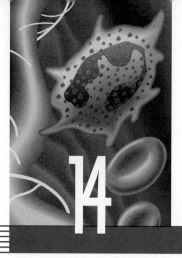

Male Reproductive System

Upon completing this chapter, you should be able to:

- Describe the male reproductive system and explain the primary functions of its organs
- Recognize, build, pronounce, and spell words that pertain to the male reproductive system
- Describe diseases, diagnostic tests, and surgical procedures that pertain to the male reproductive system

Overview   The male reproductive system, also called the male genital system, is responsible for producing, transporting, and maintaining viable sperm (the male sex cell). This system also produces the male sex hormone, testosterone, which regulates the development of a beard, pubic hair, a deep voice, and other bodily characteristics of the adult male. These functions, as well as male sexual activity, are the province of the male reproductive organs, which will be described in this chapter.

Word Elements

GENERAL TERMS – The following combining forms (CF) are used to construct general terms pertaining to masculine traits and reproduction.

CF	Meaning	Example
andr/o	male	*andro*genic = producing male traits
genit/o	reproductive	*genito*urinary = pertaining to the reproductive and urinary systems
gon/o	genitals	*gono*rrhea = type of genital infection

MALE REPRODUCTIVE ORGANS – These combining forms denote specific reproductive organs and the spermatozoa produced by these organs.

CF	Meaning	Example
balan/o	glans penis	*balano*plasty = plastic surgery of the penis
epididym/o	epididymis	*epididym*itis = inflammation of the epididymis
orch/o	testes	crypt*orch*ism = failure of a testis to descend
orchi/o	testes	*orchio*tomy = surgical incision into a testis
orchid/o	testes	*orchido*meter = instrument used to measure the testes
osche/o	scrotum	*osche*oma = tumor of the scrotum
prostat/o	prostate gland	*prostat*itis = inflammation of the prostate
semin/o	semen	*semin*uria = presence of semen in the urine
sperm/o	spermatozoa	azoo*sperm*ia = lack of spermatozoa in the semen
spermat/o	spermatozoa	*spermato*genesis = production of spermatozoa
test/o	testes	*test*algia = pain in the testes
testicul/o	testes	*testicul*ar = pertaining to a testis
vas/o	vas deferens	*vas*ectomy = surgical removal of the vas deferens
vesicul/o	seminal vesicles	*vesicul*itis = inflammation of a seminal vesicle

Anatomy and Physiology

The male reproductive system consists of the testes, the ducts that transport sperm, a number of accessory glands, and the external genitalia. These organs are illustrated in Figure 14-1 and described in the paragraphs below.

Testes

orch/o, orchi/o, orchid/o, test/o, and testicul/o = testes

The **testes** (TES-teez), also known as **testicles** (TES-tih-kulz), are a pair of egg-shaped glands suspended behind the penis in a sac called the **scrotum** (SKROE-tum). The main function of the testes is to produce **spermatozoa**

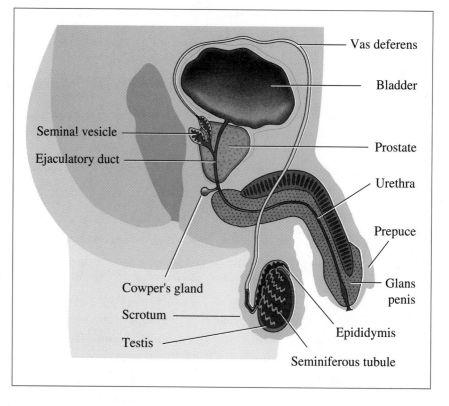

Figure 14-1:
The male reproductive system.

Vas deferens

Bladder

Seminal vesicle

Ejaculatory duct

Prostate

Urethra

Prepuce

Glans penis

Cowper's gland

Scrotum

Testis

Epididymis

Seminiferous tubule

osche/o = scrotum
sperm/o and spermat/o
= spermatozoa

(sper-MAT-uh-**ZOE**-uh), or sperm cells, which are transported to other parts of the male reproductive system via a series of ducts. A second important function of the testes is to secrete **testosterone** (tes-TOS-ter-ohn), a male sex hormone responsible for development of so-called secondary sex characteristics in men (e.g., beard, pubic hair, voice deepening, and maturation of the reproductive organs).

semin/o = semen
-iferous = producing

Each testis contains numerous tiny, winding tubes called **seminiferous tubules** (SEH-mih-**NIH**-fer-us TOO-byoolz). Spermatozoa are produced by cells lining the seminiferous tubules, while testosterone is secreted by interstitial cells in the surrounding connective tissue spaces.

Ducts

epididym/o =
epididymis

Once produced, spermatozoa pass from the seminiferous tubules in the testes through a network of ducts to the **epididymis** (EH-pih-**DIH**-dih-muss), a large tube located over the upper part of each testis. The epididymis serves as a temporary storage site for spermatozoa, and it is here that sperm cells mature and become motile.

vas/o = vas deferens

The epididymis leads to a narrow tube called the **vas deferens** (VASS DEH-fer-enz), also known as the **seminal** (SEH-mih-nul) **duct** or **ductus** (DUCK-tus) **deferens**. The vas deferens carries sperm into the pelvic region, where the seminal vesicles are located.

Associated Glands

vesicul/o = seminal vesicles

semin/o = semen

The **seminal vesicles** (VEH-sih-kulz) are a pair of glands located at the base of the bladder. They secrete a thick, sugary, yellowish fluid; when sperm from the vas deferens mix with the fluid produced by the seminal vesicles, the resulting fluid is called **semen** (SEE-men). Fluid from the seminal vesicles accounts for a large portion of the volume of semen, nourishing the highly active sperm cells. The vas deferens and the seminal vesicles join to form the **ejaculatory** (ih-**JACK**-kyoo-luh-TOR-ee) **duct**, which transports the newly formed semen to the urethra, the tube through which semen is expelled from the body during ejaculation. The urethra is also the tube through which urine leaves the body during urination.

prostat/o = prostate gland

The **prostate** (PROS-tate) **gland**, a muscular and glandular structure, is located beneath the urinary bladder and surrounds the urethra. This gland secretes an alkaline fluid that promotes sperm motility. In addition, the muscular tissue of the prostate gland aids in the expulsion of sperm during ejaculation.

Cowper's (KOW-perz) **glands**, also called the **bulbourethral** (BULL-boe-yer-**EE**-thrul) **glands**, are two pea-shaped glands located just below the prostate. They are connected by a small duct to the urethra. These glands secrete an alkaline fluid that enhances sperm viability.

Penis

balan/o = glans penis

The male external genital organ, the **penis**, is composed of erectile tissue that surrounds the urethra. The **glans** (GLANZ) **penis** is the enlarged tip of the penis where the urethral opening is located. At birth, it is covered by a flap of tissue called the **prepuce** (PREE-pyoos), or **foreskin**, which is removed if a male undergoes circumcision. During sexual activity, the penis becomes erect, and semen from the ejaculatory duct is expelled through the urethra during ejaculation.

Review Exercises

1. ***Match*** the following combining forms with their definitions.

_____	vas/o	a.	spermatozoa
_____	spermat/o	b.	glans penis
_____	orch/o	c.	seminal vesicles
_____	balan/o	d.	prostate gland
_____	prostat/o	e.	vas deferens
_____	vesicul/o	f.	testes

2. ***Define*** the following combining forms.

a. test/o _____

b. sperm/o _____

c. andr/o _____

d. orchid/o _____

e. epididym/o _____

f. osche/o _____

g. orchi/o _____

h. gon/o _____

i. testicul/o _____

j. semin/o _____

3. ***Match*** the following structures with their descriptions.

_____	prostate	a.	produce spermatozoa
_____	epididymis	b.	site of sperm storage and maturation
_____	testes	c.	secretes fluid that enhances sperm motility
_____	prepuce	d.	secrete sugary fluid that mixes with sperm, forming semen
_____	seminal vesicles	e.	covers glans penis in non-circumcised males

Terminology

The following are selected terms that pertain to pathology of the male reproductive system and to related diagnostic and therapeutic procedures. As you will see, most of the disorders listed are associated with inflammatory conditions, abnormal sperm counts, or structural abnormalities. Keeping this in mind will help you to understand other terms you may hear as well as the rationale behind treatment of male reproductive disorders.

Pathologic Conditions	Word Elements	Definition
anorchism (an-OR-kih-zum)	an = not; without orch = testes ism = condition	congenital absence of one or both testes
azoospermia (ay-ZOE-oh-**SPER**-me-uh)	a = not; without zoo = animal life sperm = spermatozoa ia = condition	condition characterized by lack of spermatozoa in the semen
balanitis (BAL-luh-**NIE**-tis)	balan = glans penis itis = inflammation	inflammation of the glans penis, usually due to infection or irritation
benign prostatic hypertrophy (pros-TAT-ick hi-PER-truh-fee)	prostat = prostate ic = pertaining to hyper = excessive trophy = growth	benign enlargement of the prostate gland, usually in men over the age of 50; also called BPH
chlamydia (kluh-MIH-dee-uh)	chlamydia = a type of bacteria	infection, usually of the urethra, by *Chlamydia trachomatis*; one of several common sexually transmitted diseases
cryptorchism (krip-TOR-kih-zum)	crypt = hidden orch = testes ism = condition	failure of one or both of the testicles to descend into the scrotum at birth
epididymitis (EH-pih-DIH-dih-**MY**-tis)	epididym = epididymis itis = inflammation	inflammation of the epididymis due to infection
gonorrhea (GON-er-**REE**-uh)	gono = genitals rrhea = discharge	infection, usually of the urethra, by *Neisseria gonorrhoeae* resulting in urethral inflammation and penile discharge; one of several common sexually transmitted diseases
gynecomastia (GIE-nuh-koe-**MASS**-stee-uh)	gyneco = female mast = breast ia = condition	abnormal enlargement of one or both of the male mammary glands (breasts)

Pathologic Conditions	Word Elements	Definition
herpes genitalis (HER-peez JEH-nih-**TAL**-lis)	herpes = a type of virus genitalis = genitals	infection of the skin and mucous membranes of the genitals by herpes simplex virus; usually transmitted by sexual contact
hydrocele (HI-droe-seel)	hydro = water cele = hernia; swelling	accumulation of fluid in a sac-like cavity, especially within the scrotum
impotence (IM-puh-tense)	im = not potence = "power"	inability to achieve or maintain a penile erection
oligospermia (OL-ih-go-**SPER**-me-uh)	oligo = scanty; few sperm = spermatozoa ia = condition	reduced number of spermatozoa in the semen; also referred to as a low sperm count
orchitis (or-KIE-tis)	orch = testes itis = inflammation	inflammation of the testes, usually due to infection
phimosis (fie-MOE-sis)	phim = "muzzle" osis = condition	narrowing of the prepuce, leading to inability of the foreskin to be retracted over the glans penis
prostatitis (PROS-tuh-**TIE**-tis)	prostat = prostate gland itis = inflammation	inflammation of the prostate gland, usually due to infection
seminoma (SEH-mih-**NO**-muh)	semin = semen oma = tumor; growth	a malignant tumor of the testes
sterility (ster-RILL-lih-tee)	sterility = "barrenness"	in males, the inability to impregnate a female
syphilis (SIH-full-lus)	no word elements	an infectious, chronic, sexually transmitted disease characterized initially by skin lesions, followed by mild flu-like symptoms and eventually serious organ damage
urethritis (YER-ree-**THRIE**-tis)	urethr = urethra itis = inflammation	inflammation of the urethra, usually due to a sexually transmitted infection such as chlamydia or gonorrhea

Diagnostic Procedures	Word Elements	Definition
FTA-ABS test	no word elements	microscopic examination of a blood or spinal fluid sample to confirm the presence of the syphilis bacterium if the RPR or VDRL test is positive
RPR test	no word elements	blood test used to determine if an individual is or has been infected with the syphilis bacterium

Diagnostic Procedures	Word Elements	Definition
semen analysis	no word elements	microscopic examination of a semen sample to count sperm cells and to evaluate their shape and motility
VDRL test	no word elements	blood test used to determine if an individual is or has been infected with the syphilis bacterium

Surgical Procedures	Word Elements	Definition
circumcision (SER-kum-**SIH**-zhun)	circum = around cision = incision	surgical removal of all or part of the prepuce (foreskin)
orchiectomy (OR-kee-**ECK**-tuh-me)	orchi = testes ectomy = surgical removal	surgical removal of one or both testes; also called orchectomy or orchidectomy
penile prosthesis (PEE-nile pros-**THEE**-sis)	pen = penis ile = pertaining to prosthesis = "an addition"	device implanted in the penis to assist in achieving penile erection
prostatectomy (PROS-tuh-**TECK**-tuh-me)	prostat = prostate gland ectomy = surgical removal	surgical removal of all or part of the prostate gland
transurethral prostatectomy (TRANZ-yer-**REE**-thrul PROS-tuh-**TECK**-tuh-me)	trans = through urethr = urethra al = pertaining to prostat = prostate gland ectomy = surgical removal	surgical removal of all or part of the prostate gland by placing a special endoscope through the urethra and removing pieces of the prostate gland through this tube; also called transurethral resection of the prostate, or TURP
vasectomy (vas-**SECK**-tuh-me)	vas = vas deferens ectomy = surgical removal	removal of all or a segment of the vas deferens

Review Exercises

4. **Match** the following terms with their definitions.

_____ sterility   a. narrowing of the prepuce

_____ chlamydia   b. inability to impregnate a female

_____ phimosis   c. malignant tumor of the testes

_____ herpes genitalis   d. accumulation of fluid in the scrotum

_____ seminoma   e. a sexually transmitted bacterial infection, usually of the urethra

_____ hydrocele   f. a viral infection of the genitals

5. **Break Down and Define** the word elements within each of the following terms, and then define the term itself.

> **Example:** prostat / itis *prostate gland / inflammation* *inflammation of the prostate gland*

a. orchidectomy

_____

b. cryptorchism

_____

c. orchiectomy

_____

d. anorchism

_____

e. orchitis

_____

f. epididymitis

_____

g. transurethral prostatectomy

_____

h. azoospermia

_____

i. prostatic hypertrophy

_____

j. gynecomastia

_____

k. testicular

_____

l. orchidoplasty

_____

m. spermotoxic

_____

n. testopathy

_____

6. ***Word Building and Spelling***. Spell out the medical term for each of the following definitions using the slashes provided to separate the word elements.

condition characterized by lack of spermatozoa   *a / sperm / ia*

a. surgical removal of the vas deferens   _____ / _____

b. inflammation of the glans penis   _____ / _____

c. scanty spermatozoa condition   _____ / _____ / _____

d. inflammation of the urethra   _____ / _____

e. surgical removal of the prostate gland   _____ / _____

f. inflammation of the seminal vesicles   _____ / _____

g. surgical repair of the scrotum   _____ / _____

Case Study. Read the case notes below. For each boldfaced term, provide a brief definition and indicate whether the term is spelled correctly; if it is misspelled, provide the correct spelling.

Example:
urithritis: *inflammation of the urethra*

Spelled correctly? ☐ Yes ✔ No *urethritis*

Patient presented as a 23-year-old male with symptoms of **urithritis**: urethral discharge and pain on urination. On questioning, patient indicated that he was sexually active, with multiple sex partners. On physical examination, patient appeared to be an otherwise healthy **circumsized** male with no genital blisters, skin rash, or other evidence of **herpes genitallis** or **syphillis**. Swabbed patient's urethra to obtain sample of discharge for analysis. Preliminary diagnosis: **gonnorhea**, possibly with concomitant **chlamidea**. Treatment plan: antibiotics to begin immediately (without waiting for test results); if test positive for gonorrhea, report case and have sexual partners come in for testing; **RPR test** or **VDRL test** to screen for syphilis.

a. circumsized: _____

    Spelled correctly? ☐ Yes ☐ No _____

b. herpes genitallis: _____

_____

    Spelled correctly? ☐ Yes ☐ No _____

c. syphillis: _____

_____

    Spelled correctly? ☐ Yes ☐ No _____

d. gonnorhea: _____

_____

Spelled correctly? ☐ Yes ☐ No _____

e. chlamidea: _____

_____

Spelled correctly? ☐ Yes ☐ No _____

f. RPR test: _____

Spelled correctly? ☐ Yes ☐ No _____

g. VDRL test: _____

Spelled correctly? ☐ Yes ☐ No _____

Listen to the section on your audiotape cassette that corresponds to this chapter and write the terms below. Be careful to spell each term correctly.

1. _____ 13. _____

2. _____ 14. _____

3. _____ 15. _____

4. _____ 16. _____

5. _____ 17. _____

6. _____ 18. _____

7. _____ 19. _____

8. _____ 20. _____

9. _____ 21. _____

10. _____ 22. _____

11. _____ 23. _____

12. _____ 24. _____

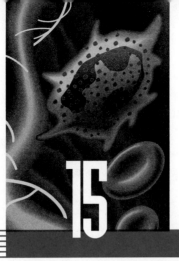

15

Female Reproductive System

Upon completing this chapter, you should be able to:

- Describe the female reproductive system and explain the primary functions of its organs
- Recognize, build, pronounce, and spell words that pertain to the female reproductive system
- Describe diseases, diagnostic tests, and surgical procedures that pertain to the female reproductive system

Overview   The female reproductive system, also known as the female genital system, is responsible for producing and transporting ova (the female sex cells), eliminating ova from the body (if they are not fertilized by sperm), nourishing and providing a place for growth of an embryo (if an ovum is fertilized by sperm), and nourishing a newborn child. The female reproductive system also produces the female sex hormones, estrogen and progesterone, which regulate the development of breasts and other bodily characteristics of the mature female. These functions, as well as female sexual activity, are the province of the female reproductive organs, which will be described in this chapter.

Word Elements

GENERAL TERMS – The following combining forms (CF) are used to construct general terms pertaining to female traits and reproductive processes.

CF	Meaning	Example
genit/o	reproductive	*genito*plasty = surgical repair of the reproductive organs
gon/o	genitals	*gono*rrhea = type of genital infection
gyn/o	woman; female	*gyno*plasty = surgical repair of the female reproductive organs
gynec/o	woman; female	*gyneco*logy = study of the female reproductive system
men/o	menstruation	*meno*pause = cessation of menstruation
menstru/o	menstruation	*menstru*al = pertaining to menstruation

PRIMARY FEMALE REPRODUCTIVE ORGANS – These combining forms are used to denote the primary organs of the female reproductive system, including the ova or eggs produced by these organs.

CF	Meaning	Example
cervic/o	cervix	*cervic*al = pertaining to the cervix
colp/o	vagina	*colpo*scopy = visual examination of the vagina
endometri/o	endometrium	*endometri*osis = growth of endometrial tissue outside of the uterus
episi/o	vulva	*episio*tomy = surgical incision in the vulva
hyster/o	uterus	*hyster*ectomy = surgical removal of the uterus
metr/o	uterus	*metro*pathy = any disease of the uterus
o/o	ovum; egg	*oo*cyte = a developing ovum
oophor/o	ovaries	*oophor*itis = inflammation of an ovary
ov/o	ovum; egg	*ov*oid = resembling an egg
ovari/o	ovaries	*ovari*an = pertaining to an ovary
ovul/o	ovum; egg	*ovul*ation = process of discharging an ovum
perine/o	perineum	*perine*al = pertaining to the perineum
salping/o	fallopian tube	*salping*ectomy = surgical removal of a fallopian tube
uter/o	uterus	*uter*ine = pertaining to the uterus
vagin/o	vagina	*vagin*itis = inflammation of the vagina
vulv/o	vulva	*vulvo*pathy = any disease of the vulva

ACCESSORY FEMALE ORGANS — These combining forms pertain to the accessory organs of the female reproductive system, the breasts.

CF	Meaning	Example
galact/o	milk	*galacto*cele = cyst formed in a milk duct
mamm/o	breast	*mammo*graphy = x-ray recording of the breasts
mast/o	breast	*mast*itis = inflammation of the breast

SUFFIXES — The following suffixes pertain to the female reproductive system.

Suffix	Meaning	Example
-arche	beginning	men*arche* = first menstrual period
-version	turning	retro*version* = tipping back of an organ

Anatomy and Physiology

The primary organs of the female reproductive system are the ovaries, fallopian tubes, uterus, vagina, and external genitalia; in addition, the mammary glands (breasts) serve as accessory organs. These structures are described in the paragraphs below.

The Ovaries

oophor/o and ovari/o = ovaries
o/o, ov/o, and ovul/o = ovum; egg

ovulation = "egg process"
corpus luteum = "yellow body"

The **ovaries** (OH-ver-reez) are a pair of almond-shaped glands located in the pelvic cavity, one on each side of the uterus. Within each ovary are thousands of vesicles, or follicles, each of which contains an immature ovum (egg). During each menstrual cycle, one follicle matures into a **graafian follicle** (GRAF-ee-en FOL-lih-kul) and ruptures to release a mature ovum in a process called **ovulation** (OV-yoo-**LAY**-shun). The ruptured follicle becomes filled with a yellow, fat-like material and is then called the **corpus luteum** (KOR-pus LOO-tee-um).

In addition to producing ova, the ovaries secrete the female sex hormones **estrogen** (ESS-troe-jen) and **progesterone** (pro-JESS-ter-ohn). During puberty, estrogen stimulates development of secondary sex characteristics, such as increased deposition of fat in the breasts, thighs, and buttocks and the growth of pubic and axillary (armpit) hair; estrogen also regulates maturation of the uterus, uterine tubes, vagina, ovaries, and breasts. In the sexually mature female, estrogen induces the process of ovulation. Progesterone is secreted by the corpus luteum. It regulates preparation of the uterus for implantation of a fertilized ovum (see discussion below). During pregnancy, progesterone inhibits ovulation and causes the breasts to enlarge and secrete milk.

Figure 15-1:
The female reproductive system (breasts not shown).

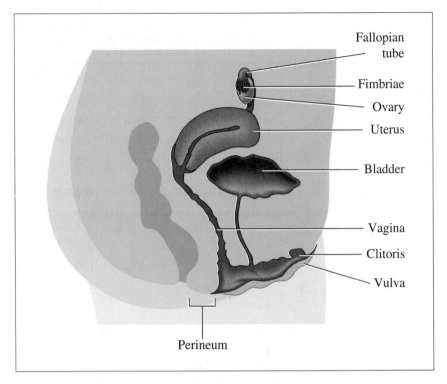

Fallopian tube

Fimbriae

Ovary

Uterus

Bladder

Vagina

Clitoris

Vulva

Perineum

Fallopian Tubes

salping/o = fallopian tube

Ova produced in the ovaries during ovulation are transported to the uterus by means of ducts called the **fallopian** (fuh-LOE-pee-en) **tubes,** also known as **uterine** (YOO-ter-in) **tubes** or **oviducts** (OH-vih-ducts). At the end closest to each ovary, the opening of each fallopian tube consists of a trumpet-shaped expansion with finger-like projections called **fimbriae** (FIM-bree-ay). When an ovum is released from an ovary, it enters the fimbriae and passes through the fallopian tube to the uterus. The fallopian tubes also provide a passageway for sperm to travel from the uterus toward the ovaries. If sperm cells are present, fertilization of an ovum generally takes place in the fallopian tube.

Uterus

hyster/o, metr/o, and uter/o = uterus

The **uterus** (YOO-ter-us) is a muscular, hollow, pear-shaped structure suspended in the pelvic cavity by bands of connective tissue called ligaments. If an ovum has been fertilized by sperm in the fallopian tubes, it becomes implanted in the uterus, which nourishes the fertilized egg as it grows into an embryo and fetus. If an ovum is not fertilized, it is not implanted in the uterus; rather, it passes through the uterus and lower reproductive organs and is eliminated from the body.

Figure 15-2: *The uterus.*

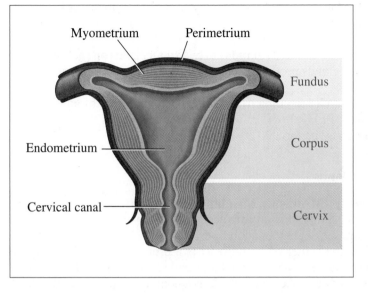

Myometrium Perimetrium

Fundus

Endometrium

Corpus

Cervical canal

Cervix

corpus = body
cervic/o = cervix

The walls of the uterus are comprised of three layers of tissue: an outer membranous layer called the **perimetrium** (PEHR-ih-**ME**-tree-um), a muscular middle layer called the **myometrium** (MY-oh-**ME**-tree-um), and a membranous inner layer called the **endometrium** (EN-doe-**ME**-tree-um). During pregnancy, it is the endometrium that provides nourishment to the growing fetus; otherwise, this lining is sloughed off and eliminated from the body during menstruation.

By convention, the upper, rounded portion of the uterus is called the **fundus** (FUN-dus), the central portion is called the **corpus** (KOR-pus), and the neck is called the **cervix** (SER-vicks). The cervix leads to the top portion of the vagina.

Vagina

colp/o and vagin/o =
vagina

The **vagina** (vuh-JIE-nuh) is a muscular tube extending from the cervix to the exterior of the body. It serves as a passageway for elimination of endometrial tissue during menstruation and for delivery of the fetus during birth.

External Genitalia

episi/o and vulv/o =
vulva

The external genital structures of the female are collectively referred to as the **vulva** (VUL-vuh). These structures include the labia majora, labia minora, and clitoris.

The **labia majora** (LAY-be-uh muh-JOR-uh) are two "large lips" of fatty tissue lying on either side of the vaginal opening. They enclose and protect the labia minora and the clitoris.

The **labia minora** (LAY-be-uh mih-NOR-uh) are "small lips" that lie underneath the labia majora. They surround and cover the openings of the urethra and vagina.

The **clitoris** (KLIH-ter-iss) is an erectile structure located just behind the juncture of the labia majora. It is a highly sensitive organ that is stimulated during sexual intercourse.

Bartholin's (BAR-toe-linz) **glands** are two small glands on each side of the vagina. These glands produce mucus, which lubricates the vagina.

perine/o = perineum

Externally, the area extending from the vaginal opening to the anus is called the **perineum** (PEHR-ih-**NEE**-um). During childbirth, the perineum is stretched and may be torn.

Mammary Glands

mamm/o and mast/o = breast

galact/o = milk

The **mammary** (MAM-mer-ee) **glands**, commonly called **breasts**, are milk-producing glands that serve as accessory organs of reproduction. Each breast is composed of glandular lobes surrounded by fibrous and fatty tissue. Externally, at the center of each breast is a protrusion called the **nipple**, which is surrounded by a pigmented area called the **areola** (EHR-ree-**OH**-luh). Each glandular lobe inside the breast contains a **milk duct** that leads to the opening in the nipple; after childbirth, the glandular activity of the breasts increases, causing the breasts to swell with milk and enabling the newborn child to receive milk through the nipples.

Menstrual Cycle

The **menstrual** (MEN-strul) **cycle** refers to the secretion of hormones and other physiologic changes that occur cyclically in women, usually every 28 days or so. After ovulation, progesterone secreted by the corpus luteum stimulates growth of the endometrium in preparation for implantation of a fertilized ovum. If fertilization and implantation do not occur, hormone levels drop and the endometrial tissue that has built up during the menstrual cycle is sloughed off in a process called **menses** (MEN-sez), or **menstruation** (MEN-stroo-**AY**-shun).

men/o and menstru/o = menstruation

-arche = beginning

In most women, the first menstrual period, called **menarche** (muh-NAR-kee), occurs at age 12 or 13. After about 35 years of menstrual cycles, estrogen secretion decreases and fewer eggs are produced by the ovaries; menses become irregular and eventually cease. The cessation of menses for the remainder of a woman's lifetime is called **menopause** (**MEH**-no-PAWZ). The term **climacteric** (klih-MACK-ter-ick) refers to the period of time in which symptoms of approaching menopause (e.g., hot flashes and irregular menses) appear.

climacteric = "a critical point in an individual's lifetime"

Review Exercises

1. **Match** the following combining forms with their definitions.

_____ mamm/o   a. vulva

_____ metr/o   b. breast

_____ episi/o   c. vagina

_____ vagin/o   d. uterus

_____ ovari/o   e. ovaries

_____ gyn/o   f. reproductive

_____ genit/o   g. menstruation

_____ men/o   h. woman; female

2. **Define** the following suffixes and combining forms.

a. mast/o _____

b. colp/o _____

c. hyster/o _____

d. gynec/o _____

e. menstru/o _____

f. ov/o _____

g. vulv/o _____

h. oophor/o _____

i. uter/o _____

j. o/o _____

k. -arche _____

l. -version _____

m. ovul/o _____

3. **Spell** the combining forms that have the following meanings.

a. cervix _____

b. endometrium _____

c. perineum _____

d. fallopian tube   _____

e. milk   _____

f. genitals   _____

4. **Match** the following terms with their definitions.

_____ vagina

_____ mammary glands

_____ ovaries

_____ endometrium

_____ progesterone

_____ cervix

_____ fallopian tubes

a. almond-shaped glands that produce ova

b. hormone that regulates preparation of the uterus for implantation of a fertilized ovum

c. ducts that transport ova to the uterus

d. portion of uterus that nourishes a fertilized egg or sloughs off during menstruation

e. portion of uterus that leads to the vagina

f. muscular passageway for the menses and for the fetus during childbirth

g. breasts

Terminology

The following are selected terms that pertain to pathology of the female reproductive system and to related diagnostic and therapeutic procedures. As you will see, most of the disorders listed are associated with inflammation or infection of the reproductive organs or with abnormal menses. Keeping this in mind will help you to understand other terms you may hear as well as the rationale behind treatment of female reproductive disorders.

Pathologic Conditions	Word Elements	Definition
amenorrhea (ay-MEN-ner-**REE**-uh)	a = without; not meno = menstruation rrhea = discharge	absence of menstruation
anteversion (AN-tee-**VER**-zhun)	ante = before; forward version = turning	tilting forward of an organ (e.g., the uterus) from its usual position
candidiasis (KAN-dih-**DIE**-uh-sis)	candid = *Candida* iasis = condition	infection, usually of the vagina, by a species of *Candida* (a fungus), resulting in itching and a white discharge; also called moniliasis (MON-nul-**LIE**-uh-sis) or yeast infection
cervicitis (SER-vih-**SIE**-tis)	cervic = cervix itis = inflammation	inflammation of the cervix, usually due to infection

Pathologic Conditions	Word Elements	Definition
chlamydia (kluh-MIH-dee-uh)	chlamydia = a type of bacteria	infection, usually of the vagina and cervix, by *Chlamydia trachomatis*; one of several common sexually transmitted diseases
dysmenorrhea (dis-MEN-ner-**REE**-uh)	dys = difficult; painful meno = menstruation rrhea = discharge	pain associated with menstruation
endometriosis (EN-doe-ME-tree-**OH**-sis)	endometri = endometrium osis = condition	growth of endometrial tissue outside the uterus
fibrocystic breast disease (FIE-broe-**SIS**-tick)	fibro = fiber; fibrous cyst = cyst ic = pertaining to	the presence of one or more fibrous cysts in the breast
galactocele (guh-LACK-toe-seel)	galacto = milk cele = hernia; swelling	cyst caused by blockage of a milk duct in the breast
genital wart	genit = reproductive al = pertaining to	soft growth (wart) occurring in the areas of the vagina and anus; caused by a sexually transmitted virus; also called condyloma acuminatum
gonorrhea (GON-er-**REE**-uh)	gono = genitals rrhea = discharge	infection, usually of the cervix, by *Neisseria gonorrhoeae* resulting in pain and a vaginal or cervical discharge; one of several common sexually transmitted diseases
herpes genitalis (HER-peez JEH-nih-**TAL**-lis)	herpes = a type of virus genitalis = genitals	infection of the skin and mucous membranes of the genitals by herpes simplex virus; usually transmitted by sexual contact
leiomyoma uteri (LIE-oh-my-**OH**-muh YOO-ter-eye)	leio = smooth my = muscle oma = tumor; growth uteri = uterus	benign tumor of the smooth muscle of the uterus; also called fibroids
leukorrhea (LOO-ker-**REE**-uh)	leuko = white rrhea = discharge	discharge of white fluid containing mucus and pus from the vagina
mastitis (mass-STIE-tis)	mast = breast itis = inflammation	inflammation of the breast, often due to infection
menorrhagia (MEH-ner-**RAY**-jee-uh)	meno = menstruation rrhagia = excessive flow	excessive uterine bleeding during menstruation

Pathologic Conditions	Word Elements	Definition
oligomenorrhea (OL-ih-go-MEH-ner-**REE**-uh)	oligo = scanty; few meno = menstruation rrhea = discharge	unusually light or infrequent menstrual flow
oophoritis (OH-uh-fer-**RIE**-tis)	oophor = ovaries itis = inflammation	inflammation of one or both ovaries, usually due to infection
ovarian cyst (oh-VEHR-ee-en SIST)	ovari = ovaries an = pertaining to	a fluid-filled sac in an ovary; may be either benign or malignant
pelvic inflammatory disease	no word elements	any inflammation and infection of the female upper reproductive organs (ovaries, fallopian tubes, or uterus); also called PID
pyosalpinx (PIE-oh-**SAL**-pinks)	pyo = pus salpinx = fallopian tube	accumulation of pus in one or both fallopian tubes
retroversion (REH-troe-**VER**-zhun)	retro = backward version = turning	tipping backward of an organ (e.g., the uterus) from its usual position
salpingitis (SAL-pin-**JIE**-tis)	salping = fallopian tube itis = inflammation	inflammation of one or both fallopian tubes, usually due to infection
sterility (ster-RILL-lih-tee)	sterility = "barrenness"	in females, the inability to become pregnant
syphilis (SIH-full-lus)	no word elements	an infectious, chronic, sexually transmitted disease characterized initially by skin lesions, followed by mild flu-like symptoms and eventually serious organ damage
toxic shock syndrome	no word elements	serious disease caused by infection by a toxin-producing strain of the bacterium *Staphylococcus aureus*; most commonly seen in young women using highly absorbent tampons during menstruation
trichomoniasis (TRIH-koe-moe-**NIE**-uh-sis)	trichomon = *Trichomonas* iasis = condition	infection, usually of the vagina, by *Trichomonas* (a protozoa); often causes vaginitis, urethritis, and cystitis
uterine prolapse (YOO-ter-in PRO-laps)	uter = uterus ine = pertaining to pro = in front of lapse = "falling; sinking"	falling or slipping of the uterus from its usual position, as when the uterine ligaments are stretched; most commonly seen in women who have given birth to several children
vaginitis (VAJ-ih-**NIE**-tis)	vagin = vagina itis = inflammation	inflammation of the vagina, usually due to infection

Diagnostic Procedures	Word Elements	Definition
colposcopy (kole-POS-kuh-pee)	colpo = vagina scopy = visual examination	examination of the vagina with a colposcope
conization (KON-ih-**ZAY**-shun)	con = "cone" ization = process	removal of a cone-shaped tissue sample from the cervix for examination and analysis
FTA-ABS test	no word elements	microscopic examination of a blood or spinal fluid sample to confirm the presence of the syphilis bacterium if the RPR or VDRL test is positive
laparoscopy (LAP-per-**OS**-kuh-pee)	laparo = abdomen scopy = visual examination	examination of the ovaries, fallopian tubes, uterus, and other organs in the abdomen using a laparoscope
mammography (muh-MOG-ruh-fee)	mammo = breast graphy = recording	x-ray recording of the breast, usually to detect tumors or other abnormal growths
Papanicolaou test (PAP-puh-NIH-koe-**LAY**-oo)	no word elements	examination of cervical cells and mucus for early detection of cervical cancer; commonly called a Pap smear
RPR test	no word elements	blood test used to determine if an individual is or has been infected with the syphilis bacterium
VDRL test	no word elements	blood test used to determine if an individual is or has been infected with the syphilis bacterium

Therapeutic Procedures	Word Elements	Definition
dilation and curettage (die-LAY-shun KYER-reh-TOZH)	dilation = "expansion" curettage = "scraping"	surgical procedure in which the cervical canal of the uterus is physically expanded to allow access to the endometrial lining, which is then scraped away for diagnostic or therapeutic purposes (e.g., to correct heavy or prolonged bleeding or to remove an embryo); commonly called a D&C
episiotomy (eh-PIZ-ee-**OT**-uh-me)	episio = vulva tomy = surgical incision	surgical incision in the vulva, usually to prevent tearing of the perineum and facilitate delivery during childbirth
hysterectomy (HISS-ter-**RECK**-tuh-me)	hyster = uterus ectomy = surgical removal	surgical removal of the uterus; surgery may be transabdominal (TAH) or vaginal
lumpectomy (lum-PECK-tuh-me)	lump = mass ectomy = surgical removal	surgical removal of a tumor from a breast without removing surrounding tissue or lymph nodes

Therapeutic Procedures	Word Elements	Definition
mammoplasty (**MAM**-moe-PLASS-tee)	mammo = breast plasty = surgical repair	surgical reconstruction of one or both breasts
mastectomy (mass-STECK-tuh-me)	mast = breast ectomy = surgical removal	surgical removal of part (simple mastectomy) or all (radical mastectomy) of the breast and surrounding tissue
oophorectomy (OH-uh-fer-**RECK**-tuh-me)	oophor = ovaries ectomy = surgical removal	surgical removal of one or both ovaries; if both ovaries and both fallopian tubes are removed, the procedure is called a bilateral salpingo-oophorectomy, or BSO
salpingectomy (SAL-pin-**JECK**-tuh-me)	salping = fallopian tube ectomy = surgical removal	surgical removal of one or both fallopian tubes
tubal ligation (TOO-bul lie-GAY-shun)	tub = tube al = pertaining to ligat = "binding" ion = process	surgical procedure in which the fallopian tubes are ligated (tied closed) in order to prevent pregnancy; a form of sterilization

Review Exercises

5. ***Break Down and Define*** the word elements within each of the following terms, and then define the term itself.

     Example: vagin / itis   *vagina / inflammation*   *inflammation of the vagina*

    a. mastitis

    _____

    b. oligomenorrhea

    _____

    c. pyosalpinx

    _____

    d. colposcopy

    _____

    e. oophorectomy

    _____

    f. anteversion

    _____

g. dysmenorrhea

_____

h. leukorrhea

_____

i. mastectomy

_____

j. menorrhagia

_____

k. oophoritis

_____

l. hysterectomy

_____

m. retroversion

_____

n. galactocele

_____

o. lumpectomy

_____

p. vaginitis

_____

6. **Match** the following terms with their definitions.

_____ toxic shock syndrome

_____ gonorrhea

_____ prolapse

_____ Pap smear

_____ trichomoniasis

_____ genital wart

_____ pelvic inflammatory disease

_____ candidiasis

_____ tubal ligation

a. sexually transmitted bacterial infection of the genitals (usually the cervix) associated with development of a vaginal discharge

b. protozoal infection, usually of the vagina

c. inflammation and infection of the ovaries, fallopian tubes, and/or uterus

d. disease associated with tampon use; caused by a bacterial toxin

e. tying of the fallopian tubes (a method of sterilization)

f. examination of cervical cells to detect cervical cancer

g. soft growth in the area of the vagina or anus, usually caused by a sexually transmitted disease

h. fungal infection of the vagina characterized by itching and a white vaginal discharge

i. slipping of the uterus from its usual position

7. ***Word Building and Spelling.*** Spell out the medical term for each of the following definitions using the slashes provided to separate the word elements.

discharge of milk (from the breast)   *galacto / rrhea*

a. surgical removal of a fallopian tube   _____ / _____

b. surgical incision in the vulva   _____ / _____

c. inflammation of the cervix   _____ / _____

d. inflammation of a fallopian tube   _____ / _____

e. without menstrual discharge   _____ / _____ / _____

f. x-ray (recording) of the breasts   _____ / _____

g. surgical repair of a breast   _____ / _____

Case Study. Read the case notes below. For each boldfaced term, provide a brief definition and indicate whether the term is spelled correctly; if it is misspelled, provide the correct spelling.

Example:

menorhagia: *excessive uterine bleeding during menstruation*

Spelled correctly?   ☐ Yes   ☑ No   *menorrhagia*

Patient presented as a 37-year-old female complaining of low back and abdominal pain which was severe during her menstrual periods. She also complained of heavy bleeding during her periods. Six months ago, the **menorhagia** was severe enough to warrant a **dilation and curretage**. Patient has no personal or family history of cervical, ovarian, or breast cancer, although she has a family history of **fibrosystic breast disease**. Pelvic examination suggestive of **lyomyoma uteri**, symptoms suggestive of **endometreosis**. Ordered an ultrasound, which confirmed presence of lyomyoma uteri, but also showed evidence of a mass around the right ovary. Appearance consistent with an **ovarian cyst**, but inconclusive. Performed a **laparoscopy**: found endometrial tissue near the right ovary, removed an endometrial cyst through the laparoscope. Diagnosis: lyomyoma uteri and endometreosis. Treatment plan: referral to fertility specialist for consult on options, since patient wishes to conceive.

a. dilation and curretage: _____

_____

Spelled correctly?   ☐ Yes   ☐ No _____

b. fibrosystic breast disease: _____

Spelled correctly?   ☐ Yes   ☐ No _____

c. lyomyoma uteri: _____

_____

Spelled correctly? ☐ Yes ☐ No _____

d. endometreosis: _____

Spelled correctly? ☐ Yes ☐ No _____

e. ovarian cyst: _____

_____

Spelled correctly? ☐ Yes ☐ No _____

f. laparoscopy: _____

_____

Spelled correctly? ☐ Yes ☐ No _____

Listen to the section on your audiotape cassette that corresponds to this chapter and write the terms below. Be careful to spell each term correctly.

1. _____   13. _____

2. _____   14. _____

3. _____   15. _____

4. _____   16. _____

5. _____   17. _____

6. _____   18. _____

7. _____   19. _____

8. _____   20. _____

9. _____   21. _____

10. _____ 22. _____

11. _____ 23. _____

12. _____ 24. _____

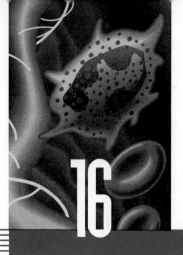

Skeletal System

Upon completing this chapter, you should be able to:

- Describe the skeletal system and explain its primary functions
- Recognize, build, pronounce, and spell words that pertain to the skeletal system
- Describe diseases, diagnostic tests, and therapeutic procedures that pertain to the skeletal system

Overview   The skeletal system consists of all of the bones of the body and the joints formed by these bones. Bones support the body, giving it shape; by surrounding many of the body's internal organs, bones also serve a protective function, helping to prevent trauma to delicate internal organs such as the brain. In addition, bones serve as storage sites for certain minerals (calcium and phosphorus) and as production sites for blood cells. Joints, the places at which two or more bones meet, provide flexibility to the skeletal system, permitting the skeleton and thus the body to move.

Word Elements

BONE AND CARTILAGE – The following combining forms (CF) refer to bone and cartilage. Some are general, while others denote specific bones.

CF	Meaning	Example
chondr/o	cartilage	*chondro*malacia = softening of the cartilage
crani/o	skull	*cranio*tomy = surgical incision in the skull
lumb/o	loin; waist	*lumb*ar = pertaining to the waist
myel/o	bone marrow*	*myel*oid = resembling bone marrow
oste/o	bone	*osteo*tomy = surgical incision in a bone
spondyl/o	vertebrae	*spondyl*itis = inflammation of the vertebrae
vertebr/o	vertebrae	*vertebr*al = pertaining to a vertebra

JOINTS – These combining forms refer to joints and related structures, such as those that support or protect joints.

CF	Meaning	Example
arthr/o	joint	*arthr*itis = inflammation of a joint
articul/o	joint	*articul*ar = pertaining to a joint
burs/o	bursa	*burs*itis = inflammation of a bursa
ligament/o	ligament	*ligament*ous = pertaining to a ligament
synov/o	synovial fluid; synovial membrane	*synov*ectomy = surgical removal of a synovial membrane
ten/o	tendon	*teno*desis = surgical binding or fixation of a tendon
tend/o	tendon	*tendo*plasty = surgical repair of a tendon
tendin/o	tendon	*tendin*itis = inflammation of a tendon

PATHOLOGIC CONDITIONS – These combining forms describe pathologic conditions resulting from abnormal fusion, sliding, or curvature of bones.

CF	Meaning	Example
ankyl/o	crooked; stiff	*ankyl*osis = fusion and stiffening of a joint
kyph/o	humpback	*kyph*osis = humpback posture
lord/o	curve; swayback	*lord*osis = swayback posture
lux/o	to slide	sub*lux*ation = partial dislocation of a bone from the joint
scoli/o	crooked; bent	*scoli*osis = abnormal curvature of the spine

*NOTE: Depending on the context, myel/o can also refer to the spinal cord (see Chapter 12).

SUFFIXES – The following suffixes pertain to the skeletal system. They describe processes that occur naturally or via therapeutic intervention.

Suffix	Meaning	Example
-clasia	to break	arthro*clasia* = breaking of a joint
-desis	to bind together	arthro*desis* = binding together of a joint
-physis	to grow	epi*physis* = upper, growing part of a bone
-porosis	becoming porous or less dense	osteo*porosis* = disease in which the bones become porous and brittle

Anatomy and Physiology

The adult skeleton consists of 206 bones and numerous joints. Because many bone disorders involve breaks in bones or abnormal bone formation, it is important not only to know the names of the major bones, but also to understand how they develop. Thus, this section describes the formation and structure of bones as well as the anatomy of the skeletal system.

Bone Formation

chondr/o = cartilage

In the fetus, bones are composed of a soft, flexible tissue called **cartilage** (KAR-tul-lej). As the fetus develops, cartilage is replaced with bone tissue in a process called **ossification** (OS-sih-fih-**KAY**-shun), or bone formation.

oste/o = bone
-blasts = immature cells
-cytes = cells

Ossification begins when cartilage is replaced by immature bone cells called **osteoblasts** (**OS**-tee-oh-BLASTS). In the forming bone, osteoblasts develop into mature bone cells, called **osteocytes** (**OS**-tee-oh-SITES). At the same time, osteoblasts produce an enzyme that causes calcium and phosphorus in the area to combine into a hard substance called calcium phosphate, giving the bone its characteristic hardness. A fully formed bone is composed of osteocytes cemented together with calcium phosphate deposits.

-clasts = cells that break (-clasia = to break)
myel/o = bone marrow

Throughout life, osteocytes in fully formed bone are continually renewed and replaced by maturing osteoblasts. As maturing osteoblasts are added to the bone, cells called **osteoclasts** (**OS**-tee-oh-KLASTS) digest older osteocytes, thereby preventing the bone from growing too large or heavy. Osteoclasts also serve to smooth and shape the bone and to hollow out a cavity inside the bone; this cavity is filled with **bone marrow,** a soft tissue containing a rich supply of blood vessels and nerves.

Bone Structure

Although all bones are formed in the same way (in the process described above), bones vary widely in their shape and size. Based on their shape and size, bones are classified into five groups:

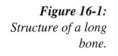

Figure 16-1:
Structure of a long bone.

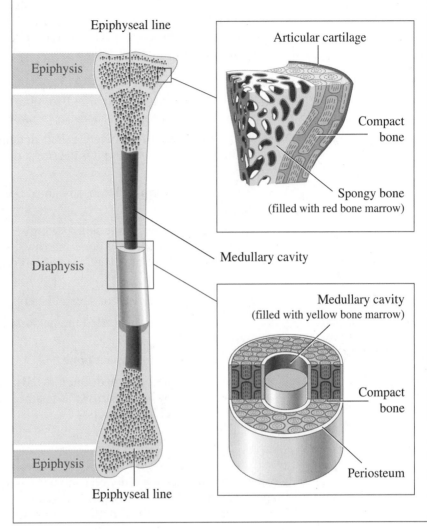

Epiphyseal line

Epiphysis

Articular cartilage

Compact bone

Spongy bone
(filled with red bone marrow)

Diaphysis

Medullary cavity

Medullary cavity
(filled with yellow bone marrow)

Compact bone

Epiphysis

Periosteum

Epiphyseal line

- **long bones**, the strong bones of the arms and legs
- **short bones**, the irregularly shaped structures in the wrists, ankles, and toes
- **flat bones**, the broad bones found in the shoulder, skull, and ribs
- **sesamoid** (SEH-suh-moyd) **bones**, the very small bones found near joints
- **irregular bones**, those that do not fall neatly into the first four categories, such as the vertebrae and the bones of the ear

sesamoid = "resembling a sesame seed"

epi- = above
-physis = to grow
dia- = through

Because long bones have regular, well-defined shapes, most discussions of bone structure focus on these bones. As Figure 16-1 shows, each end of the bone is called an **epiphysis** (uh-PIH-fuh-sis), while the long central portion is called the **diaphysis** (die-AF-fuh-sis).

In children, the epiphysis contains cartilage, allowing the bone to grow longer. In adults, this cartilage is ossified, forming the **epiphyseal** (EH-pih-**FIH**-zee-ul) **line**. Each epiphysis consists of three layers of tissue:

articul/o = joint

- a thin outer layer of cartilage, called **articular** (ar-TIH-kyoo-ler) **cartilage**, so named because it is the site at which bones meet to form joints

- a thick layer of **compact bone**, so named because of its hard, dense nature

- an inner area of porous tissue called **spongy** or **cancellous** (KAN-sull-luss) **bone** filled with "red bone marrow," so named because it is comprised mainly of blood cells in various stages of development

The diaphysis is also comprised of several layers of tissue:

peri- = surrounding
oste/o = bone
-um = thing

- a sturdy outer membrane called the **periosteum** (PEHR-ee-**OS**-tee-um)

- a thick layer of hard **compact bone**

- an inner area called the **medullary** (**MEH**-dyoo-LEHR-ee) **cavity** filled with "yellow bone marrow," so named because it is composed mainly of fat and blood vessels

The Axial Skeleton

By convention, the skeleton is divided into two parts: the axial skeleton and the appendicular skeleton. The **axial** (AX-ee-ul) **skeleton** consists of the 80 bones that form the skull, vertebral column, ribs, and sternum.

crani/o = skull

The **skull** consists of a total of 29 bones, including those that make up the cranium, the face, and the ears. The **cranium** (KRAY-nee-um) is the structure that surrounds the brain, protecting it from injury.

spondyl/o and
vertebr/o = vertebrae

The **vertebral** (VER-teh-brul) **column** consists of 26 bones called **vertebrae** (VER-tuh-bray) separated and cushioned by flat, round, shock-absorbing structures called **vertebral disks**. The vertebrae are named and numbered according to their location (see insert in Figure 16-2):

cervic/o = neck

- the 7 **cervical** (SER-vih-kul) vertebrae, C1-C7, are located in the neck region

thorac/o = chest
- the 12 **thoracic** (ther-RASS-ick) vertebrae, T1-T12, are located in the chest region

lumb/o = loin; waist
- the 5 **lumbar** (LUM-bar) vertebrae, L1-L5, are located in the lower back region

sacr/o = lower back
- the **sacrum** (SAY-krum), a single bone consisting of five fused vertebrae, is located in the "sacral" region just above the tail bone

coccyx = tail bone
- the tail bone or **coccyx** (KOCK-sicks), a single bone consisting of four fused vertebrae, is located in the tail region

Together, these bones form a protective column around the spinal cord, which is an important component of the central nervous system.

sternum = breast bone
The **ribs** are 12 pairs of bones connected to the vertebral column in the back and to the **sternum** (STER-num) in the front, forming a protective cage around the heart and lungs.

The Appendicular Skeleton

The **appendicular** (AP-pen-**DICK**-kyoo-ler) **skeleton** consists of the 126 bones that make up the upper and lower extremities. In effect, these bones are appendages to the axial skeleton. Note that the upper and lower extremities consist of several pairs of bones, one set on each side of the body. For example, the upper extremities include a pair of shoulder blades: one shoulder blade on the right side of the body, and one on the left.

The upper extremities consist of 64 bones (32 pairs):

- the **clavicle** (KLAV-ih-kul), or collarbone
- the **scapula** (SKAP-yoo-luh), or shoulder blade
- the **humerus** (HYOO-mer-us), or upper arm bone
- the **radius** (RAY-dee-us) and **ulna** (ULL-nuh), or forearm bones
- the **carpals** (KAR-pulz), or wrist bones
- the **metacarpals** (MEH-tuh-**KAR**-pulz), or hand bones
- the **phalanges** (full-LAN-jeez), or finger bones

The lower extremities consist of 62 bones (31 pairs):

- the three bones of the **pelvic girdle**, or hip bone: the **ilium** (ILL-lee-um), **ischium** (ISS-kee-um), and **pubis** (PYOO-biss)
- the **femur** (FEE-mer), or thigh bone
- the **patella** (puh-TELL-uh), or kneecap
- the **tibia** (TIH-bee-uh) and **fibula** (FIH-byoo-luh), or lower leg bones

Figure 16-2: *The axial and appendicular skeleton.*

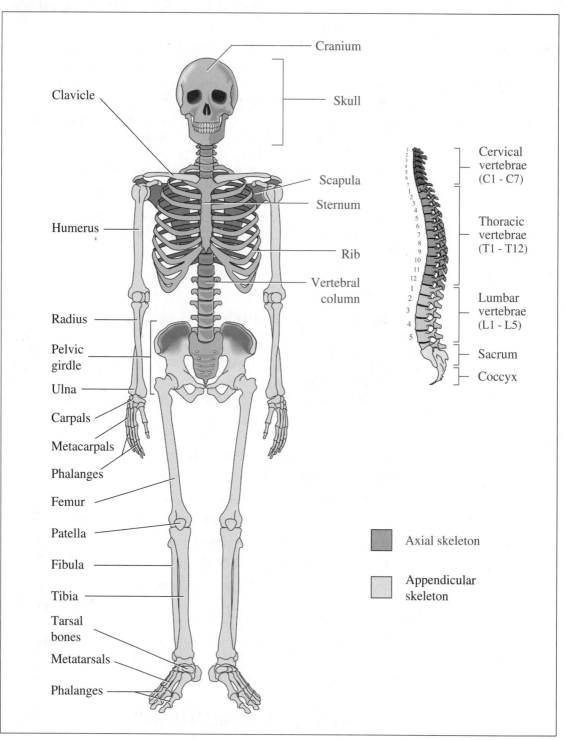

Figure 16-3: *Internal (A) and external (B) views of a typical diarthrosis.*

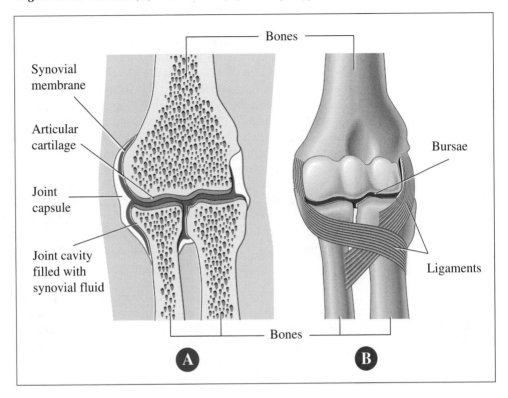

Bones

Synovial
membrane

Articular
cartilage

Joint
capsule

Joint cavity
filled with
synovial fluid

Bursae

Ligaments

Bones

A   **B**

• the **tarsal** (TAR-sul) bones, or ankle bones

• the **metatarsals** (MEH-tuh-**TAR**-sulz), or feet bones

• the **phalanges** (full-LAN-jeez), or toe bones

Joints

*arthr/o and
articul/o = joint*

The bones of the axial and appendicular skeletons come together to form **joints**, which are also called **arthroses** (ar-THROE-seez) or **articulations** (ar-TIH-kyoo-**LAY**-shunz). Joints vary widely in the degree of movement they afford. Some joints are constructed in such a way that little or no movement is possible. Most, however, are somewhat or freely movable, allowing us a wide range of motion; joints in the fingers, for example, afford very precise movements, such as those that enable surgeons to perform very delicate surgical procedures. The three types of joints are:

*syn- = together;
united*

• immovable joints, or **synarthroses** (SIN-ar-**THROE**-seez), such as the joints between the skull bones

*amphi- = both sides;
double*

• somewhat movable joints, or **amphiarthroses** (AM-fee-ar-**THROE**-seez), such as the joints between the vertebrae

diarthrosis = "mov-
able joint"

- freely movable joints, or **diarthroses** (DIE-ar-**THROE**-seez), such as those in the shoulders, fingers, and knees

A typical diarthrosis is shown in Figure 16-3. You should keep in mind that its structure is designed to minimize friction between the bones as they move. The surfaces of the bones are covered with **articular cartilage**, which is very smooth and slippery. The **joint cavity** (the area between the bones) is lined with the **synovial** (sih-NO-vee-ul) **membrane** and is filled with **synovial fluid**, a clear, sticky substance produced by the synovial membrane to nourish and lubricate the joint. Because of the important role of the synovial membrane and fluid in the movement of joints, diarthroses are often called synovial joints. The entire joint is sealed in a sturdy, cartilaginous structure called the **joint capsule**. Bands of connective tissue called **ligaments** (LIH-guh-ments) surround the joint capsule, connecting the bones and strengthening the joint. Located in the spaces between the ligaments and the joint are sacs of synovial fluid similar to that in the joint cavity; these sacs, called **bursae** (BER-say), act as cushions and help prevent injury.

synov/o = synovial
fluid; synovial
membrane

ligament/o = ligament

burs/o = bursa

Movement of a joint is controlled largely by muscles. Bands of connective tissue called **tendons** (TEN-dunz) bind muscles to the bones on either side of the joint; contraction of these muscles forces the bones in the joint to move. Bursae are found in the spaces between tendons and joints as well as in the spaces between ligaments and joints.

ten/o, tend/o, and
tendin/o = tendon

Review Exercises

1. **Match** the following suffixes and combining forms with their definitions.

   g -physis   a. vertebrae

   f -porosis   b. bone

   c ten/o   c. tendon

   a spondyl/o   d. joint

   e ankyl/o   e. crooked; stiff

   d arthr/o   f. becoming porous or less dense

   b oste/o   g. to grow

2. **Define** the following suffixes and combining forms.

   a. articul/o   joint

b. vertebr/o _____ *vertebrae* _____

c. tendin/o _____ *tendon* _____

d. synov/o _____ *synovial fluid* _____

e. tend/o _____ *tendon* _____

f. scoli/o _____ *curvature* _____

g. -desis _____ *fusion* _____

h. -clasia _____ *break* _____

3. **Spell** the combining forms that have the following meanings.

a. skull _____ *cranio* _____

b. cartilage _____ ~~cartho~~ *chrondr* _____

c. bursa _____ *bursae* _____

d. ligament _____ *ligamento* _____

e. curve; swayback _____ *lord* _____

f. bone marrow _____ *myleo* _____

g. humpback _____ *kyph* _____

4. **Write** the common or alternative name for each of the following terms.

a. osteocyte _____ *bone cell* _____

b. cranium _____ *skull* _____

c. sternum _____ *breast bone* _____

d. arthrosis _____ *inflammation bone formation of joint* _____

e. coccyx _____ *tail bone* _____

f. articulation _____ *formation of joint* _____

Terminology

The following are selected terms that pertain to pathology of the skeletal system and to related diagnostic and therapeutic procedures. As you will see, most of the disorders listed are associated with breakage, inflammation, abnormal formation, dislocation, or the abnormal shape of a bone or joint. Keeping this in mind will help you to understand other terms you may hear as well as the rationale behind treatment of bone and joint disorders.

Pathologic Conditions	Word Elements	Definition
ankylosing spondylitis (ANG-kull-**LOE**-sing SPON-dull-**LIE**-tis)	ankyl = crooked; stiff osing = condition spondyl = vertebrae itis = inflammation	chronic inflammatory disease of the spine characterized by fusion and loss of mobility of two or more vertebrae
ankylosis (ANG-kull-**LOE**-sis)	ankyl = crooked; stiff osis = condition	stiffening and immobility of a joint due to fusion of the bones across the joint cavity; usually associated with arthritis
arthralgia (ar-THRAL-juh)	arthr = joint algia = pain	pain in a joint
arthritis (ar-THRIE-tis)	arthr = joint itis = inflammation	inflammation of a joint
arthropathy (ar-THROP-uh-thee)	arthro = joint pathy = disease	any disease of the joints
bursitis (ber-SIE-tis)	burs = bursa itis = inflammation	inflammation of the bursae, usually occurring in association with arthritis
chondromalacia patellae (KON-droe-muh-**LAY**-shuh puh-TELL-lay)	chondro = cartilage malacia = softening patellae = kneecap	condition characterized by damage to the cartilage of the kneecap, resulting in pain; most commonly found in adolescents
comminuted fracture (**KOM**-ih-NYOO-ted FRACK-sher)	com = together minuted = "diminished" fracture = "to break"	splintered or crushed bone
compound fracture (FRACK-sher)	com = together pound = "to place" fracture = "to break"	a break in a bone accompanied by an open wound in the skin; also called an open fracture
compression fracture (FRACK-sher)	com = together pression = "squeeze" fracture = "to break"	a break in a bone resulting from compression; usually involves one or more vertebrae
fracture (FRACK-sher)	fracture = "to break"	any break in a bone
gouty arthritis (GOW-tee ar-THRIE-tis)	arthr = joint itis = inflammation	inflammation of the joints caused by gout (a disease involving abnormal uric acid metabolism); most commonly affects the big toe
greenstick fracture (FRACK-sher)	fracture = "to break"	condition in which a bone is partially bent and partially broken, as when a green stick breaks

Pathologic Conditions	Word Elements	Definition
herniated disk (**HER**-nee-AY-ted)	herni = hernia; protrusion ated = subjected to	protrusion of a vertebral disk into the center of the vertebral column, irritating the spinal nerves and causing pain
impacted fracture (FRACK-sher)	fracture = "to break"	a break in a bone in which one fragment is wedged into the other
kyphosis (kie-FOE-sis)	kyph = humpback osis = condition	increased curvature of the thoracic region of the vertebral column, leading to a humpback posture; may be caused by arthritis, poor posture, osteomalacia, or chronic respiratory disease
lordosis (lor-DOE-sis)	lord = curve; swayback osis = condition	forward curvature of the lumbar region of the vertebral column, leading to a swayback posture; usually caused by increased weight in the abdomen, as during pregnancy
luxation (luck-SAY-shun)	lux = to slide ation = process	displacement of a bone from its joint; commonly called dislocation
osteoarthritis (OS-tee-oh-ar-**THRIE**-tis)	osteo = bone arthr = joint itis = inflammation	chronic inflammatory disease characterized by destruction of articular cartilage and overgrowth of bone in the weight-bearing joints; often called OA or DJD (degenerative joint disease)
osteomalacia (OS-tee-oh-muh-**LAY**-shuh)	osteo = bone malacia = softening	softening and weakening of the bones, usually due to vitamin D deficiency; in children, the condition is called rickets
osteomyelitis (OS-tee-oh-MY-ull-**LIE**-tis)	osteo = bone myel = bone marrow itis = inflammation	inflammation of the bone and bone marrow, usually due to infection
osteoporosis (OS-tee-oh-por-**OH**-sis)	osteo = bone porosis = becoming porous or less dense	loss of calcium and bone tissue, causing the bone to become porous, brittle, and easily fractured; most commonly seen in post-menopausal women
Paget's disease (PAJ-ets)	no word elements	disease characterized by weakened, thickened, deformed bones; most commonly seen in middle-aged and elderly adults
periostitis (PEHR-ee-OST-**EYE**-tis)	peri = surrounding ost = bone itis = inflammation	inflammation of the periosteum, usually due to a blow to the bone
rheumatoid arthritis (ROO-muh-toyd ar-THRIE-tis)	rheumat = watery flow oid = resembling arthr = joint itis = inflammation	chronic joint disease characterized by inflammation, pain, stiffness, and eventually deformity of the affected joints due to inflammation of the synovial membrane; commonly called RA

Pathologic Conditions	Word Elements	Definition
scoliosis (SKOLE-lee-**OH**-sis)	scoli = crooked; bent osis = condition	abnormal curvature of the vertebral column, eventually causing back pain, disk disease, or arthritis; often a congenital disease, but sometimes results from poor posture
simple fracture (FRACK-sher)	fracture = "to break"	a break in a bone without an external wound (with no break in the skin); also called a closed fracture
spina bifida (SPY-nuh BIH-fih-duh)	spina = spine bifida = "clefted; branched"	congenital disorder characterized by malformation of the spine due to abnormal formation and joining of the vertebrae
sprain (sprane)	no word elements	twisting of a joint, resulting in pain, swelling, and injury to the ligaments
subluxation (SUB-luck-**SAY**-shun)	sub = under; beneath lux = to slide ation = process	partial displacement of a bone from its joint; commonly called partial dislocation
synovitis (SIH-no-**VIE**-tis)	synov = synovial membrane itis = inflammation	inflammation of the synovial membrane, usually resulting from injury, infection, or arthritis

Diagnostic Procedures	Word Elements	Definition
arthrocentesis (AR-throe-sen-**TEE**-sis)	arthro = joint centesis = puncture	use of a needle to puncture a joint, usually to remove synovial fluid for analysis
arthrography (ar-THROG-ruh-fee)	arthro = joint graphy = recording	x-ray recording of a joint following injection of a contrast agent
arthroscopy (ar-THROS-kuh-pee)	arthro = joint scopy = visual examination	visual examination of a joint using an arthroscope
bone scan	no word elements	method of visualizing a bone by using a special scanner to record the radioactivity emitted from bones following intravenous injection of a radioactive substance
rheumatoid factor test (ROO-muh-toyd)	rheumat = watery flow oid = resembling	test used to detect a substance (rheumatoid factor) present in the blood of patients with rheumatoid arthritis

Therapeutic Procedures	Word Elements	Definition
amputation (AM-pyoo-**TAY**-shun)	amputation = "process of pruning or cutting off"	surgical removal of all or part of a limb
arthrectomy (ar-**THRECK**-tuh-me)	arthr = joint ectomy = surgical removal	surgical removal of a joint, often to replace it with an artificial joint
arthroclasia (AR-throe-**KLAY**-zhuh)	arthro = joint clasia = to break	deliberate breaking of a fused joint to permit movement
arthrodesis (AR-throe-**DEE**-sis)	arthro = joint desis = to bind together	surgical fixation or binding together of bones to immobilize a joint
arthroplasty (**AR**-throe-PLASS-tee)	arthro = joint plasty = surgical repair	surgical repair or replacement of a joint
bursectomy (ber-**SECK**-tuh-me)	burs = bursa ectomy = surgical removal	surgical removal of one or more bursae
craniotomy (KRAY-nee-**OT**-uh-me)	cranio = skull tomy = surgical incision	surgical incision in the skull, usually to relieve pressure or to perform brain surgery
osteotomy (OS-tee-**OT**-uh-me)	osteo = bone tomy = surgical incision	surgical incision in a bone, usually removing a portion in order to change its alignment or to shorten it
synovectomy (SIH-no-**VECK**-tuh-me)	synov = synovial fluid; synovial membrane ectomy = surgical removal	surgical removal of a synovial membrane, usually to treat chronic inflammation of a joint in patients with rheumatoid arthritis

Review Exercises

5. **Break Down and Define** the word elements within each of the following terms, and then define the term itself.

> **Example:** arthr / itis   *joint / inflammation*   *inflammation of a joint*

a. arthralgia   arthr/algia   joint pain

b. chondromalacia   chondro/malacia   softening of cartilage

c. kyphosis   kyph/osis   humpback condition

d. arthrocentesis _joint puncture_ _removal of fluid from joint_

e. synovectomy _removal of synovial fluid (sac)_

f. bursitis _inflamation of bursa sac_

g. arthroscopy _scope into joint_

h. scoliosis _abnormal curvature of spine_

i. ankylosis _condition of stiffness_

j. ankylosing spondylitis _stiffness + inflamation of cloth_

k. osteomyelitis

l. osteoporosis

m. arthrography

n. arthroclasia

o. arthrodesis

p. bursectomy

q. osteotomy

6. **Define** the following terms.

a. Paget's disease

b. gouty arthritis

c. spina bifida _____

_____

d. luxation _____

_____

e. subluxation _____

_____

f. herniated disk _____

_____

g. bone scan _____

_____

7. **Match** the following terms with their definitions.

_____ fracture   a. break in a bone accompanied by an open wound

_____ compound fracture   b. break in a bone without an external wound

_____ compression fracture   c. break with one bone fragment wedged into another

_____ greenstick fracture   d. partially bent, partially broken bone

_____ impacted fracture   e. any break in a bone

_____ simple fracture   f. break in a bone resulting from compression

8. **Word Building and Spelling**. Spell out the medical term for each of the following definitions using the slashes provided to separate the word elements.

inflammation of a bone   *oste / itis*

a. inflammation of the synovial membrane   _____ / _____

b. swayback condition   _____ / _____

c. surgical incision in the skull   _____ / _____

d. inflammation of a bone and joint   _____ / _____ / _____

e. surgical repair of a joint   _____ / _____

f. surgical removal of a joint   _____ / _____

g. softening of the bones   _____ / _____

h. any disease of the joints   _____ / _____

Case Study. Read the case notes below. For each boldfaced term, provide a brief definition and indicate whether the term is spelled correctly; if it is misspelled, provide the correct spelling.

> **ostioporosis:** *brittle, porous bones due to calcium and bone tissue loss*
>
> ***Example:***
>
> *Spelled correctly?*   ☐ Yes   ✔ No   *osteoporosis*

Patient presented as a 46-year-old perimenopausal female concerned about **ostioporosis** due to a family history of the disease. Tests showed adequate bone density. Due to patient's high risk, prescribed estrogen to slow postmenopausal bone loss. Patient to return yearly for repeat bone density tests.

One-year follow-up: Patient's bone density is approximately the same (total bone mass loss < 2%). However, patient complained of **arthralgia** in both shoulders, hands, and knees. On examination, some type of **arthroputhy** was apparent: joints were reddened, warm, and inflamed. Patient reported that the pain had developed over a few weeks and was accompanied by a general feeling of sickness, fatigue, unexplained weight loss, and a low-grade fever. Suspect **rhumatoid arthritis**. To confirm diagnosis and rule out **osteoarthritis** or other disease, ordered x-rays, aspiration of synovial fluid for analysis, **reumatoid factor test**, sed rate, and red blood cell count. Results confirmed diagnosis of RA. Treatment plan: NSAIDs, heat and cold applications, program of exercise and rest; **arthragraphy** at next follow-up to monitor progression.

a. arthralgia: _____

_____

Spelled correctly?   ☐ Yes   ☐ No _____

b. arthroputhy: _____

_____

Spelled correctly?   ☐ Yes   ☐ No _____

c. rhumatoid arthritis: _____

_____

Spelled correctly?   ☐ Yes   ☐ No _____

d. osteoarthritis: _____

_____

Spelled correctly?   ☐ Yes   ☐ No _____

e. reumatoid factor test: _____

_____

Spelled correctly? ☐ Yes ☐ No _____

f. arthragraphy: _____

_____

Spelled correctly? ☐ Yes ☐ No _____

Listen to the section on your audiotape cassette that corresponds to this chapter and write the terms below. Be careful to spell each term correctly.

1. _____   14. _____

2. _____   15. _____

3. _____   16. _____

4. _____   17. _____

5. _____   18. _____

6. _____   19. _____

7. _____   20. _____

8. _____   21. _____

9. _____   22. _____

10. _____   23. _____

11. _____   24. _____

12. _____   25. _____

13. _____

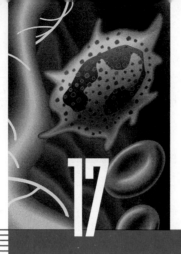

Muscular System

Upon completing this chapter, you should be able to:

- Describe the muscular system and explain its primary functions
- Recognize, build, pronounce, and spell words that pertain to the muscular system
- Describe diseases, diagnostic tests, and therapeutic procedures that pertain to the muscular system

Overview

The muscular system consists of all of the muscles in the body, and is responsible for all types of movement. Muscles are responsible both for moving bones – allowing us to adjust our posture, walk, run, turn, twist, shake, lift, etc. – and for moving internal organs – causing food to be pushed through the digestive tract, blood to be pushed through vessels, urine to be eliminated from the bladder, etc. All of these movements are accomplished by the contraction and relaxation of muscles attached to bones or internal organs. In addition to causing movement, contraction and relaxation of muscles also serve to generate body heat; shivering when cold, for example, helps to heat the body. Thus, muscles function in locomotion, internal processes, and heat production.

Word Elements

– The following combining forms (CF) pertain to structures of the muscular system. Some are used to refer to muscle, while others denote tissues that support muscle.

CF	Meaning	Example
fasci/o	fascia	*fascio*tomy = surgical incision in a fascia
fibr/o	fiber; fibrous	*fibro*myositis = inflammation of fibrous muscle tissue
my/o	muscle	*my*algia = muscle pain
myos/o	muscle	*myos*itis = inflammation of a muscle
ten/o	tendon	*teno*lysis = surgical separation of a tendon from adhesions
tend/o	tendon	*tendo*lysis = another name for tenolysis
tendin/o	tendon	*tendino*plasty = surgical repair of a tendon

PROPERTIES OF MUSCLES – These combining forms describe properties or activities of muscles. Except for flex/o, they are most often used to construct terms describing pathologic conditions.

CF	Meaning	Example
clon/o	turmoil	myo*clon*us = uncontrollable muscle twitching
flex/o	to bend	*flex*ion = the act of bending
sthen/o	strength	mya*sthen*ia = lack of muscle strength (muscle weakness)
ton/o	tension	*ton*ic = characterized by [muscle] tension

SUFFIX – The following suffix pertains to the muscular system. It is most often used in terms describing abnormal muscle development.

Suffix	Meaning	Example
-trophy	nourishment; growth	a*trophy* = without growth; degeneration

Anatomy and Physiology

The muscular system consists of three different types of muscles, each of which serves somewhat different functions. Although all three types will be described, this chapter will focus on skeletal muscles, which are responsible for voluntary movement. Since many muscle diseases involve abnormal muscle development or restricted muscle movement, this section will explain the structure and movements of skeletal muscles as well as conventions for naming them.

Types of Muscle

my/o and myos/o = muscle

The three types of muscle in the body are called skeletal, smooth, and cardiac.

Skeletal muscles are attached to bones and are responsible for movement of the body through space, including such activities as walking, running, bending, and lifting. Skeletal muscles respond to both conscious (voluntary) and unconscious (involuntary) control, and are therefore called **voluntary muscles** by some physicians. Other physicians refer to skeletal muscles as **striated** (STRIE-ay-ted) **muscles** because of their striped appearance on microscopic examination. Inside the body, these muscles are enclosed and separated by **fasciae** (**FASH**-shee-ee), connective tissues that help protect against injury.

fasci/o = fascia

Smooth muscles lack the striped appearance of skeletal muscles. They are found in the walls of many internal (visceral) organs and blood vessels, and are mainly responsible for assisting internal processes such as digestion and circulation. Because smooth muscles are located in visceral organs and respond only to unconscious (involuntary) control, they are often called **visceral** (VIH-ser-ul) or **involuntary muscles**.

viscer/o = internal organs

Cardiac (KAR-dee-ack) **muscle** is a specialized type of muscle located only in the walls of the heart, where it forms the **myocardium** (MY-oh-**KAR**-dee-um). Cardiac muscle is responsible for the pumping action of the heart. Cardiac muscle is somewhat similar in appearance to skeletal muscle. However, like smooth muscle, it is not under conscious control: the heart pumps whether we think about it or not.

cardi/o = heart

Mechanics of Movement

fibr/o = fiber; fibrous
ten/o, tend/o, and tendin/o = tendon
ton/o = tension

Muscles are connected to bones by bands of fibrous connective tissue called **tendons** (TEN-dunz). When a muscle contracts (shortens or tenses), it pulls on the attached bones, causing at least one of them to move. The coordinated actions of many muscles on many bones result in movements such as bending, turning, and lifting. Although contraction of different muscles may pull a bone in different directions, the overall effect is usually a smooth motion.

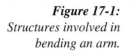

Figure 17-1:
Structures involved in
bending an arm.

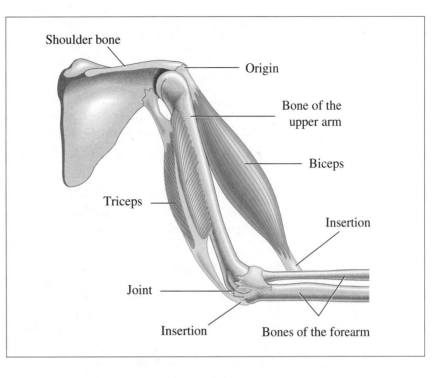

To see how a relatively simple movement is accomplished, examine Figure 17-1. Two muscles are involved in bending and straightening the arm: the biceps and the triceps. Each of these muscles is attached at one end of the bone of the upper arm at a point called the **origin**. This is the point toward which the forearm will be pulled. The other end of each muscle, called the **insertion**, is attached to the movable bones of the forearm. When the biceps contract, the forearm is pulled from the insertion toward the origin, causing the forearm to bend up. When the biceps relax, however, the forearm does not fall back into its original position; instead, it must be pulled back down by contraction of the triceps. This is why several muscles are needed to coordinate the motion of bones around a joint: the action of one muscle (e.g., to bend an arm) must be counteracted by that of another muscle (e.g., to straighten the arm).

Types of Movement

Muscles are arranged around bones in several different ways, allowing several different types of movement. As in the bending and straightening of an arm, most of these movements occur in pairs, one opposing the other. The main types of movement afforded by the actions of muscles on bones and joints are:

flex/o = to bend

- **flexion** (FLECK-shun) and **extension** (eck-STEN-shun), the bending and straightening of a limb
- **abduction** (ab-DUCK-shun) and **adduction** (ad-DUCK-shun), movement away from and toward the torso
- **pronation** (pro-NAY-shun) and **supination** (SOO-pih-**NAY**-shun), the turning of a hand to a palm down or palm up position (or the turning of the body to a face down or face up position when lying down)
- **dorsiflexion** (DOR-sih-**FLECK**-shun) and **plantar** (PLAN-tar) **flexion**, the bending of the foot upward and downward
- **rotation**, turning in a circular motion around an axis
- **circumduction** (SIR-kum-**DUCK**-shun), swinging a limb or moving the eyes in a circular motion

Naming of Muscles

sthen/o = strength

A great many muscles are needed to perform the types of movements described above. In fact, most exercise programs are designed to include a wide range of motions in order to strengthen as many muscles as possible while increasing flexibility. Some of the major muscles used to flex, extend, abduct, adduct, rotate, and circumduct various parts of the body are shown in Figure 17-2.

The names of these muscles may seem intimidating at first, especially since many different conventions can be used to identify muscles. In general, muscles are named for their location in the body, for the type of movement they cause, and/or for their size, appearance, or shape. In addition, some muscles are actually groups of muscles or have more than one origin or insertion; many of these muscles are named for the number of components that make up the muscle. To illustrate these conventions, let's examine the muscles labeled in color in Figure 17-2.

Muscle Name	Meaning	Convention
pectoralis (PECK-ter-**AL**-iss) major (MAY-jer)	pertaining to the breast/chest important; big	location size
biceps (BY-seps)	two heads	number of origins
triceps (TRY-seps)	three heads	number of origins
trapezius (truh-PEE-zee-us)	irregular four-sided figure	shape
deltoid (DELL-toyd)	resembling a triangle	shape

Continued on page 245

Figure 17-2a: *Major muscles of the body (anterior view).*

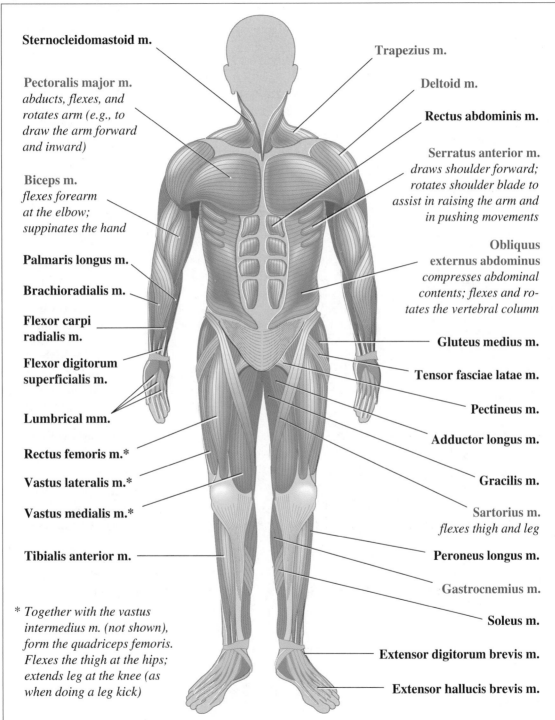

Sternocleidomastoid m.

Pectoralis major m.
abducts, flexes, and rotates arm (e.g., to draw the arm forward and inward)

Biceps m.
flexes forearm at the elbow; suppinates the hand

Palmaris longus m.

Brachioradialis m.

Flexor carpi radialis m.

Flexor digitorum superficialis m.

Lumbrical mm.

Rectus femoris m.*

Vastus lateralis m.*

Vastus medialis m.*

Tibialis anterior m.

* Together with the vastus intermedius m. (not shown), form the quadriceps femoris. Flexes the thigh at the hips; extends leg at the knee (as when doing a leg kick)

Trapezius m.

Deltoid m.

Rectus abdominis m.

Serratus anterior m.
draws shoulder forward; rotates shoulder blade to assist in raising the arm and in pushing movements

Obliquus externus abdominus
compresses abdominal contents; flexes and rotates the vertebral column

Gluteus medius m.

Tensor fasciae latae m.

Pectineus m.

Adductor longus m.

Gracilis m.

Sartorius m.
flexes thigh and leg

Peroneus longus m.

Gastrocnemius m.

Soleus m.

Extensor digitorum brevis m.

Extensor hallucis brevis m.

Figure 17-2b: *Major muscles of the body (posterior view).*

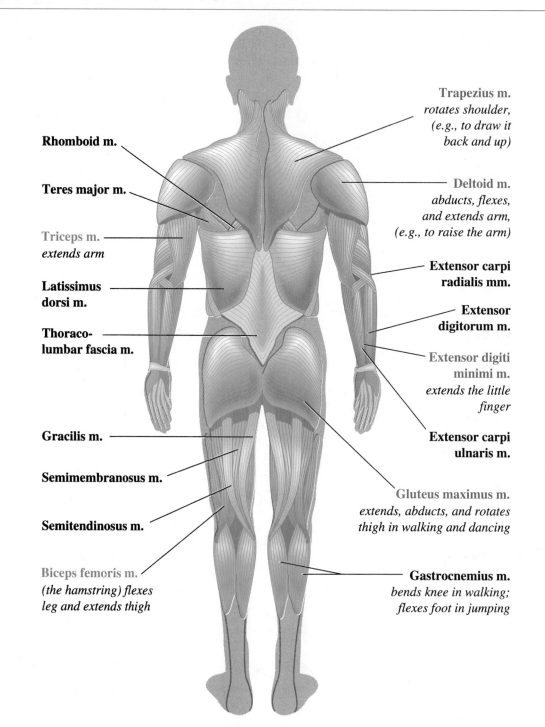

Rhomboid m.

Teres major m.

Triceps m.
extends arm

Latissimus dorsi m.

Thoraco-lumbar fascia m.

Gracilis m.

Semimembranosus m.

Semitendinosus m.

Biceps femoris m.
(the hamstring) flexes leg and extends thigh

Trapezius m.
rotates shoulder, (e.g., to draw it back and up)

Deltoid m.
abducts, flexes, and extends arm, (e.g., to raise the arm)

Extensor carpi radialis mm.

Extensor digitorum m.

Extensor digiti minimi m.
extends the little finger

Extensor carpi ulnaris m.

Gluteus maximus m.
extends, abducts, and rotates thigh in walking and dancing

Gastrocnemius m.
bends knee in walking; flexes foot in jumping

Muscle Name	Meaning	Convention
serratus (SEHR-uh-tus)	serrated	appearance
anterior (an-TEER-ee-er)	front	location
extensor (eck-STEN-ser)	extension	type of movement
digiti minimi (DIH-jih-tee MIH-nih-me)	little finger	location
obliquus (uh-BLEE-kwuss)	slanting	appearance
externus (eck-STER-nus)	external	location
abdominus (ub-DOM-ih-nus)	abdomen	location
gluteus (GLOO-tee-us)	pertaining to the buttocks	location
maximus (MACK-sih-mus)	greatest; biggest	size
quadriceps (KWOD-ruh-seps)	four heads	number of origins
femoris (FEH-mer-iss)	thigh	location
sartorius (sar-TOR-ee-us)	tailor; ribbon	shape
biceps (BY-seps)	two heads	number of origins
femoris (FEH-mer-iss)	thigh	location
gastrocnemius (GAS-truck-NEE-me-us)	stomach-leg	shape-location

Review Exercises

1. **Match** the following suffix and combining forms with their definitions.

   _____ -trophy   a. turmoil

   _____ tendin/o   b. tendon

   _____ myos/o   c. tension

   _____ ton/o   d. muscle

   _____ clon/o   e. nourishment; growth

2. **Define** the following combining forms and compound combining forms.

   a. my/o   _____

   b. fibr/o   _____

c. myofibr/o _____

d. sthen/o _____

e. asthen/o _____

f. ten/o _____

g. fasci/o _____

h. flex/o _____

i. tend/o _____

3. **Match** the following types of muscle, types of movement, and examples of muscles with their definitions.

_____ flexion

_____ skeletal muscle

_____ pronation

_____ gluteus maximus

_____ pectoralis major

_____ abduction

_____ smooth muscle

_____ cardiac muscle

a. type of muscle that is attached to bones; also called striated or voluntary muscle

b. type of muscle found only in the heart; forms the myocardium

c. type of muscle found in the walls of the internal organs and blood vessels; also called visceral or involuntary muscle

d. the bending of a limb

e. turning to a palm down or face down position

f. movement away from the torso

g. important/large muscle found in the breast/chest

h. biggest muscle in the buttocks

Terminology

The following are selected terms that pertain to pathology of the muscular system and to related diagnostic and therapeutic procedures. As you will see, most of the disorders listed are associated with degeneration, pain, or abnormal movement of a muscle. Keeping this in mind will help you to understand other terms you may hear as well as the rationale behind treatment of muscle disorders.

Pathologic Conditions	Word Elements	Definition
atonia (ay-TOE-nee-uh)	a = not; without ton = tension ia = condition	complete lack of tension in a muscle, so that it is flaccid or floppy
dystonia (dis-TOE-nee-uh)	dys = difficult; painful ton = tension ia = condition	abnormal tension in a muscle, resulting in muscle rigidity and pain

Pathologic Conditions	Word Elements	Definition
muscle atrophy (AT-troe-fee)	a = not; without trophy = nourishment; growth	wasting away or degeneration of muscle tissue
muscular dystrophy (DIS-troe-fee)	dys = difficult; painful trophy = nourishment; growth	group of hereditary diseases characterized by progressive degeneration of the muscles, leading to increasing weakness and debilitation
myalgia (my-AL-jyuh)	my = muscle algia = pain	muscle pain
myasthenia gravis (MY-uh-**STHEE**-nee-uh GRAV-iss)	my = muscle a = not; without sthen = strength ia = condition	chronic condition characterized by muscle weakness and droopiness, especially in the eyes, face, throat, and limbs
myoclonus (MY-oh-**KLOE**-nus)	myo = muscle clon = turmoil us = thing	rapid, uncontrollable twitching of a muscle or group of muscles; may be occasional or frequent
myodiastasis (MY-oh-DIE-uh-**STAY**-sis)	myo = muscle diastasis = separation	separation of muscles or muscle fibers, usually due to excessive stretching as sometimes occurs to the abdominal muscles of pregnant women
myosarcoma (MY-oh-sar-**KOE**-muh)	myo = muscle sarc = flesh; muscle oma = tumor; growth	malignant tumor arising from muscle cells; it is called rhabdomyosarcoma (RAB-doe-MY-oh-sar-**KOE**-muh) if it involves skeletal muscle, or leiomyosarcoma (LIE-oh-MY-oh-sar-**KOE**-muh) if it involves smooth muscle
myositis (MY-oh-**SIE**-tis)	myos = muscle itis = inflammation	inflammation of a muscle due to infection or other type of damage or injury; also called myitis (my-EYE-tis)
paralysis (per-RAL-luh-sis)	paralysis = "beyond loose"	loss of voluntary motion due to an inability to contract one or more muscles
polymyositis (POL-ee-MY-oh-**SIE**-tis)	poly = many myos = muscle itis = inflammation	inflammation of muscles throughout the body, usually as a result of an autoimmune disease
tendinitis (TEN-dih-**NIE**-tis)	tendin = tendon itis = inflammation	inflammation of a tendon, usually as a result of injury
tremor (TREH-mer)	tremor = "to shake"	involuntary trembling or quivering of a body part due to rapid contraction and relaxation of the muscles in the affected area

Diagnostic Procedures	Word Elements	Definition
electromyography (ih-LECK-troe-my-**OG**-ruh-fee)	electro = electricity myo = muscle graphy = recording	procedure used to record and analyze the electrical activity in a muscle to identify possible nerve or muscle disorders; called EMG, for short
muscle biopsy (BY-op-see)	bi = life opsy = view	surgical removal of muscle tissue for microscopic examination

Therapeutic Procedures	Word Elements	Definition
fasciotomy (FASH-shee-**OT**-uh-me)	fascio = fascia tomy = surgical incision	process of making a surgical incision in a fascia, usually to relieve pressure on the muscle it surrounds
myorrhaphy (my-OR-ruh-fee)	myo = muscle rrhaphy = suture; stitch	suturing (stitching together) of a muscle wound
myotomy (my-OT-uh-me)	myo = muscle tomy = surgical incision	cutting or dissection of a muscle
tendolysis (ten-DOL-uh-sis)	tendo = tendon lysis = separation; dissolution	surgical procedure used to free a tendon from fibrous connective tissue (called adhesions) restricting its movement; also called tenolysis
tendoplasty (**TEN**-doe-PLASS-tee)	tendo = tendon plasty = surgical repair	surgical repair of an injured tendon; also called tendinoplasty or tenoplasty
tenodesis (teh-NOD-uh-sis)	teno = tendon desis = to bind together	surgical binding or fixation of a tendon to a bone, usually by transferring the tendon to a new point of attachment

Review Exercises

4. **Match** the following terms with their definitions.

_____ tremor

_____ tendolysis

_____ electromyography

_____ dystonia

_____ muscular dystrophy

a. procedure used to record the electrical activity in a muscle

b. group of hereditary diseases characterized by progressive degeneration of the muscles

c. surgical procedure used to free a tendon from fibrous connective tissue restricting its movement

d. involuntary quivering of a body part

e. abnormal tension in a muscle, resulting in muscle rigidity and pain

5. ***Break Down and Define*** the word elements within each of the following terms, and then define the term itself.

    Example: myo / tomy   *muscle / surgical incision*   *surgical incision in a muscle*

  a. tendoplasty

_____

  b. myalgia

_____

  c. myositis

_____

  d. polymyositis

_____

  e. tendinitis

_____

  f. fasciotomy

_____

  g. myodiastasis

_____

  h. atonia

_____

  i. myorrhaphy

_____

  j. tenodesis

_____

  k. electromyography

_____

6. ***Word Building and Spelling.*** Spell out the medical term for each of the following definitions using the slashes provided to separate the word elements.

    muscle protein   *myo / globin*

  a. muscle turmoil   _____ / _____

  b. tumor arising from muscle flesh   _____ / _____ / _____

  c. any disease of the muscles   _____ / _____

d. condition characterized by muscles
   without strength   _____ / _____ / _____ / _____

e. inflammation of a fascia   _____ / _____

f. surgical repair of a fascia   _____ / _____

g. pain arising from fibrous tissue and muscle   _____ / _____ / _____

h. softening of the muscles   _____ / _____

7. ***Choose and Construct.*** Choose the appropriate word elements from the list provided to construct terms for the following.

blast/o	my/o	ton/o	-oma
fibr/o	ten/o	-ia	-plasty

surgical repair of a muscle   *myo* **/** *plasty*

a. tumor of a muscle   _____ / _____

b. tumor of immature muscle cells   _____ / _____ / _____

c. tumor of muscle and fibrous tissue _____ / _____ / _____

d. surgical repair of a tendon   _____ / _____

e. surgical repair of a tendon and muscle   _____ / _____ / _____

f. condition of muscle tension   _____ / _____ / _____

Case Study. Read the case notes below. For each boldfaced term, provide a brief definition and indicate whether the term is spelled correctly; if it is misspelled, provide the correct spelling.

Example: **myastheenia:** *muscle weakness*

Spelled correctly?   ☐ Yes   ☑ No   *myasthenia*

Patient presented as a 5-year-old boy brought in by his mother. She was concerned that the boy learned to sit up and walk much later than her first child and now has a waddling gait. He cannot run easily, has difficulty climbing stairs, and falls down often. On examination, the boy had enlarged but weak muscles. The **myastheenia** and bulkiness were most pronounced in the calf muscles. The boy did not complain of **myalgia**, and there was no evidence of **myoklonus** or other irregular muscle activity. A **muscle biopsy** revealed **muscle attrophy** with fat and connective tissue deposits. **Electromiography** showed short, weak bursts of electrical activity and intact nerves, ruling out atrophy of neurologic origin. Blood tests revealed elevated creatinine phospho-kinase levels. Diagnosis: **muscular distruphy** (Duchenne type). Treatment plan: orthopedic appliances, physical therapy, and genetic counselling for family.

a. myalgia: _____

Spelled correctly? ☐ Yes ☐ No _____

b. myoklonus: _____

_____

Spelled correctly? ☐ Yes ☐ No _____

c. muscle biopsy: _____

_____

Spelled correctly? ☐ Yes ☐ No _____

d. muscle attrophy: _____

_____

Spelled correctly? ☐ Yes ☐ No _____

e. electromiography: _____

_____

Spelled correctly? ☐ Yes ☐ No _____

f. muscular distruphy: _____

_____

Spelled correctly? ☐ Yes ☐ No _____

 Listen to the section on your audiotape cassette that corresponds to this chapter and write the terms below. Be careful to spell each term correctly.

1. _____   7. _____

2. _____   8. _____

3. _____   9. _____

4. _____   10. _____

5. _____   11. _____

6. _____   12. _____

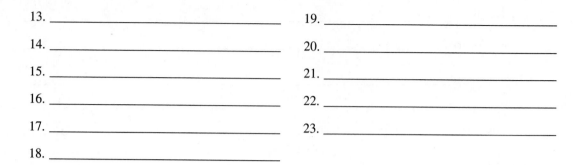

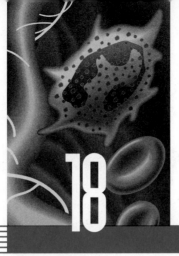

The Skin

Upon completing this chapter, you should be able to:

- Describe the skin and explain its primary functions
- Recognize, build, pronounce, and spell words that pertain to the skin
- Describe diseases, diagnostic tests, and therapeutic procedures that pertain to the skin

Overview   The skin is a protective organ consisting of several layers of tissue and a number of accessory organs, including nails, hair follicles, oil glands, and sweat glands. Together, these structures serve a wide range of protective and regulatory functions. The skin and its accessory organs help provide protection against injury, bacterial invasion, dehydration, and harmful ultraviolet rays. In addition, these structures play an important role in the regulation of body temperature and in the excretion of certain types of waste products formed in the body. The skin also contains many nerve endings and serves as a sensory receptor for pain, temperature, pressure, and touch.

Word Elements

SKIN CELLS AND STRUCTURES – The following combining forms (CF) pertain to the skin. They refer to various types of skin cells and structures, including accessory skin organs and secretions.

CF	Meaning	Example
cutane/o	skin	sub*cutane*ous = pertaining to beneath the skin
derm/o	skin	*derm*al = pertaining to the skin
dermat/o	skin	*dermat*ology = study of the skin
hidr/o	sweat	hyper*hidr*osis = excessive sweating
kerat/o	hard; horn-like	*kerat*osis = any horny growth on the skin
lip/o	fat	*lip*oma = growth made up of fatty tissue
melan/o	black	*melan*oma = tumor of the dark pigment cells
onych/o	nail	*onych*omalacia = softening of the fingernails
pil/o	hair	*pil*oerection = hair "standing on end"
seb/o	sebum	*seb*orrhea = excessive secretion of sebum
squam/o	scale-like	*squam*ous = pertaining to scale-like [cells]
sud/o	sweat	*sud*orific = promoting the flow of sweat

SUFFIX – The following suffix is used to denote the skin. It is used mainly in terms describing pathologic skin conditions.

Suffix	Meaning	Example
-derma	skin	pyo*derma* = pus-producing skin infection

Anatomy and Physiology

The skin is a surprisingly complex organ consisting of three layers of tissue: the epidermis, dermis, and subcutaneous tissue. Embedded in or on these layers of skin are several accessory organs: nails, hair, and the oil and sweat glands. These structures are illustrated in Figure 18-1 and described in the paragraphs below.

Layers of the Skin

derm/o, dermat/o, and cutane/o = skin
squam/o = scale-like

The **epidermis** (EH-pih-**DER**-miss), the outermost layer of the skin, is itself composed of many layers; it consists of layer upon layer of flat, scale-like cells called **squamous epithelial** (**SKWOM**-us EH-pih-**THEEL**-ee-ul)

Figure 18-1: *The skin and its accessory organs.*

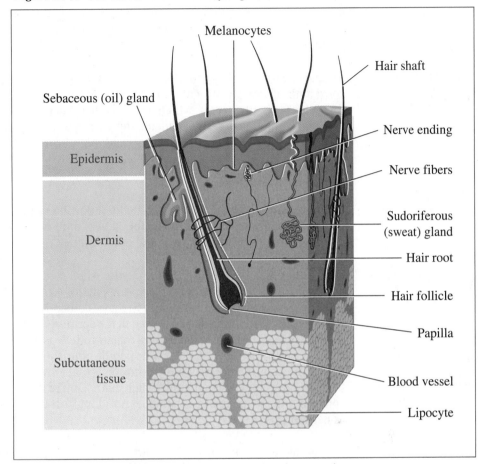

Melanocytes

Hair shaft

Sebaceous (oil) gland

Nerve ending

Epidermis

Nerve fibers

Dermis

Sudoriferous
(sweat) gland

Hair root

Hair follicle

Papilla

Subcutaneous
tissue

Blood vessel

Lipocyte

*kerat/o = hard; horn-
like*
*basal = pertaining to
the base*

melan/o = black
-cytes = cells

cells. The top layer of the epidermis consists of dead cells filled with a hard, "horn-like" protein called **keratin** (KEHR-uh-tin); these so-called "horny cells" serve as protective covering. The deepest layer, called the **basal** layer, consists of new and growing cells. In addition to squamous epithelial cells, the basal layer of the epidermis contains pigment-producing cells, called **melanocytes** (mel-LAN-no-sites). The pigment produced by these cells, called **melanin** (MEL-luh-nin), gives color to the skin.

Unlike the dermis and subcutaneous tissue, the epidermis does not contain blood vessels, lymphatic vessels, or nerve endings. The new, growing cells of the basal layer receive their nourishment from nutrients that seep up from the dermis. As these new cells grow and mature, they are pushed upward, replacing the dead cells of the outer layer.

corium = "hide"

The **dermis** (DER-miss), or **corium** (KOR-ee-um), lies immediately under the epidermis. The dermis consists mainly of dense connective tissue. Embedded in this tissue are numerous blood and lymph vessels, nerve endings, oil and sweat glands, and hair follicles.

subcutaneous = below the skin

lip/o = fat

Subcutaneous (SUB-kyoo-**TAY**-nee-us) **tissue** is a cushion-like layer consisting of loosely structured connective tissue and a large number of **lipocytes** (LIH-poe-sites), which are cells that manufacture and store fat. The main functions of subcutaneous tissue are to protect the tissues and organs underneath it (inside the body) and to prevent heat loss.

Accessory Skin Organs

onych/o = nail

Nails are hard plates of keratin that cover a portion of the skin on the top surface of the fingers and toes. The function of nails is to protect the tips of the fingers and toes from bruises and other injuries.

pil/o = hair

papill/o = nipple-like; can also refer to tiny protrusions in other parts of the body

Hair fibers are composed of horny cells filled with hard keratin. The portion of a hair fiber that protrudes through the skin and is visible to the eye is called the hair shaft, while the portion that is embedded in the skin is called the hair root. The hair root is anchored in the dermis by a sac called the **hair follicle** (FOL-lih-kull). Just below each hair follicle is a loop of capillaries, called the **papilla** (puh-PIL-luh). The papilla nourishes a bulb of cells at the base of the hair follicle, producing horny cells that move up through the hair follicle and add to the length of the hair shaft. Unlike the soft keratin of the epidermis, the hard keratin of hair does not slough off easily and must be cut as needed.

Hair is normally found on all body surfaces except the palms and soles of the feet. In certain areas of the body, hair serves a protective function. Eyelashes and eyebrows, for example, protect the eyes; similarly, nostril hairs help prevent inhalation of dust particles.

seb/o = sebum

Sebaceous (suh-BAY-shus) **glands**, or oil glands, secrete an oily substance called **sebum** (SEE-bum). These glands are located in the dermis, near hair follicles. Sebum lubricates the skin and hair and helps prevent infection by destroying harmful organisms on the surface of the skin.

sud/o and hidr/o = sweat

Sudoriferous (SOO-der-**RIF**-er-us) **glands**, commonly called **sweat glands**, are small coiled glands that produce sweat (perspiration). They open as pores on the surface of the skin and are especially abundant on the palms, soles, forehead, and armpits. The main functions of these glands are to cool the body by evaporation, to excrete waste products through the pores of the skin, and to moisturize surface cells.

Review Exercises

1. **Match** the following suffix and combining forms with their definitions.

_____ seb/o   a. scale-like

_____ -derma   b. nail

_____ pil/o   c. sebum

_____ onych/o   d. hair

_____ kerat/o   e. skin

_____ squam/o   f. hard; horn-like

_____ sud/o   g. sweat

2. **Define** the following combining forms.

a. cutane/o   _____

b. hidr/o   _____

c. dermat/o   _____

d. lip/o   _____

e. melan/o   _____

f. derm/o   _____

3. **Match** the following terms with their alternative forms.

_____ sebaceous gland   a. sweat gland

_____ sudoriferous gland   b. fat cell

_____ dermis   c. oil gland

_____ lipocyte   d. corium

_____ melanocyte   e. pigment cell

Terminology

The following are selected terms that pertain to pathology of the skin and to related diagnostic and therapeutic procedures. As you will see, most of the disorders listed are associated with inflammation or infection, abnormal growth, or abnormal glandular secretion. Keeping this in mind will help you to understand other terms you may hear as well as the rationale behind treatment of skin disorders.

Pathologic Conditions	Word Elements	Definition
acne (ACK-nee)	no word elements	pus-filled eruption of the skin due to infection or to the build-up of sebum and keratin in the pores
actinic keratosis (ack-TIN-ick KEHR-uh-**TOE**-sis)	actinic = "pertaining to radiation" kerat = hard; horn-like osis = condition	thickening of the outer keratin-filled layers of the skin due to excessive exposure to the sun
alopecia (AL-oh-**PEE**-shuh)	alopecia = "fox mange"	partial or complete loss of hair; commonly called baldness
anhidrosis (AN-hi-**DROE**-sis)	an = without; not hidr = sweat osis = condition	condition characterized by little or no sweat production (i.e., inadequate perspiration)
basal cell carcinoma (BAY-zul SELL KAR-sih-**NO**-muh)	carcin = cancer oma = tumor; growth	malignant tumor arising from the basal layer of the epidermis
bulla (BULL-uh)	no word elements	a large, fluid-filled blister
burn, first-degree	no word elements	mild burn affecting the epidermis; characterized by redness, pain, and no blisters
burn, second-degree	no word elements	burn affecting both the epidermis and dermis; characterized by redness, blistering, and pain
burn, third-degree	no word elements	severe burn characterized by destruction of the epidermis and dermis and damage to the subcutaneous layer, leaving charred, white tissue
carbuncle (KAR-bunk-ul)	carbuncle = "little coal"	large, deep boil or group of boils usually involving subcutaneous tissue
cellulitis (SELL-yoo-**LIE**-tis)	cellul = "living cell" itis = inflammation	inflammation and infection of all layers of skin, especially the loose tissues within the subcutaneous layer of the skin
comedo (KOE-meh-doe)	no word elements	a blackhead; a sebum plug within the opening of a hair follicle
contusion (kun-TOO-zhun)	no word elements	a bruise; bleeding underneath the skin caused by injury, but without a break in the skin
cyst (SIST)	cyst = "sac"	a fluid-filled or solid sac in or under the skin

Pathologic Conditions	Word Elements	Definition
dermatitis (DER-muh-**TIE**-tis)	dermat = skin itis = inflammation	inflammation of the skin
dermatomycosis (DER-muh-toe-my-**KOE**-sis)	dermato = skin mycosis = fungal infection	fungal infection of the skin
ecchymosis (EH-kih-**MOE**-sis)	ec = out chym = to pour osis = condition	black-and-blue mark on the skin caused by leakage of blood from blood vessels underneath the skin; commonly called a bruise
eczema (EGG-zeh-muh)	eczema = "boiled out"	inflammatory condition of the skin characterized by redness, itching, and blisters
erythema (EHR-ih-**THEE**-muh)	erythem = redness a = condition	redness of the skin caused by swelling of the capillaries
erythroderma (uh-RITH-roe-**DER**-muh)	erythro = red derma = skin	red discoloration of the skin
furuncle (FYUR-unk-ul)	no word elements	bacterial infection of a hair follicle and/or sebaceous gland, producing a pus-filled lesion commonly called a boil
granuloma (GRAN-yoo-**LOE**-muh)	granul = granules oma = tumor; growth	a benign mass of granulation tissue (soft, fleshy projections that form during the healing process)
hirsutism (**HER**-soo-TIH-zum)	hirsutism = "shagginess"	excessive body hair, usually in the male pattern of hair distribution (i.e., on the face and chest as well as scalp)
hyperhidrosis (HI-per-hi-**DROE**-sis)	hyper = excessive hidr = sweat osis = condition	condition characterized by excessive sweat production (i.e., excessive perspiration)
impetigo (IM-puh-**TIE**-go or IM-puh-**TEE**-go)	no word elements	a spreading bacterial skin infection characterized by the formation of abundant pus-producing vesicles; most common in children
keratosis (KEHR-uh-**TOE**-sis)	kerat = hard; horn-like osis = condition	any horny growth on the skin (e.g., a wart or callus)
laceration (LASS-er-**AY**-shun)	laceration = "process of tearing"	a cut
lesion (LEE-zhun)	lesion = "hurt place"	a wound, injury, or other pathologic change in the skin or other body tissue

Pathologic Conditions	Word Elements	Definition
lipoma (lih-POE-muh)	lip = fat oma = tumor; growth	a benign growth made up of fatty tissue
macule (MACK-yool)	macule = "spot"	a small spot on the skin that is colored or thickened, but not raised (e.g., a petechia or flat nevus)
maculopapular lesion (MACK-yoo-loe-**PAP**-pyoo-ler)	maculo = "spot" papul = "pimple" ar = pertaining to	lesion consisting of both macules and papules
malignant melanoma (MEL-luh-**NO**-muh)	melan = black oma = tumor; growth	malignant tumor of the pigment cells (melanocytes)
nevus (NEE-vuss)	nevus = "birthmark"	pigmented lesion of the skin, such as a mole; occasionally progress to malignant melanoma
papillary carcinoma (**PAP**-pul-LEHR-ee KAR-sih-**NO**-muh)	papill = nipple-like ary = pertaining to carcinoma = malignant epithelial tumor	malignant tumor of epithelial tissue characterized by many finger-like or nipple-like projections
papilloma (PAP-pul-**LOE**-muh)	papill = nipple-like oma = tumor; growth	a benign growth arising from the epithelial cells of the skin; often resembles a wart
papule (PAP-pyool)	papule = "pimple"	small, solid, red, raised area on the skin (e.g., as seen in eczema and measles)
petechia (puh-TEE-kee-uh)	petechia = "skin spot"	a pinpoint hemorrhage under the skin (a small ecchymosis)
pruritus (prer-RYE-tis)	pruritis = "itch thing"	itching
psoriasis (sir-RYE-uh-sis)	psor = itching iasis = condition	chronic skin disease characterized by itchy red patches covered with silvery scales
pustule (PUS-tyool)	pustule = "blister"	a raised, pus-filled vesicle or sac within or just beneath the epidermis
pyoderma (PIE-oh-**DER**-muh)	pyo = pus derma = skin	any of several skin diseases characterized by pus-producing lesions, usually caused by bacterial infection
scabies (SKAY-beez)	scabies = "scratch things"	contagious parasitic infection of the skin characterized by the formation of small, raised, itchy lesions

Pathologic Conditions	Word Elements	Definition
sebaceous cyst (seh-BAY-shus SIST)	seb = sebum aceous = pertaining to cyst = "sac"	a walled collection of sebum arising from a sebaceous gland; the cyst may enlarge as sebum collects and may become infected
seborrhea (SEH-ber-**REE**-uh)	sebo = sebum rrhea = discharge	excessive secretion of sebum by the sebaceous glands
squamous cell carcinoma (SKWOM-us SELL KAR-sih-**NO**-muh)	carcinoma = malignant epithelial tumor	malignant tumor of the squamous epithelial cells
tinea (TIH-nee-uh)	tinea = "a grub, larva, or worm"	contagious fungal infection of the skin causing severe itching; commonly called ringworm
urticaria (ER-tih-**KEHR**-ee-uh)	urticaria = "stinging nettle"	skin reaction characterized by the formation of smooth, raised, itchy patches; commonly called hives
wheal	no word elements	smooth, slightly elevated area that is slightly redder or paler than the surrounding skin; if itchy, wheals are called hives
xeroderma (ZEER-oh-**DER**-muh)	xero = dry derma = skin	dry skin

Diagnostic Procedures	Word Elements	Definition
excisional biopsy (eck-SIH-zhun-null BY-op-see)	ex = out cision = incision al = pertaining to bi = life opsy = view	use of a sharp instrument to remove an entire tumor or lesion plus surrounding normal tissue for examination
exfoliative cytology (eks-FOE-lee-uh-tiv sie-TOL-uh-jee)	ex = out foliative = "leaf; layer" cyto = cell logy = study of	microscopic examination of desquamated (sloughed off) skin cells obtained by aspirating, scraping, or washing a skin lesion
incisional biopsy (in-SIH-zhun-null BY-op-see)	in = in; into cision = incision al = pertaining to bi = life opsy = view	use of a sharp instrument to remove a portion of a tumor or other lesion for examination
needle biopsy (BY-op-see)	bi = life opsy = view	insertion of a hollow needle into the skin to draw off a sample of diseased tissue for examination

Diagnostic Procedures	Word Elements	Definition
punch biopsy (BY-op-see)	bi = life opsy = view	removal of the core of a skin lesion or tumor for examination; generally performed when complete excision of the diseased area is not possible
skin biopsy (BY-op-see)	bi = life opsy = view	removal of skin tissue (usually diseased) for microscopic examination and analysis

Therapeutic Procedures	Word Elements	Definition
abrasion (uh-BRAY-zhun)	abrasion = "scraping"	scraping away of a scarred or diseased area
chemabrasion (KEM-uh-BRAY-zhun)	chem = chemical abrasion = "scraping"	application of chemicals to remove surface layers of scarred or diseased skin cells
cryosurgery (KRIE-oh-SER-jer-ee)	cryo = cold surgery = surgery	use of subfreezing temperature (usually liquid nitrogen) to destroy diseased tissue
debridement (dih-BREED-ment or day-breed-MAWN)	debridement = "to unbridle"	removal of dirt, foreign objects, damaged tissue, or cellular debris from a wound or burn to prevent infection and to promote healing
dermabrasion (DERM-uh-BRAY-zhun)	derm = skin abrasion = "scraping"	use of revolving brushes or sand paper to remove scars or lesions from the skin
electrodesiccation (ih-LECK-troe-DEH-sih-KAY-shun)	electro = electricity desiccation = "process of drying"	use of a high-frequency electrical spark to dehydrate and destroy diseased tissue
irrigation (EER-rih-GAY-shun)	irrigation = "process of carrying water into"	use of water or other fluids to cleanse a skin lesion or deep wound
lipectomy (lih-PECK-tuh-me)	lip = fat ectomy = surgical removal	surgical removal of subcutaneous fat; if suction is used, the procedure is called suction lipectomy or liposuction

Review Exercises

4. *Define* the following terms.

   a. actinic keratosis _____

   b. cellulitis _____

c. hirsutism _____

d. erythema _____

e. wheal _____

f. scabies _____

5. **Match** the following terms with their definitions.

_____ tinea   a. a blackhead

_____ bulla   b. itching

_____ furuncle   c. ringworm

_____ alopecia   d. partial or complete hair loss (baldness)

_____ urticaria   e. group of boils

_____ comedo   f. a boil

_____ carbuncle   g. hives

_____ pruritus   h. a large, fluid-filled blister

_____ nevus   i. mole or other pigmented skin lesion

6. **Circle** the choices below that will make each statement true.

a. A (contusion/laceration) is a cut, while a (contusion/laceration) is an injury without a break in the skin.

b. (Ecchymosis/Petechia) is the technical term for a bruise, while (ecchymosis/petechia) is a pinpoint bruise.

c. A (macule/papule) is a small, colored or thickened, flat spot on the skin, while a (macule/papule) is a small, red, raised area on the skin.

d. (Debridement/Irrigation) is the use of fluids to cleanse a wound, while (debridement/irrigation) is the surgical removal of foreign matter or damaged tissue from a wound.

7. **Break Down and Define** the word elements within each of the following terms, and then define the term itself.

     Example: cryo/ surgery   *cold / surgery*   *cold surgery*

a. dermatitis

_____

b. anhidrosis

_____

c. dermatomycosis

_____

d. melanoma

_____

e. chemabrasion

_____

f. erythroderma

_____

g. seborrhea

_____

h. psoriasis

_____

i. keratosis

_____

j. sebaceous cyst

_____

k. dermabrasion

_____

l. dermatology

_____

m. subcutaneous

_____

n. transdermal

_____

o. intradermal

_____

8. **_Word Building and Spelling_**. Spell out the medical term for each of the following definitions using the slashes provided to separate the word elements.

inflammation of the skin   _dermat_ / _itis_

a. surgical removal of fat   _____ / _____

b. tumor arising from fat   _____ / _____

c. condition characterized by excessive sweating _____ / _____ / _____

d. dry skin _____ / _____

e. fungal infection of the nails _____ / _____

f. destroying or dissolving keratin _____ / _____

g. condition characterized by reduced sweating _____ / _____ / _____

Case Study. Read the case notes below. For each boldfaced term, provide a brief definition and indicate whether the term is spelled correctly; if it is misspelled, provide the correct spelling.

> **leasions:** *pathologic changes of any type in the skin or other tissue*
>
> *Example:*   *Spelled correctly?*   ☐ Yes   ✔ No   *lesions*

Patient presented as an 8-year-old boy with **leasions** on his face, neck, shoulders, arms, and legs. They included a combination of **mackulopapular lesions** and weeping **pustules.** The lesions had progressed from red **makules** on the face to spreading, weeping pustules within a couple of days. Patient had a history of **exzema**, but no other type of **pyoderma** or **dermatitis**. Diagnosis: **impatigo**. Treatment plan: antibiotics, with frequent washing of affected areas; no sharing of linens.

a. mackulopapular lesions: _____

    Spelled correctly?   ☐ Yes   ☐ No _____

b. pustules: _____

    Spelled correctly?   ☐ Yes   ☐ No _____

c. makules: _____

    Spelled correctly?   ☐ Yes   ☐ No _____

d. exzema: _____

    Spelled correctly?   ☐ Yes   ☐ No _____

e. pyoderma: _____

_____

    Spelled correctly?   ☐ Yes   ☐ No _____

f. dermatitis: _____

   Spelled correctly?   ☐ Yes   ☐ No _____

g. impatigo: _____

   _____

   Spelled correctly?   ☐ Yes   ☐ No _____

Listen to the section on your audiotape cassette that corresponds to this chapter and write the terms below. Be careful to spell each term correctly.

1. _____   21. _____

2. _____   22. _____

3. _____   23. _____

4. _____   24. _____

5. _____   25. _____

6. _____   26. _____

7. _____   27. _____

8. _____   28. _____

9. _____   29. _____

10. _____   30. _____

11. _____   31. _____

12. _____   32. _____

13. _____   33. _____

14. _____   34. _____

15. _____   35. _____

16. _____   36. _____

17. _____   37. _____

18. _____   38. _____

19. _____   39. _____

20. _____   40. _____

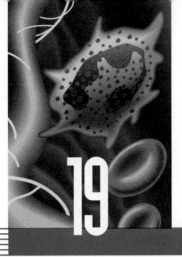

Special Senses: The Eyes

Upon completing this chapter, you should be able to:

- Describe the primary functions of the structures that make up the eyes
- Recognize, build, pronounce, and spell words that pertain to the eyes
- Describe diseases, diagnostic tests, and therapeutic procedures that pertain to the eyes

Overview   The eyes function as the body's organs of sight. Like other sensory organs, the eyes are designed to detect stimuli in the environment and to convey information about these stimuli to the brain. Sensory receptors in the eye respond to light and to shadings of darkness and light. Within each eye, specialized structures use the shadings in reflected light to generate a point-by-point reproduction of objects in the visual field. Vision results from the interaction of these structures with a network of nerve cells that convert light energy into electrical impulses for transmission to the brain. In the brain, the two-dimensional reproductions generated by each eye are integrated to produce a single, three-dimensional image of objects in the environment.

Word Elements

STRUCTURES OF THE EYE – The following combining forms (CF) pertain to the eyes. Some are used to refer to the eye as a whole, while others are used to denote the main structures of the eye.

CF	Meaning	Example
choroid/o	choroid	*choroid*itis = inflammation of the choroid
cili/o	ciliary body	*cili*ectomy = surgical removal of a portion of the ciliary body
cor/o	pupil	*coro*diastasis = dilation of the pupil
corne/o	cornea	*corne*al = pertaining to the cornea
cycl/o	ciliary body	*cyclo*plegia = paralysis of the ciliary body
ir/o	iris	*ir*itis = inflammation of the iris
irid/o	iris	*irido*malacia = softening of the iris
kerat/o	cornea*	*kerat*itis = inflammation of the cornea
ocul/o	eye	*ocul*ar = pertaining to the eyes
ophthalm/o	eye	*ophthalmo*logy = study of the eyes
opt/o	eye	*opto*metry = measurement of the eyes and vision
papill/o	optic disk*	*papill*edema = swelling of the optic disk
phak/o	lens	a*phak*ia = absence of the lens
pupill/o	pupil	*pupill*ary = pertaining to the pupil
retin/o	retina	*retino*pathy = any disease of the retina
scler/o	sclera	*scler*itis = inflammation of the sclera
uve/o	uvea	*uve*itis = inflammation of the uvea
vitre/o	glass	*vitre*ous = glass-like substance

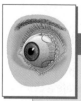

ACCESSORY STRUCTURES – These combining forms refer to accessory structures that support or protect the eyes.

CF	Meaning	Example
blephar/o	eyelids	*blepharo*spasm = twitching of the eyelid
conjunctiv/o	conjunctiva	*conjunctiv*itis = inflammation of the conjunctiva
dacry/o	tear duct	*dacry*oma = swelling of a blocked tear duct
lacrim/o	tear	*lacrim*al = pertaining to tears

*NOTE: Depending on the context, papill/o can also refer to tiny protrusions in other parts of the body, including the skin, the tongue, and the kidney. Similarly, kerat/o can also refer to hard or horn-like substances, such as those found on the skin (see Chapter 18).

CONDITIONS AFFECTING THE EYE — These combining forms pertain to conditions that affect the eyes, especially their visual functioning.

CF	Meaning	Example
ambly/o	dull; dim	*ambly*opia = dulled vision
phot/o	light	*photo*sensitivity = sensitivity to light
scot/o	darkness	*scot*oma = area of darkness in the visual field
xer/o	dry	*xer*ophthalmia = dryness of the conjunctiva

SUFFIXES — The following suffixes pertain to vision. They are generally used in terms having to do with vision abnormalities.

Suffix	Meaning	Example
-opia	vision	ambly*opia* = dulled vision
-opsia	vision	heter*opsia* = unequal vision in the two eyes

Anatomy and Physiology

ocul/o, ophthalm/o, and opt/o = eye

The adult human eyes are globe-shaped structures, each approximately one inch in diameter. Both eyes are set in bony sockets, called **orbits**, in the skull. Each eye consists of layers of specialized tissue surrounding two liquid-filled cavities. The main structures of the eye are illustrated in Figure 19-1 and described in the paragraphs below.

The Sclera

scler/o = sclera

The white outer layer of the eyeball is called the **sclera** (SKLEHR-uh). Composed of collagen and other connective tissue, the sclera forms a tough outer surface that protects the inner structures of the eye from injury. At the front of the eye, the sclera forms a transparent, domed structure called the **cornea** (KOR-nee-uh). The cornea has a curved surface that serves to focus light coming into the eye. In addition, the cornea protects the front portion of the eye from injury.

corne/o and kerat/o = cornea

The Uvea

uve/o = uvea

Lying immediately below the sclera is the vascular layer of the eye, which is called the **uvea** (YOO-vee-uh). In addition to supplying blood to muscles and nerves within the eye, the pigmented tissues of the uvea also give the eyes their color. Three structures make up the uvea: the choroid, the ciliary body, and the iris.

Figure 19-1: *The eye.*

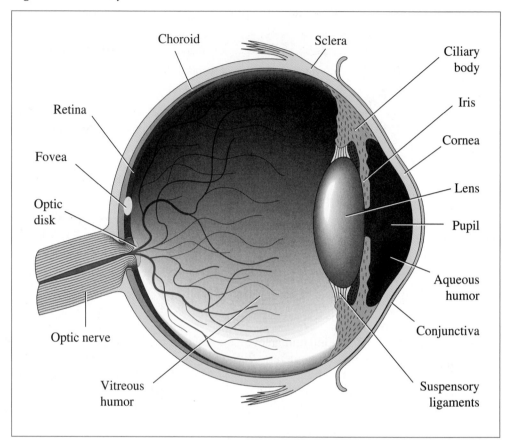

choroid/o = choroid

The **choroid** (KOR-oyd) is a layer of darkly pigmented tissue that lies just below the sclera. In addition to housing the many tiny blood vessels that deliver nutrients to tissues throughout the eye, the dark surface of the choroid also acts to absorb light within the eye. This prevents the blurring of visual images by light present within the eye.

cycl/o and cili/o = ciliary body

Just below the junction of the sclera and cornea, the choroid becomes thicker, forming a structure known as the **ciliary** (**SILL**-ee-EHR-ee) **body**. As you will see below, smooth muscles that are embedded in the ciliary body adjust the shape of the lens to enable the eye to focus on objects at varying distances.

ir/o and irid/o = iris

pupill/o and cor/o = pupil

Another extension of the choroid is the **iris**, a ring of pigmented tissue that protrudes into the cavity of the eye. The pigmentation of the iris is what determines eye color. The opening in the center of the iris is called the **pupil**. By regulating the size of the pupil, tiny muscles in the iris control the amount of light entering the eye. In bright light, muscles in the iris contract, causing the pupils to shrink. In dimmer light, these muscles relax, causing the pupils to dilate. Contraction of the pupils is referred to as **miosis** (my-OH-sis), while dilation of the pupils is called **mydriasis** (mih-DRY-uh-sis). In healthy individuals, both pupils are roughly the same size.

mi/o = less; smaller
mydr/o = widen; enlarge

Refractory Media

Light entering the eye passes through several liquid and solid structures that refract (bend) the light rays slightly, bringing them into sharper focus. These refractory structures include the crystalline lens and the fluids that fill the internal chambers of the eyeball.

phak/o = lens

The crystalline **lens** is suspended from the ciliary body just behind the pupil. The lens is a transparent, elastic disk which is attached to the ciliary body by tiny fibers called **suspensory ligaments**. When the eye is focusing on closer objects, muscles in the ciliary body cause the lens to take on a roughly spherical shape. To focus on more distant objects, ciliary muscles flatten the lens slightly. The process by which the ciliary body adjusts the curvature of the lens, allowing it to focus on nearer or more distant objects, is called **accommodation**. Age-related changes in the efficiency of this process are the reason most older people require glasses for near vision.

aque/o = water
vitre/o = glass
humor = liquid

The lens and the suspensory ligaments divide the inner eyeball cavity into two chambers. The chamber between the cornea and the lens is filled with a watery fluid called the **aqueous** (AY-kwee-us) **humor**. The chamber behind the lens is filled with a more gelatinous fluid called the **vitreous** (VIH-tree-us) **humor**. In addition to its refractory function, the vitreous humor maintains pressure within the eyeball, preventing it from collapsing inward.

The Retina

retin/o = retina

Light-sensitive receptor cells in the eye are located in the **retina** (REH-tih-nuh), a thin layer of tissue located on the inner surface of the choroid. Based on their microscopic appearance, retinal cells are classified as **rods** and **cones**. Rods, which are most concentrated on the periphery of the retina, detect shades of gray at all levels of light. Cones, which are found mainly in the central area of the retina, detect color but operate only at high light levels. Both rods and cones contain light-sensitive molecules called **photopigments** (FOE-toe-**PIG**-ments) that are capable of converting light energy into an electrical impulse that can be transmitted to the brain for interpretation. Although rods are far more numerous than cones, cones generally detect visual stimuli with greater precision. Thus, maximal visual acuity occurs in a cone-rich area of the retina known as the **fovea** (FOE-vee-uh).

phot/o = light

fove/o = fovea

The Optic Nerve

papill/o = optic disk

Nerve fibers (and blood vessels) enter and leave the retina through an area called the **optic disk**. Because the optic disk has no rods or cones, it is also referred to as the **blind spot**. Beyond the optic disk, fibers from each eye join to form the **optic nerve**. The optic nerve carries impulses from the retina to areas of the brain that are responsible for processing visual information.

Supporting Structures

blephar/o = eyelids

Although not directly involved in vision, other structures help protect the eye from injury. The **eyelids**, for example, are folds of skin that protect the eyeball from physical trauma by closing reflexively in response to any sudden movement toward the eye. Additional protection is provided by the **eyelashes**, two or three rows of fine hairs which curve outward from the front edge of each eyelid.

conjunctiv/o = conjunctiva

The inside of each eyelid is lined by a thin, usually transparent membrane known as the **conjunctiva** (KON-junk-**TIE**-vuh), which also extends over the white of the eye. Irritation of the conjunctiva by dust or smoke can cause blood vessels in the membrane to swell, producing the condition commonly known as "bloodshot eyes."

Figure 19-2:
Supporting structures of the eye.

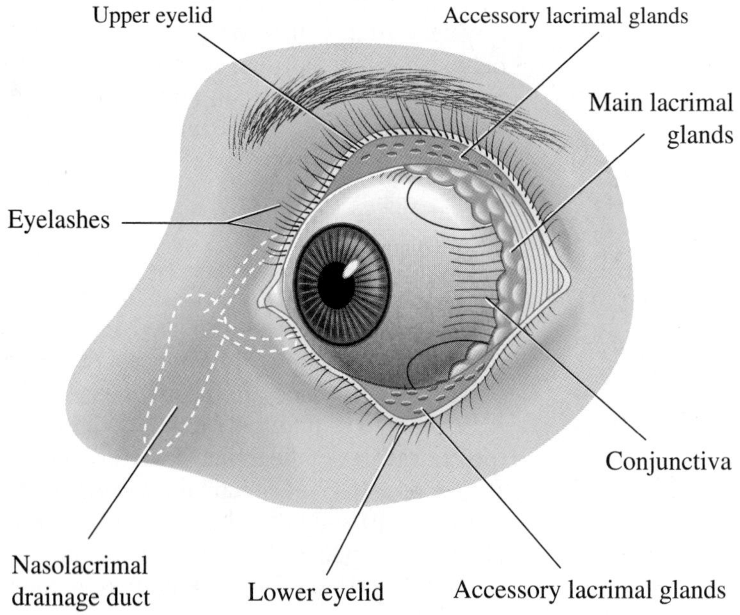

Upper eyelid

Accessory lacrimal glands

Main lacrimal glands

Eyelashes

Conjunctiva

Nasolacrimal drainage duct

Lower eyelid

Accessory lacrimal glands

lacrim/o = tear
dacry/o = tear duct

Closely associated with the conjunctiva is the **lacrimal** (LACK-rih-mul) **apparatus**, the glandular system that produces and drains tears. The main lacrimal glands secrete tears during crying and when the eye is injured. The accessory glands, which lie within the conjunctiva, constantly produce a smaller volume of tears, lubricating the conjunctiva and the cornea with each blink of the eyes. Once produced, tears collect at the edges of the eyes, where they pass through **nasolacrimal** (NAY-zoe-**LACK**-rih-mul) **drainage ducts** into the nose.

nas/o = nose

Review Exercises

1. **Match** the following combining forms with their definitions.

_____	irid/o	a.	optic disk
_____	blephar/o	b.	cornea
_____	choroid/o	c.	choroid
_____	ophthalm/o	d.	ciliary body
_____	kerat/o	e.	eyelids
_____	papill/o	f.	iris
_____	pupill/o	g.	pupil
_____	cili/o	h.	eye

2. **Define** the following suffixes and combining forms.

a. uve/o _____

b. ocul/o _____

c. cor/o _____

d. corne/o _____

e. -opia _____

f. opt/o _____

g. ir/o _____

h. phak/o _____

i. conjunctiv/o _____

j. -opsia _____

k. vitre/o _____

l. xer/o _____

3. **Spell** the combining forms that have the following meanings.

a. tear   _____

b. retina   _____

c. light   _____

d. darkness   _____

e. dull; dim   _____

f. ciliary body   _____

g. sclera   _____

h. tear duct   _____

4. **Match** the following structures with their descriptions.

_____ choroid

_____ optic disc

_____ lens

_____ retina

_____ sclera

_____ ciliary body

_____ vitreous humor

_____ iris

a. tough, white outer layer of eyeball

b. layer of darkly pigmented tissue that contains blood vessels supplying the eye

c. transparent, elastic disk suspended just behind the pupil

d. ring of pigmented tissue that controls the amount of light entering the eye

e. gelatinous fluid that maintains pressure within the eyeball

f. area through which blood vessels and nerve fibers leave the retina

g. choroid structure containing muscles responsible for adjusting the curvature of the lens

h. thin layer of tissue that contains light-sensitive rods and cones

Terminology

The following are selected terms that pertain to pathology of the eyes and to related diagnostic and therapeutic procedures. As you will see, most of the disorders listed result from structural abnormalities that interfere with the ability of the eye to detect or refract light. Keeping this in mind will help you to understand other terms you may hear as well as the rationale behind treatment of visual disorders.

Pathologic Conditions	Word Elements	Definition
achromatopsia (ay-KROE-muh-**TOP**-see-uh)	a = without; not chromat = color opsia = vision	color blindness

Pathologic Conditions	Word Elements	Definition
amblyopia (AM-blee-**OH**-pee-uh)	ambly = dim; dull opia = vision	reduced or dulled vision
ametropia (AM-eh-**TROE**-pee-uh)	a = not; without metr = measure opia = vision	general term for any error of refraction in which light is not properly focused on the retina
anisocoria (an-EYE-so-**KOR**-ee-uh)	aniso = unequal cor = pupil ia = condition	inequality in the size of the pupils; often a sign of neurologic disease
astigmatism (uh-**STIG**-muh-**TIZ**-um)	a = not; without stigmat = point ism = condition	refractive disorder in which excessive curvature of the cornea or lens causes light to be scattered over the retina rather than focused on a single point
blepharoptosis (BLEF-er-oh-**TOE**-sis)	blepharo = eyelids ptosis = drooping	drooping of the upper eyelid; often called ptosis for short
cataract (KAT-er-act)	cataract = "waterfall"	condition in which the crystalline lens becomes cloudy or opaque as a result of protein deposits on its surface
conjunctivitis (kun-JUNK-tih-**VIE**-tis)	conjunctiv = conjunctiva itis = inflammation	inflammation of the conjunctiva, usually due to infection or allergy; also called pink-eye
dacryocystitis (DACK-ree-oh-sih-**STIE**-tis)	dacryo = tear duct cyst = sac itis = inflammation	inflammation or swelling of a lacrimal duct, usually as a result of a blockage
diabetic retinopathy (DIE-uh-**BEH**-tick REH-tih-**NOP**-uh-thee)	retino = retina pathy = disease	damage to the retina resulting from vascular abnormalities in the eyes of patients with diabetes; leading cause of blindness in adults
diplopia (dih-PLOE-pee-uh)	dipl = double opia = vision	double vision
glaucoma (glaw-KOE-muh)	glauc = gray oma = tumor; growth	condition in which intraocular pressure increases, potentially causing damage to the retina and/or optic nerve and irreversible loss of vision
hemianopia (HEH-me-uh-**NO**-pee-uh)	hemi = half an = not; without opia = vision	blindness in one half of the visual field
hyperopia (HI-per-**OH**-pee-uh)	hyper = excessive opia = vision	farsightedness; refractive disorder in which light is focused on a point behind the retina

Pathologic Conditions	Word Elements	Definition
keratitis (KEHR-uh-**TIE**-tis)	kerat = cornea itis = inflammation	inflammation of the cornea, usually due to infection or other type of damage
myopia (my-OH-pee-uh)	my = "to shut; squint" opia = vision	nearsightedness; refractive disorder in which light is focused on a point in front of the retina
nyctalopia (NICK-tull-**LOE**-pee-uh)	nyct = night al = blindness opia = vision	night blindness; reduced vision in dim light or at night, often as a result of vitamin A deficiency
nystagmus (nih-STAG-muss)	nystagmus = "to nod"	constant rhythmic oscillation (movement back and forth) of the eyeball
papilledema (PAP-ul-eh-**DEE**-muh)	papill = optic disk edema = swelling	swelling of the optic disk; often a sign of dangerously high pressure within the skull; also called "choked disk"
presbyopia (PREZ-bee-**OH**-pee-uh)	presby = old age opia = vision	reduced ability of the eye to focus on nearby objects due to age-related reductions in the elasticity of the crystalline lens
retinal detachment (REH-tin-ul)	retin = retina al = pertaining to	separation of the retina from the choroid; usually occurs as a result of trauma or disease
retinitis pigmentosa (REH-tih-**NIE**-tis PIG-men-TOE-suh)	retin = retina itis = inflammation pigment = pigment osa = condition	hereditary disease involving progressive degeneration of the rods and cones of the retina; initial night blindness and loss of peripheral vision gradually progress to total blindness
retinopathy (REH-tin-**NOP**-uh-thee)	retino = retina pathy = disease	general term for any disease of the retina
scleritis (skler-EYE-tis)	scler = sclera itis = inflammation	inflammation of the sclera; usually occurs in conjunction with rheumatoid arthritis and other collagen diseases
scotoma (skoe-TOE-muh)	scot = darkness oma = tumor; growth	an area of darkness in an otherwise normal field of vision; usually results from localized damage to the retina or optic nerve
strabismus (struh-BIZ-muss)	stabismus = "squinting"	any disorder in which both eyes cannot focus on the same point; also called lazy eye or dysconjugate gaze
stye (STY)	stye = "to rise"	inflammation of a gland within the eyelid

Pathologic Conditions	Word Elements	Definition
uveitis (YOO-vee-**EYE**-tis)	uve = uvea itis = inflammation	inflammation of the iris, ciliary body, and/or choroid, often as a result of an autoimmune reaction
xerophthalmia (ZEER-off-**THAL**-me-uh)	xer = dry ophthalm = eye ia = condition	dryness of the conjunctiva, often as a result of vitamin A deficiency

Diagnostic Procedures	Word Elements	Definition
fundoscopy (fun-DOS-kuh-pee)	fundo = hollow interior scopy = visual examination	use of a funduscope (ophthalmoscope) to examine the innermost structures of the eye, particularly the blood vessels supplying the retina and the optic disk
gonioscopy (GO-nee-**OS**-kuh-pee)	gonio = angle scopy = visual examination	measurement of the angle of the anterior chamber of the eye; used to monitor the drainage of aqueous humor from the eye in patients at risk for glaucoma
ophthalmoscopy (OFF-thul-**MOS**-kuh-pee)	ophthalmo = eye scopy = visual examination	visual examination of the interior of the eye using an ophthalmoscope
retinoscopy (REH-tih-**NOS**-kuh-pee)	retino = retina scopy = visual examination	technique in which a beam of light is shone on the retina to determine if errors of refraction occur
Snellen's chart (SNELL-unz)	no word elements	standard test of visual acuity in which a subject is asked to read letters and numbers on a chart 20 feet away; also called an "E" chart
tonometry (tuh-NOM-eh-tree)	tono = tension; pressure metry = measurement	measurement of pressure within the eye; used to detect glaucoma

Therapeutic Procedures	Word Elements	Definition
cataract surgery	cataract = "waterfall"	procedure in which an opaque or clouded lens is removed and an artificial lens is inserted in its place
iridectomy (EER-ih-**DECK**-tuh-me)	irid = iris ectomy = surgical removal	surgical removal of a portion of the iris, usually to create an opening through which aqueous humor can drain (to relieve pressure in patients with glaucoma)
keratoplasty (**KEHR**-uh-toe-PLASS-tee)	kerato = cornea plasty = surgical repair	procedure in which an opaque section of the cornea is replaced with normal tissue; also called a corneal transplant

Therapeutic Procedures	Word Elements	Definition
orthoptic training (or-THOP-tick)	orth = straight opt = eye ic = pertaining to	exercise program designed to restore normal coordination to the eye muscles in patients with strabismus
radial keratotomy (RAY-dee-ul KEHR-uh-**TOT**-uh-me)	radial = "extending out from the center" kerato = cornea tomy = surgical incision	procedure in which a series of shallow, spoke-like incisions are made to flatten the cornea, correcting an error of refraction commonly associated with nearsightedness

Review Exercises

5. ***Break Down and Define*** the word elements within each of the following terms, and then define the term itself.

      Example: scler/ itis   *sclera / inflammation*   *inflammation of the sclera*

a. nyctalopia

_____

b. fundoscopy

_____

c. amblyopia

_____

d. xerophthalmia

_____

e. hemianopia

_____

f. anisocoria

_____

g. tonometry

_____

h. blepharoptosis

_____

i. ametropia

_____

j. astigmatism

_____

k. achromatopsia

_____

l. dacryocystitis

_____

m. gonioscopy

_____

6. **_Choose and Construct._** Choose the appropriate word elements from the list provided to construct terms for the following.

hyper-	kerat/o	-itis	-tomy
dipl/o	ophthalm/o	-logy	cycl/o
irid/o	-ectomy	-opia	-scopy

    inflammation of the cornea   _kerat / itis_

a. surgical incision in the cornea   _____ / _____

b. study of the eyes   _____ / _____

c. surgical removal of the iris   _____ / _____

d. surgical incision in the iris   _____ / _____

e. inflammation of the iris and ciliary body   _____ / _____ / _____

f. visual examination of the eyes   _____ / _____

g. double vision   _____ / _____

h. excessive vision (farsightedness)   _____ / _____

7. **_Word Building and Spelling._** Spell out the medical term for each of the following definitions using the slashes provided to separate the word elements.

    any disease of the retina   _retino / pathy_

a. inflammation of the cornea   _____ / _____

b. surgical incision into the cornea   _____ / _____

c. inflammation of the conjunctiva   _____ / _____

d. poor vision in old age   _____ / _____

e. inflammation of the uvea   _____ / _____

f. swelling of the optic disk   _____ / _____

g. any disease of the retina   _____ / _____

h. inflammation of the sclera   _____ / _____

8. **Match** the following terms with their definitions.

_____ nystagmus	a. constant rhythmic oscillation of the eyeball
_____ keratoplasty	b. hereditary condition in which degeneration of the retina results in gradually diminishing vision
_____ myopia	
_____ glaucoma	c. separation of the retina from the choroid
_____ retinitis pigmentosa	d. condition characterized by increased pressure within the eye
_____ scotoma	e. nearsightedness
_____ stye	f. inflammation of a gland in the eyelid
_____ diabetic retinopathy	g. corneal transplant
_____ cataract	h. damage to the retina resulting from vascular abnormalities in individuals with diabetes
_____ retinal detachment	i. area of darkness in an otherwise normal visual field
_____ retinoscopy	j. technique in which a light is shone on the retina to determine whether errors of refraction occur
	k. condition in which the lens becomes clouded or opaque

Case Study. Read the case notes below. For each boldfaced term, provide a brief definition and indicate whether the term is spelled correctly; if it is misspelled, provide the correct spelling.

Example:

dipplopia: *double vision*

Spelled correctly? ☐ Yes ☑ No *diplopia*

Patient presented as a 4-year-old girl with **dipplopia**. On examination, convergent **strabizmus** was immediately obvious. Motion of the left eye was limited, and **ambliopia** of this eye was evident on testing with the **Snelen's chart**. Testing also revealed **hyperopia**, a probable contributing factor to the strabizmus. There was no evidence of retinal or optic nerve pathology on **opthalmoscopy** or **retinascopy**. Treatment plan: corrective glasses, **orthoptic training**; follow-up through age 10.

a. strabizmus: _____

_____

Spelled correctly? ☐ Yes ☐ No _____

b. ambliopia: _____

Spelled correctly? ☐ Yes ☐ No _____

c. Snelen's chart: _____

_____

Spelled correctly? ☐ Yes ☐ No _____

d. hyperopia: _____

_____

Spelled correctly? ☐ Yes ☐ No _____

e. opthalmoscopy: _____

_____

Spelled correctly? ☐ Yes ☐ No _____

f. retinascopy: _____

_____

Spelled correctly? ☐ Yes ☐ No _____

g. orthoptic training: _____

_____

Spelled correctly? ☐ Yes ☐ No _____

Listen to the section on your audiotape cassette that corresponds to this chapter and write the terms below. Be careful to spell each term correctly.

1. _____   4. _____

2. _____   5. _____

3. _____   6. _____

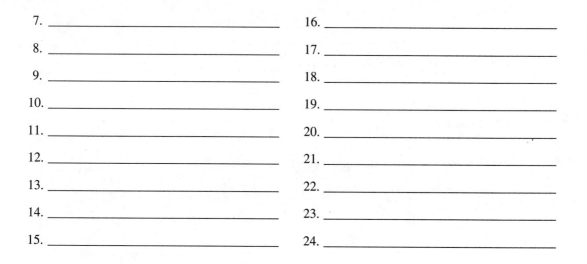

7. _____

8. _____

9. _____

10. _____

11. _____

12. _____

13. _____

14. _____

15. _____

16. _____

17. _____

18. _____

19. _____

20. _____

21. _____

22. _____

23. _____

24. _____

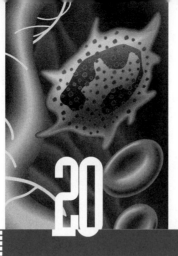

Special Senses: The Ears

Upon completing this chapter, you should be able to:

- Describe the primary functions of the structures that make up the ears
- Recognize, build, pronounce, and spell words that pertain to the ears
- Describe diseases, diagnostic tests, and surgical procedures that pertain to the ears

Overview   The ears function as the body's organs of hearing and equilibrium. Sound energy is transmitted through the environment in the form of pressure waves of varying intensity. For hearing to occur, specialized structures within the ears must convert the energy in sound waves into electrical signals that can be transmitted to and interpreted by the brain. In addition to detecting auditory stimuli in the environment, the ears also contain specialized structures that monitor the position of the body in space, maintaining a sense of balance and equilibrium despite changes in the position of the body.

Word Elements

STRUCTURES OF THE EAR – The following combining forms (CF) pertain to the ears. They are used to refer to the ear as a whole or to the structures that make up the ear.

CF	Meaning	Example
aur/o	external ear	*aur*al = pertaining to the ear
cochle/o	cochlea	*cochle*ar = pertaining to the cochlea
labyrinth/o	inner ear	*labyrinth*itis = inflammation of the inner ear
mastoid/o	mastoid process	*mastoid*ectomy = surgical removal of the mastoid process
myring/o	eardrum	*myring*otomy = surgical incision in the eardrum
ot/o	ear	*oto*scopy = visual examination of the ear
staped/o	stapes	*staped*ectomy = surgical replacement of the stapes
tympan/o	eardrum	*tympan*ostomy = placement of a tube into the eardrum
vestibul/o	vestibular apparatus	*vestibulo*tomy = surgical incision into the vestibular apparatus

SOUND AND HEARING – These combining forms refer to sound and hearing. As you might expect, they are used in terms pertaining to function and assessment.

CF	Meaning	Example
acoust/o	sound	*acoust*ic = pertaining to sound or the perception of sound
audi/o	hearing	*audio*metry = measurement of hearing

SUFFIXES – The following suffixes pertain to the ears. They are generally used to refer to pathologic conditions, either anatomic or functional.

Suffix	Meaning	Example
-cusis	hearing	ana*cusis* = complete hearing loss
-otia	condition of the ear	macr*otia* = unusually large ears

Anatomy and Physiology

ot/o = ear
mastoid/o = mastoid process
temporal = near the temple

In addition to their fleshy external appendages, the ears are made up of a series of intricate membranes and bony structures nestled within the **mastoid** (MASS-toyd) **process**, a honeycomb-like extension of the **temporal** (TEM-per-ul) **bone** of the skull. Each ear has three main subdivisions: the outer ear, which conducts sound waves by displacement of air; the middle ear, which conducts the sound through a series of small bones; and the inner ear, which conducts the sound through liquid and transforms its energy into an electrical impulse that can be transmitted to the brain. The divisions of the ear are illustrated in Figure 20-1 and described in the paragraphs below.

The Outer Ear

aur/o = external ear

The outermost structure of the ear is the visible portion, which is called the **auricle** (OR-ih-kull) or **pinna** (PIN-uh). The auricles are composed of folds of cartilage, covered with skin that produces a waxy yellow substance called **cerumen** (ser-ROO-men). Cerumen functions as a filter for the outer ear, trapping dust and other foreign substances and preventing them from entering internal structures. As a result of their broad, indented shape, the

Figure 20-1: *The ear.*

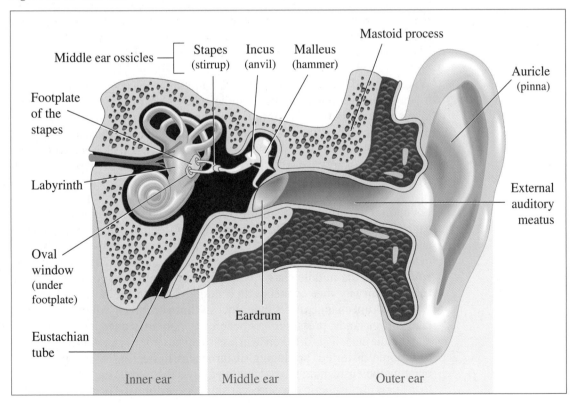

auricles act as highly effective receivers, intercepting sound waves from many different directions and channeling them toward the inner structures of the ear.

audi/o = hearing
acoust/o = sound
tympan/o and myring/o
= eardrum

Sound waves that are picked up by the auricles enter the ear by way of the **external auditory meatus** (**A**W-dih-TOR-ee me-AY-tuss), a tubular structure also known as the **acoustic** (uh-KOOS-tick) **meatus** or **external ear canal**. The external auditory meatus ends at the **tympanic** (tim-PAN-ick) **membrane**, a thin, circular membrane stretched across the end of the canal. This membrane is the structure commonly referred to as the **eardrum**. When sound waves reach the end of the external auditory meatus, they push against the eardrum, causing it to vibrate. The strength of the vibration in the eardrum depends on the force of the air molecules hitting it, which in turn depends on the loudness of the sound being transmitted.

The Middle Ear

The middle ear extends from the tympanic membrane to the **oval window**, the membrane-covered opening to the inner ear. Between the tympanic membrane and the oval window are a series of three tiny bones named for their characteristic shapes: the **malleus** (MAL-lee-us), or "hammer;" the **incus** (ING-kus) or "anvil;" and the **stapes** (STAY-peez) or "stirrup." These three bones are known collectively as the **ossicles** (OS-ih-kulls).

staped/o = stapes
ossicle = "little bone"

When a sound wave causes the eardrum to vibrate, its energy is transferred to the movable bones of the middle ear. In a manner similar to the displacement of the eardrum by airborne sound waves, the resulting movement of the ossicles displaces the footplate of the stapes, causing it to press against the oval window. Also as in the case of the eardrum, the amount of pressure exerted on the oval window by the stapes depends on the frequency and intensity of the incoming sound.

For auditory stimuli to be faithfully reproduced, pressure within the middle ear must be maintained at a level approximately equal to that in the external auditory meatus. Because it is exposed to the external environment, the outer ear is always at atmospheric pressure. Atmospheric pressure is conveyed to the middle ear by way of the **eustachian** (yoo-STAY-shun) **tube**, an airway that connects the middle ear with the nose and throat. During abrupt changes in altitude, such as those occurring when an airplane takes off or lands, pressure may become temporarily unequal in the outer and middle ears. This difference in pressure causes the tympanic membrane to become distorted, producing disturbances in hearing and/or pain. By opening the eustachian tube, yawning allows the middle ear to equilibrate to the new atmospheric pressure, causing the eardrum to "pop" back into its normal position.

Figure 20-2:
Structures of the inner ear.

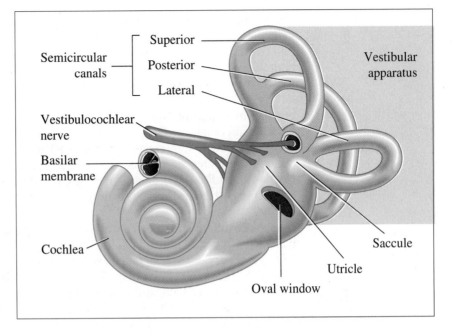

The Inner Ear

labyrinth/o = inner ear

cochle/o = cochlea

vestibul/o = vestibular apparatus

The Inner Ear

The inner ear consists of a series of fluid-filled passages known collectively as the labyrinth (LAB-er-rinth). The structures that make up the labyrinth are illustrated in Figure 20-2. The front portion, called the **cochlea** (KOCK-lee-uh or KOKE-lee-uh), is the part of the inner ear involved in hearing. The rear portion, called the **vestibular** (veh-STIH-byoo-ler) **apparatus**, is the part of the inner ear involved in the maintenance of equilibrium and balance.

Structurally, the cochlea is a long, tightly wound tube that looks somewhat like a snail's shell. The interior of the cochlea is divided lengthwise by a structure known as the **basilar** (BAZ-ull-ler) **membrane**. Embedded in the basilar membrane are the receptive cells of the inner ear, which are known as **hair cells** because of their tiny hairlike projections. Hair cells extend from the basilar membrane, toward a second membrane known as the **tectorial** (teck-TOR-ee-ul) **membrane**. Together, the basilar membrane, hair cells, and tectorial membrane are known as the **organ of Corti** (KOR-tee).

Sound waves enter the inner ear by way of the oval window. As the oval window is displaced by the motion of the stapes, it generates a tiny wave within the fluid of the cochlea. This wave, in turn, causes a portion of the basilar membrane to vibrate. Hair cells embedded in the membrane "ride" this wave, and are moved closer to the tectorial membrane. If the deflection is strong enough to cause contact between the hair cells and the tectorial membrane, the brushing action generates an electrical signal within the hair cells. Tones of different frequencies cause different portions of the basilar membrane to vibrate and different hair cells to be stimulated. The strength, pattern, and site of initiation of the resulting electrical signal all provide information to the brain about the nature of the incoming sound.

Similar mechanisms are used by the vestibular apparatus to generate information about the body's position in space. The vestibular apparatus consists of three **semicircular** (SEH-me-**SIR**-kyoo-ler) **canals** and two bulging structures known as the **saccule** (SACK-yool) and the **utricle** (YOO-trih-kull). All of these structures are filled with a specialized fluid called the **endolymph** (EN-doe-limf).

semi- = half

endo- = within

Like the basilar membrane, the walls of the semicircular canals contain tiny hair cells. When the head moves, fluid within the canals stimulates these cells, causing them to generate an electrical signal. The speed and magnitude of the movement are reflected in the degree of bending in the hair cells and the number of cells stimulated. Because they are positioned at right angles to one another, the semicircular canals can detect motion of the head in all three dimensions. The saccule and utricle use similar mechanisms to generate information about the position of the body in relation to the force of gravity. Both structures contain tiny stones known as **otoliths** (OH-toe-liths). If the position of the head changes with respect to gravity, these tiny stones begin to roll, stimulating hair cells in their path.

The Vestibulocochlear Nerve

Impulses generated by the hair cells in the inner ear and vestibular apparatus are conveyed to the brain by way of the **vestibulocochlear** (veh-STIH-byoo-loe-**KOCK**-lee-er) **nerve**, which is also called the **eighth cranial** (KRAY-nee-ul) **nerve** or, less commonly, the **auditory nerve**. In the brain, differences in the pattern or strength of signals from the individual ears are used to localize sound in space. Similarly, the structures of the vestibular apparatus provide the information that the brain uses to generate reflex responses to falling or other sudden changes in the body's position. This information is also used to coordinate the activity of muscles in the eyes, allowing the eyes to remain focused despite movement of the head.

Review Exercises

1. **Match** the following combining forms with their definitions.

   _____ tympan/o   a. inner ear

   _____ cochle/o   b. sound

   _____ acoust/o   c. stapes

   _____ staped/o   d. cochlea

   _____ ot/o   e. ear

   _____ labyrinth/o   f. eardrum

2. **Match** the following structures with their descriptions.

   _____ cerumen

   _____ endolymph

   _____ utricle

   _____ eustachian tube

   _____ auricle

   _____ external auditory
   meatus

   _____ basilar
   membrane

   _____ tympanic
   membrane

   a. membrane extending the length of the cochlea in which hair cells are embedded

   b. visible portion of the ear, also called the pinna

   c. thin, circular membrane that stretches across the end of the external auditory meatus

   d. one of the vestibular structures; contains otoliths that detect the direction of gravity

   e. waxy substance produced in the outer ear

   f. specialized fluid found in structures of the inner ear

   g. passageway between the outer and middle ear

   h. tubular airway that connects the middle ear with the nose and throat

3. **Define** the following suffixes and combining forms.

   a. mastoid/o   _____

   b. -otia   _____

   c. audi/o   _____

   d. vestibul/o   _____

   e. -cusis   _____

   f. myring/o   _____

   g. aur/o   _____

Terminology

The following are selected terms that pertain to pathology of the ears and to related diagnostic and surgical procedures. As you will see, most of the disorders listed result from inflammation or from structural changes that diminish the ability of the ear to detect or transmit sound. Keeping this in mind will help you to understand other terms you may hear as well as the rationale behind treatment of auditory and vestibular disorders.

Pathologic Conditions	Word Elements	Definition
anacusis (AN-nuh-**KYOO**-sis)	ana = without; not cusis = hearing	complete hearing loss; total deafness
conductive hearing loss (kun-DUCK-tiv)	no word elements	hearing loss due to an impairment in the transmission of sound because of damage to the eardrum or ossicles or obstruction of the ear canal
labyrinthitis (LAB-er-rin-**THIE**-tis)	labyrinth = inner ear itis = inflammation	inflammation of the inner ear, usually due to viral infection
mastoiditis (MASS-toyd-**EYE**-tis)	mastoid = mastoid process itis = inflammation	inflammation of the air cells of the mastoid process, usually as a result of bacterial infection
Meniere's disease (MAY-nee-**EHRZ**)	no word elements	rare disorder characterized by progressive deafness, vertigo, and tinnitus, possibly due to swelling of membranous structures within the labyrinth
myringitis (MEER-in-**JIE**-tis)	myring = eardrum itis = inflammation	inflammation of the eardrum
otitis externa (oh-TIE-tis eck-STER-nuh)	ot = ear itis = inflammation externa = outer	inflammation of the external auditory meatus and/or auricle, usually as a result of bacterial infection; also called swimmer's ear
otitis media (oh-TIE-tis ME-dee-uh)	ot = ear itis = inflammation media = middle	inflammation of the middle ear, usually as a result of bacterial infection; most commonly seen in young children
otodynia (OH-toe-**DIE**-nyuh)	oto = ear dynia = pain	pain in the ear; earache; also called otalgia (oh-TAL-jyuh)
otomycosis (OH-toe-my-**KOE**-sis)	oto = ear mycosis = fungal infection	fungal infection of the external auditory meatus
otopathy (oh-TOP-uh-thee)	oto = ear pathy = disease	general term for any disease of the ear

Pathologic Conditions	Word Elements	Definition
otopyorrhea (OH-toe-pie-er-**REE**-uh)	oto = ear pyo = pus rrhea = discharge	discharge of pus from the ear, usually as a result of recurrent otitis media and perforation of the eardrum
otosclerosis (OH-toe-skler-**OH**-sis)	oto = ear sclerosis = hardening	hereditary disorder in which hardening of the bone around the oval window impedes movement of the stapes; most common form of conductive hearing loss; ultimately leads to deafness
presbycusis (PREZ-bee-**KYOO**-sis)	presby = old age cusis = hearing	loss of hearing with age due to degeneration of hair cells in the organ of Corti; most common form of sensorineural hearing loss
sensorineural hearing loss (SEN-ser-ree-**NYER**-rull)	sensori = sensation neur = nerve al = pertaining to	hearing loss due to an impairment in the transmission of sound from the inner ear to the brain, usually involving damage to inner ear structures (usually the cochlea) or to the auditory nerve
tinnitus (tih-NIE-tuss or TIH-nih-tuss)	tinnitus = "tinkling"	subjective sensation of ringing or tinkling sounds in the ear; usually results from damage to inner ear structures associated with hearing
vertigo (VER-tih-go)	vertigo = "turning around"	subjective sensation that either the self or the surroundings are spinning; usually results from damage to inner ear structures associated with balance and equilibrium

Diagnostic Procedures	Word Elements	Definition
audiometry (AW-dee-**OM**-eh-tree)	audio = hearing metry = measurement	measurement of a patient's ability to detect tones of different frequencies that are transmitted through a headset
otoscopy (oh-TOS-kuh-pee)	oto = ear scopy = visual examination	visual examination of the ear (especially the eardrum) using an otoscope
pneumatic otoscopy (noo-MAT-ick oh-TOS-kuh-pee)	pneum = air atic = pertaining to oto = ear scopy = visual examination	procedure in which movement of the tympanic membrane is observed as puffs of air are blown into the external auditory meatus; used to assess the function of the eardrum
Rinne test (RIH-nee)	no word elements	procedure in which a tuning fork placed first on the mastoid process and then at the opening of the external auditory meatus is used to distinguish conductive from sensorineural hearing losses

Surgical Procedures	Word Elements	Definition
cochlear implant (KOCK-lee-er or KOKE-lee-er)	cochle = cochlea ar = pertaining to	experimental procedure in which an electronic transmitter is implanted within the middle ear; performed to restore hearing in patients with sensorineural hearing loss
fenestration (FEH-neh-**STRAY**-shun)	fenestra = "window" tion = process	surgical procedure in which an artificial opening is created in the oval window; performed mainly to treat otosclerosis
labyrinthotomy (LAB-er-rin-**THOT**-uh-me)	labyrintho = inner ear tomy = surgical incision	surgical incision into one or more structures of the inner ear
mastoidectomy (MASS-toyd-**ECK**-tuh-me)	mastoid = mastoid process ectomy = surgical removal	surgical removal of mastoid cells
myringotomy (MEER-in-**GOT**-uh-me)	myringo = eardrum tomy = surgical incision	surgical incision into the eardrum to drain fluid from the middle ear to relieve pressure; also called tympanotomy
otoplasty (**OH**-toe-PLASS-tee)	oto = ear plasty = surgical repair	plastic surgery to alter the size or shape of the auricles
stapedectomy (STAY-pih-**DECK**-tuh-me)	staped = stapes ectomy = surgical removal	surgical replacement of the stapes with a prosthetic device; performed mainly to treat advanced otosclerosis
tympanectomy (TIM-pan-**NECK**-tuh-me)	tympan = eardrum ectomy = surgical removal	surgical removal of the eardrum; also called myringectomy (MEER-in-**JECK**-tuh-me)
tympanostomy (TIM-pan-**NOS**-tuh-me)	tympano = eardrum stomy = surgical opening	procedure in which plastic tubes are placed in one or both ears to allow drainage of the middle ear across the tympanic membrane; usually performed to treat recurrent otitis media in young children

Review Exercises

4. ***Break Down and Define*** the word elements within each of the following terms, and then define the term itself.

    Example: oto / scopy   *ear / visual examination*   *visual examination of the ear*

  a. myringotomy

b. otoplasty

_____

c. audiometry

_____

d. tympanectomy

_____

e. otopyorrhea

_____

f. anacusis

_____

g. labyrinthitis

_____

h. otodynia

_____

i. otitis media

_____

j. otitis externa

_____

k. presbycusis

_____

l. myringitis

_____

m. otosclerosis

_____

n. otomycosis

_____

5. *Word Building and Spelling*. Spell out the medical term for each of the following definitions using the slashes provided to separate the word elements.

surgical removal of the mastoid process	*mastoid / ectomy*
a. inflammation of the mastoid process	_____ / _____
b. inflammation of the ear	_____ / _____

c. any disease of the ear   _____ / _____

d. surgical removal of the eardrum   _____ / _____

e. surgical opening into the eardrum   _____ / _____

f. surgical removal of the stapes   _____ / _____

g. surgical incision in the inner ear   _____ / _____

h. visual examination of the ear   _____ / _____

6. **Match** the following terms with their definitions.

_____ cochlear implant

_____ fenestration

_____ conductive hearing loss

_____ pneumatic otoscopy

_____ vertigo

_____ tympanostomy

_____ stapedectomy

_____ sensorineural hearing loss

_____ Rinne test

_____ Meniere's disease

_____ tinnitus

a. implantation of an electronic transmitter in the middle ear

b. procedure in which plastic tubes are inserted through the eardrum(s) to drain the middle ear

c. test that uses a tuning fork to distinguish between conductive and sensorineural hearing losses

d. surgical replacement of the stapes with a prosthetic device

e. hearing loss due to impairment in the transmission of sound from the outer to inner ear

f. hearing loss due to impairment in the transmission of sound from the inner ear to the brain

g. procedure in which movement of the tympanic membrane is observed as puffs of air are blown into the external auditory meatus

h. subjective sensation of ringing or tinkling in the ears

i. subjective sensation that either the self or the surroundings are spinning

j. rare disorder involving progressive deafness, vertigo, and tinnitus

k. surgical procedure in which an artificial opening is created in the oval window

 Case Study. Read the case notes below. For each boldfaced term, provide a brief definition and indicate whether the term is spelled correctly; if it is misspelled, provide the correct spelling.

Example:

ottitis medea: *inflammation of the middle ear, usually due to infection*

Spelled correctly? ☐ Yes ☑ No   *otitis media*

Patient presented as a 3-year-old boy with signs and symptoms of **ottitis medea**. His initial symptoms, sudden onset of prolonged crying and ear tugging, were consistent with **otodynia**. He was also feverish and fussy. The crying and ear tugging subsided, but the parents noted a sticky discharge from the ear. On examination, **otopyoria** was immediately evident. Sent a swab of the discharge to the laboratory for culture and analysis. On **otoscopy**, the tympanic membrane of the affected ear was clearly infected. **Adiometry** revealed hearing loss. Diagnosis: acute otitis media. Treatment plan: antibiotics with follow-up in one week; **miringotomy** if infection has not cleared by that time.

a. otodynia: _____

_____

Spelled correctly? ☐ Yes ☐ No _____

b. otopyoria: _____

_____

Spelled correctly? ☐ Yes ☐ No _____

c. otoscopy: _____

_____

Spelled correctly? ☐ Yes ☐ No _____

d. adiometry: _____

_____

Spelled correctly? ☐ Yes ☐ No _____

e. miringotomy: _____

_____

Spelled correctly? ☐ Yes ☐ No _____

Listen to the section on your audiotape cassette that corresponds to this chapter and write the terms below. Be careful to spell each term correctly.

1. _____   4. _____

2. _____   5. _____

3. _____   6. _____

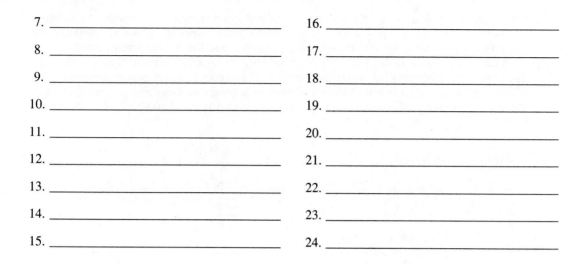

7. _____   16. _____

8. _____   17. _____

9. _____   18. _____

10. _____   19. _____

11. _____   20. _____

12. _____   21. _____

13. _____   22. _____

14. _____   23. _____

15. _____   24. _____

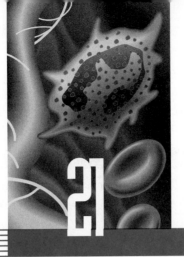

21

Oncology

Upon completing this chapter, you should be able to:

- Describe the general characteristics of benign and malignant tumors
- Explain how tumors are classified based on their histogenesis, staging, grading, and appearance
- Recognize, build, pronounce, and spell terms that pertain to oncology
- Describe diagnostic tests and therapeutic procedures that pertain to oncology

Overview   Oncology is the study of tumors, abnormal masses that form when cells reproduce at an unusually high rate. Such growths can form in any area of the body, and can be either benign or malignant. Much has been learned about tumors in recent decades, and many once-fatal illnesses are now treatable. As the field of oncology has grown, specialized terminology has been developed to describe the diseases and diagnostic and therapeutic processes involved in the field. This chapter will introduce this terminology.

Word Elements

TUMORS – The following combining forms (CF) pertain to oncology. They are used to refer to cancerous and benign tumors, including their development in previously normal cells and tissues.

CF	Meaning	Example
blast/o	immature	neuro*blast*oma = tumor of immature nerve tissue
carcin/o	cancer	*carcino*genic = producing cancer
hist/o	tissue	*histo*genesis = production of tissue
mut/a	genetic change	*muta*genic = producing genetic change
ne/o	new	*neo*plasm = a new growth (tumor)
onc/o	tumor; mass	*onco*logy = study of tumors
plas/o	growth; development	dys*plas*ia = condition of abnormal tissue development

TUMOR TREATMENT – The following combining forms pertain to methods of treating tumors, especially cancerous tumors.

CF	Meaning	Example
cauter/o	burn; heat	*cauter*ization = use of heat to destroy tissue
chem/o	chemical; drug	*chemo*therapy = drug treatment
cry/o	cold	*cryo*surgery = use of cold temperature to destroy tissue

SUFFIXES – The following suffixes pertain to oncology. Those denoting tumor types are often added to the names of tissues to build terms describing pathologic conditions.

Suffix	Meaning	Example
-carcinoma	malignant epithelial tumor	adeno*carcinoma* = malignant tumor of a gland
-oma	tumor	lymph*oma* = tumor of lymph tissue
-plasm	growth; development	neo*plasm* = a new growth (tumor)
-sarcoma	malignant connective tissue tumor	chondro*sarcoma* = malignant tumor of cartilage
-therapy	treatment	radio*therapy* = radiation treatment

Characteristics of Tumors

-oma = tumor
ne/o = new
-plasm = growth;
development

onc/o = tumor; mass

Throughout life, new tissue cells are continually produced to replace older cells that become worn out or destroyed. This is usually an orderly process, in which new cells are produced at roughly the same pace as older cells become worn. Occasionally, however, new cells grow at an excessive, uncontrolled pace, creating abnormal masses of tissue known as **tumors** or **neoplasms** (**NEE**-oh-**PLAZ**-ums).

Tumors can grow in any body tissue and are made up of the same general types of cells as the tissue in which they form. They can be either **benign** (contained and not life-threatening) or **malignant** (cancerous, life-endangering). Benign and malignant tumors have very different characteristics (see Table 21-1). Although oncology is the study of both benign and malignant tumors, far more attention is devoted to malignancies due to their potentially life-threatening nature. Accordingly, this chapter will focus primarily on cancerous tumors.

Table 21–1:
Characteristics of benign and malignant tumors.

Benign Tumors	Malignant (Cancerous) Tumors
grow slowly	grow rapidly
usually encapsulated (contained in a fibrous capsule) and non-infiltrating	non-encapsulated; have projections that invade and infiltrate the surrounding tissue
composed of normal, specialized cells similar to those in normal tissue	composed of cells that have lost their specialized structure and become immature
do not spread to other sites sites	left untreated, can spread to remote sites
usually not serious, causing harm only if pressure is placed on surrounding tissue	left untreated, usually pose serious threat to patients' health

Development of Malignant Tumors

mut/a = genetic
change

All cells reproduce according to instructions contained within their genetic material, or DNA. If something acts to change a cell's DNA, the cell will develop, grow, and reproduce according to the new instructions. Occasionally, a genetic change (**mutation**) will cause a cell to become malignant. When the malignant cell reproduces, it passes the malignant trait to its daughter cells, which in turn grow and reproduce as malignant cells.

The pattern of growth of malignant cells is quite different from that of normal cells. Normal cells develop in a highly organized ways. They have specialized (**differentiated**) structures and functions, and they align them-

Figure 21–1: *Malignant cell growth and metastasis.*

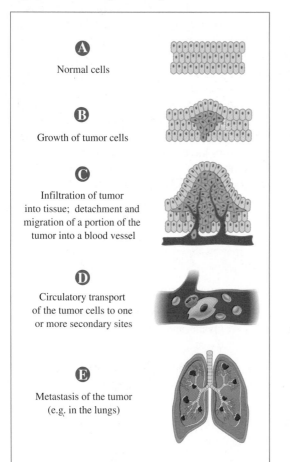

Ⓐ Normal cells

Ⓑ Growth of tumor cells

Ⓒ Infiltration of tumor into tissue; detachment and migration of a portion of the tumor into a blood vessel

Ⓓ Circulatory transport of the tumor cells to one or more secondary sites

Ⓔ Metastasis of the tumor (e.g. in the lungs)

selves in very orderly arrangements. Malignant cells, in contrast, grow in very disorganized ways. Instead of developing into specialized cells, they revert to immature (**dedifferentiated**) cells. Dedifferentiated cells are also referred to as **anaplastic** (AN-nuh-**PLASS**-tick), and the phenomenon in which cells become dedifferentiated or anaplastic is called **anaplasia** (AN-nuh-**PLAY**-zhuh). In addition to being anaplastic, malignant cells grow in disorderly patterns. They reproduce very quickly, pile up on each other, invade the underlying tissue, and detach and travel to other sites (see Figure 21-1). The spread of a malignant tumor from the site of origin to another part of the body is called **metastasis** (meh-TASS-tuh-sis). Eventually, such tumors invade, spread, and take over enough tissue to cause serious harm.

Malignant tumors (cancers) result from cellular mutations. Only some mutations lead to cancer, however. Some mutations lead to other types of diseases, and some are relatively harmless. Anything that has the ability to cause mutations, whether cancer-causing or not, is referred to as **mutagenic** (MYOO-tuh-**JEN**-nick). Those mutagens that have the ability to cause cancer are referred to as **carcinogenic** (KAR-sin-no-**JEN**-nick). Examples of carcinogens include tobacco smoke, radiation, and some types of industrial solvents and by-products (benzene, hydrocarbons, etc.).

Classification and Description of Tumors

Because tumors can arise from all types of tissues in all areas of the body, classifying them in various ways can make it easier to convey the nature of a tumor being observed. Tumors are often classified and described according to:

- the types of tissue in which they originate (histogenesis)
- their appearance
- the degree to which their cells are differentiated or dedifferentiated (grading)
- the extent to which they have grown and metastasized (staging)

Histogenesis

hist/o = tissue

Tumors are classified first according to the type of tissue in which they arise: their **histogenesis** (HIS-toe-**JEN**-neh-sis). Tumors may arise from epithelial, connective, hematopoietic, or nervous tissue, or they may be of mixed-tissue origin.

Epithelial tissue is the tissue that lines the surfaces of the body. This includes the skin and the tissues that line the internal organs and body cavities. Malignant tumors of epithelial origin are generally named by adding **carcinoma** (KAR-sih-**NO**-muh) to the name of the tissue in which the tumor is seen (see Table 21-2). The majority of malignant tumors (about 85%) are carcinomas.

-carcinoma = malignant epithelial tumor

-sarcoma = malignant connective tissue tumor

Connective tissue is any type of tissue that connects one tissue to another or that serves to support body structures. This includes fibrous tissue, fat, muscle, bone, cartilage, and vascular tissue. Malignant tumors of connective tissue origin are named by adding **sarcoma** (sar-KOE-muh) to the name of the tissue in which the tumor is seen (see Table 21-2).

hemat/o = blood
-poietic = forming

leuk/o = white
myel/o = bone marrow
lymph/o = lymph
-oma = tumor

Hematopoietic (heh-MAT-oh-poy-**ET**-tick) tissue consists of the blood and lymphatic systems, including the tissues that produce blood cells. There is no single term that is used to name tumors of hematopoietic origin. Cancers arising from white blood cells are called leukemias, for example, while some cancers arising from the bone marrow are called myelomas (MY-ul-**LOE**-muhs) and many cancers of lymphatic origin are called lymphomas. Note that some hematopoietic tissue is considered connective tissue; thus, some malignant tumors of hematopoietic origin are called sarcomas.

Nervous tissue consists of all of the tissues that make up the nervous system, including nerves, glia, and meninges (see Chapter 12). There are no well-defined rules for naming tumors of nervous tissue origin. There are also no well-defined rules for naming mixed-tissue tumors (see Table 21-2).

-oma = tumor

This discussion has focused on the naming of malignant tumors. Benign tumors are also named according to the tissue in which they originate. In many cases, the suffix **-oma** is used to denote a benign tumor. For example, a benign tumor of epithelial origin is called a papilloma (PAP-ull-**LOE**-muh), while a benign tumor of glandular origin is called an adenoma (AD-dih-**NO**-muh). Similarly, tumors originating in cartilage, bone, fat, vessels, skeletal muscle, or nerve sheaths are called chondromas (kon-DROE-muhs), osteomas (OS-tee-**OH**-muhs), lipomas (lih-POE-muhs), angiomas (AN-jee-**OH**-muhs), rhabdomyomas (RAB-doe-my-**OH**-muhs), or neurofibromas (NOOR-oh-fie-**BROE**-muhs), respectively. As Table 21-2 indicates, however, -oma is also used in the names of some malignant tumors.

Table 21–2:
Classification of tumors
by histogenesis.

Tissue Type	Example	Malignant Tumor Name
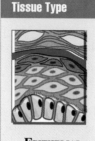 **EPITHELIAL**	epithelial cells squamous cells basal cells melanocytes pancreas breast glandular tissue glandular stomach tissue glandular lung tissue glandular colon tissue ovarian tissue	papillocarcinoma squamous cell carcinoma basal cell carcinoma malignant melanoma pancreatic carcinoma adenocarcinoma of the breast adenocarcinoma gastric adenocarcinoma adenocarcinoma of the lungs adenocarcinoma of the colon cystadenocarcinoma of the ovaries
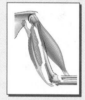 **CONNECTIVE**	fibrous tissue fat smooth muscle skeletal muscle bone cartilage blood vessel tissue lymph vessel tissue	fibrosarcoma liposarcoma leiomyosarcoma rhabdomyosarcoma osteosarcoma chondrosarcoma hemangiosarcoma angiosarcoma, lymphangiosarcoma
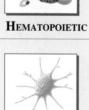 **HEMATOPOIETIC**	white blood cells red and white blood cells bone marrow cells lymphatic tissue	leukemia erythroleukemia multiple myeloma lymphoma, Hodgkin's disease
 NERVOUS	glia retina immature nerve tissue nerve sheaths	glioma, astrocytoma retinoblastoma neuroblastoma neurofibrosarcoma

Tissue Type	Example	Malignant Tumor Name
MIXED-TISSUE	breast kidney bone/muscle/skin/gland/etc.	cystosarcoma phyllodes nephroblastoma teratoma choriocarcinoma, malignant teratoma

Appearance

Tumors that have been detected in the tissues are immediately examined with the naked eye (if possible), by palpation (if possible), and under the microscope (following a biopsy). They are then described according to their appearance and texture. Many terms can be used to describe tumors. A few of the most commonly used are:

- **alveolar** (al-VEE-oh-ler), forming microscopic sacs
- **annular** (AN-nyoo-ler), ring-shaped or circular
- **cystic** (SIS-tick), forming fluid-filled sacs
- **diffuse,** spreading evenly throughout a tissue
- **dysplastic** (dis-PLASS-tick), abnormal but not clearly cancerous in appearance (usually "precancerous")
- **follicular** (ful-LICK-yoo-ler), forming tiny follicle- or gland-like sacs
- **fungating** (FUNG-gate-ing), having a mushrooming pattern of growth
- **medullary** (**MED**-yoo-LEHR-ee), having a large, soft consistency
- **necrotic** (neh-KROT-ick), containing dead tissue
- **nodular,** forming discrete nodules
- **papillary** (**PAP**-pull-LEHR-ee), forming finger-like projections
- **polypoid,** resembling a polyp (finger-like projection extending from central base)
- **scirrhous** (SKEHR-russ), having a hard and packed consistency
- **serous** (SEER-russ), containing a thin, watery fluid
- **ulcerating,** having an open lesion
- **verrucous** (VEHR-roo-kuss), resembling a wart

Table 21–3: *The TNM staging system.*

Component	Designation	Meaning
TUMOR	T_0	no evidence of primary tumor
	T_{IS}	tumor **in situ** (in SIE-too), confined to the site of origin
	T_1, T_2, T_3, T_4	designation of T_1 - T_4 indicates increasing size and degree of involvement of tumor, T_1 being smallest and T_4 being largest
	T_x	tumor cannot be assessed
NODE	N_0	regional lymph nodes not demonstrably abnormal
	N_1, N_2, N_3, N_4	designation of N_1 - N_4 indicates increasing degree (number and distance) of lymph node abnormality, N_1 being smallest and N_4 being largest
	N_x	regional lymph nodes cannot be assessed clinically
METASTASIS	M_0	no evidence of metastasis
	M_1, M_2, M_3	designation of M_1 - M_3 indicates increasing degree or distance of metastasis, M_1 being smallest and M_3 being largest

Grading

Grading is the classification of tumors according to their histologic composition: specifically, the extent to which their cells are differentiated or dedifferentiated. Grade 1 tumors have well differentiated cells that closely resemble normal tissue cells. Grade 2 tumors are somewhat less differentiated, Grade 3 tumors are relatively dedifferentiated, and Grade 4 tumors are highly dedifferentiated or anaplastic. Grading can be useful in evaluating a patient's prognosis. In general, patients with Grade 1 tumors have the best prognosis, while those with Grade 4 tumors have very poor prognoses.

Staging

The classification of tumors according to the extent to which they have grown and metastasized is called **staging.** The TNM system is commonly used to stage tumors. In this system, T describes the size and local spread of the tumor, N describes the number and/or distance of lymph nodes that have been affected by the tumor, and M describes the extent to which the tumor has metastasized. A subscript is used to indicate the size or spread of the tumor (see Table 21-3). For example, the designation $T_1N_0M_0$ describes a small tumor (T_1) with no evidence of lymph node involvement (N_0) and no evidence of metastasis (M_0).

Tumor staging can have significant treatment implications. Whereas a small, highly localized tumor with no evidence of spread may be successfully treated with surgery, for example, a larger spreading tumor may require more aggressive treatment with a combination of surgery, radiation, and chemotherapy.

chem/o = chemical; drug
-therapy = treatment

Review Exercises

1. **Define** the following suffixes and combining forms.

 a. onc/o _____

 b. -oma _____

 c. -carcinoma _____

 d. -sarcoma _____

 e. -plasm _____

 f. plas/o _____

 g. chem/o _____

 h. -therapy _____

 i. cry/o _____

 j. cauter/o _____

 k. blast/o _____

 l. hist/o _____

 m. ne/o _____

 n. mut/a _____

 o. carcin/o _____

2. **Circle** the choices that will make each statement true.

 a. (Grading/Staging) is the classification of tumors according to their histologic composition, while (grading/staging) is the classification of tumors according to their degree of spread.

 b. Cells in a Grade 1 tumor are relatively (well differentiated/anaplastic), while cells in a Grade 4 tumor are (well differentiated/anaplastic).

 c. In the TNM staging system, a subscript of 0 denotes (no/extensive) tumor involvement, lymph node involvement, or metastatic spread, while a subscript of 3 or 4 indicates (no/extensive) tumor involvement, lymph node involvement, or metastatic spread.

3. **Match** the following descriptions with the type of tumor they characterize.

_____ grow slowly   a. benign tumors

_____ grow rapidly   b. malignant tumors

_____ usually encapsulated

_____ non-encapsulated

_____ infiltrate surrounding tissue

_____ usually do not infiltrate surrounding tissue

_____ cells are differentiated

_____ cells are dedifferentiated (anaplastic)

_____ usually spread to other sites

_____ do not spread to other sites

_____ generally cause serious illness

_____ generally do not cause serious illness

4. **Match** the following terms with their definitions.

_____ forming fluid-filled sacs   a. alveolar

_____ forming discrete nodules   b. cystic

_____ forming finger-like projections   c. follicular

_____ resembling a polyp   d. papillary

_____ spreading evenly throughout a tissue   e. polypoid

_____ forming tiny follicle- or gland-like sacs   f. nodular

_____ having a mushrooming growth pattern   g. fungating

_____ forming microscopic sacs   h. verrucous

_____ resembling a wart   i. diffuse

5. **Define** the following terms.

a. annular   _____

b. dysplastic   _____

c. medullary   _____

d. necrotic   _____

e. scirrhous   _____

f. serous

g. ulcerating

h. in situ

Terminology

The following are selected diagnostic and therapeutic procedures commonly used in the field of oncology. Diseases are not listed here, since specific tumors are generally named by combining the word elements introduced in this chapter with terms listed in previous chapters. You will have the opportunity to analyze and construct such terms – as well as diagnostic and therapeutic terms – in the exercises following these tables.

Diagnostic Procedures	Word Elements	Definition
acid phosphatase test (FOS-fuh-tase)	no word elements	blood test measuring the level of an enzyme that is elevated in patients with prostate cancer
alpha-fetoprotein test (FEE-toe-**PROE**-teen)	no word elements	blood test used to detect a protein found in patients with liver or testicular cancer
bone marrow biopsy (BY-op-see)	bi = life opsy = view	use of a needle to extract bone marrow for examination and evaluation
CEA test	no word elements	blood test used to detect a substance that is elevated in patients with some types of gastrointestinal cancer (especially colon cancer)
estradiol receptor assay (ESS-truh-**DIE**-ol)	no word elements	test measuring the responsiveness of tumor cells to estradiol (a type of estrogen); predicts responsiveness to anti-estrogen hormone therapy
excisional biopsy (eck-SIH-zhun-nul BY-op-see)	ex = out cision = incision al = pertaining to	use of a sharp instrument to remove an entire tumor plus the surrounding normal tissue for examination
exfoliative cytology (eks-FOE-lee-uh-tiv sie-TOL-uh-jee)	ex = out foliative = "leaf; layer" cyto = cell logy = study of	microscopic examination of desquamated (sloughed off) cells obtained by aspirating, scraping, or washing a tissue
incisional biopsy (in-SIH-zhun-null BY-op-see)	in = in; into cision = incision al = pertaining to	use of a sharp instrument to remove a portion of a tumor for examination

Diagnostic Procedures	Word Elements	Definition
needle biopsy (BY-op-see)	bi = life opsy = view	insertion of a hollow needle into the skin to suction out a sample of tissue for examination
progesterone receptor assay (pro-JESS-ter-ohn)	no word elements	test measuring the responsiveness of tumor cells to progesterone (a female hormone); predicts responsiveness to hormone therapy
prostate-specific antigen test	no word elements	blood test used to measure the level of a protein produced by prostate cancer cells
radionuclide scan (RAY-dee-oh-**NOO**-klide)	radio = radioactivity nuclide = a type of atom	test in which pictures (scans) of organs are taken after the injection of a radioactive substance; used to detect certain types of tumors
staging laparotomy (LAP-er-**OT**-uh-me)	laparo = abdomen tomy = surgical incision	creation of a large incision in order to examine the abdomen and assess the extent of tumor growth

Therapeutic Procedures	Word Elements	Definition
adjuvant therapy (AD-joo-vent)	adjuvant = "to aid"	treatment (often drug treatment) used to assist or enhance the main mode of treatment
alkaloids (AL-kul-loydz)	alkal = alkaline oid = resembling	alkaline chemicals found in plants that are pharmacologically active; used in chemotherapy
alkylating agents (**AL**-kul-LAY-ting)	no word elements	chemicals that readily attach to vital cell molecules, thereby blocking cell growth; used in chemotherapy
antibiotic therapy (AN-tih-bie-**OT**-ick)	anti = against biot = life ic = pertaining to	treatment with antibiotics (substances that inhibit cell growth); used in chemotherapy
antimetabolites (AN-tih-meh-**TAB**-bull-lites)	anti = against metabolite = substance created by metabolism	chemicals that inhibit cell growth by blocking the use of substances needed for growth; used in chemotherapy
biological therapy	bio = life log = study ical = pertaining to	use of drugs that stimulate the body's own defenses to fight disease
chemotherapy	chemo = chemical; drug therapy = treatment	use of drugs to treat a disease
cryosurgery (KRIE-oh-**SER**-jer-ee)	cryo = cold surgery = surgery	use of freezing temperature to destroy diseased tissue

Therapeutic Procedures	Word Elements	Definition
cytotoxic agents (SIE-toe-**TOCK**-sick)	cyto = cell toxic = poisonous	chemicals that kill dividing cells (e.g., antimetabolites and alkylating agents); used in chemotherapy
electrocauterization (ih-LECK-troe-KOT-er-ih-**ZAY**-shun)	electro = electricity cauter = burn; heat ization = process	use of an electrically activated instrument to burn off and destroy diseased tissue
en bloc resection (en block ree-SECK-shun)	en bloc = as a whole	removal of a tumor as a whole, plus a large area of surrounding tissue
exenteration (eck-SEN-ter-**AY**-shun)	ex = out enter = small intestine ation = process	surgical removal of all of the organs and soft tissue in a body cavity
radiation therapy	radi = radioactivity ation = process	use of ionizing radiation (e.g., x-rays) to destroy diseased tissue
steroids	no word elements	chemicals that resemble (or are identical to) steroid hormones; used in chemotherapy
surgical excision (eck-SIH-zhun)	ex = out cision = incision	process of surgically cutting out a tumor (or other piece of tissue)

Review Exercises

6. ***Break Down and Define*** the word elements within each of the following terms, and then define the term itself.

> *Example:* cyto / logy   *cell / study of*   *study of cells*

   a. neoplasm

   _____

   b. antineoplastic

   _____

   c. dysplasia

   _____

   d. anaplasia

   _____

   e. chemotherapy

   _____

f. cytotoxic

_____

g. electrocauterization

_____

h. laparotomy

_____

i. neurofibroma

_____

j. neurofibrosarcoma

_____

k. adenocarcinoma

_____

7. ***Choose and Construct.*** Choose the appropriate word elements from the list provided to construct terms for the following.

blast/o	hist/o	neur/o	retin/o	-oma
carcin/o	lymph/o	onc/o	-genesis	-carcinoma
cholangi/o	nephr/o	papill/o	-logy	

study of tumors   *onco* **/** *logy*

a. production of tumors   _____ **/** _____

b. production of cancer   _____ **/** _____

c. production of tissue   _____ **/** _____

d. study of tissues   _____ **/** _____

e. tumor of immature retinal tissue   _____ **/** _____ **/** _____

f. tumor of immature nerve tissue   _____ **/** _____ **/** _____

g. tumor of lymph tissue   _____ **/** _____

h. tumor of immature kidney tissue   _____ **/** _____ **/** _____

i. malignant tumor of epithelial cells _____ **/** _____

j. malignant epithelial tumor of the bile ducts _____ **/** _____

8. **Word Building and Spelling**. Spell out terms for benign and malignant tumors of the following connective tissues using the suffixes -oma and -sarcoma. Use the slashes provided to separate the word elements. Some word elements have been added to assist you.

fat	*lip / oma*	*lipo / sarcoma*
a. vessel tissue	_____ / _oma_ ___	_____ / _sarcoma_ ___
b. blood vessels	_hem_ / _____ / _____	_____ / _____ / _____
c. lymph vessels	_____ / _____ / _____	_____ / _____ / _____
d. fibrous tissue	_____ / _____	_____ / _____
e. smooth muscle	_leio_ / _____ / _____	_____ / _____ / _____
f. skeletal muscle	_rhabdo_ / _____ / _____	_____ / _____ / _____
g. bone	_____ / _____	_____ / _____
h. cartilage	_chondr_ / _____	_____ / _____

Case Study. Read the case notes below. For each boldfaced term, provide a brief definition and indicate whether the term is spelled correctly; if it is misspelled, provide the correct spelling.

Example:
carsinoma: *malignant epithelial tumor*
Spelled correctly? ☐ Yes ☑ No *carcinoma*

Patient presented as a 45-year-old female with a painless lump in her right breast and a family history of **carsinoma**. On palpation, the mass was firm, about 3 cm in diameter, located just underneath and 2 cm to the left of the nipple, with possible skin involvement. A single movable mass in the right armpit was also palpated, indicating possible axillary lymph node involvement. A mammogram showed a single tumorous mass in the right breast. Performed an **excisional biopsy** of the tumor and palpable lymph node, and a biopsy of the other right axillary lymph nodes. Microscopic examination of the tumor revealed a **scirous** carcinoma. Cells were somewhat differentiated, with some evidence of **aniplasia**. The excised lymph node was positive histologically, but no evidence of tumor was found in any of the other lymph nodes and there was no evidence of **metastasis**. **Estradiole receptor assay** and **projesterone receptor assay** were positive. Diagnosis: $T_2N_1M_0$ Stage 2 Grade 2 carcinoma of the right breast. Treatment plan: **radiation therapy** with **adjuvent chemotherapy.**

a. excisional biopsy: _____

_____

Spelled correctly? ☐ Yes ☐ No _____

b. scirous: _____

_____

Spelled correctly? ☐ Yes ☐ No _____

c. aniplasia: _____

_____

Spelled correctly? ☐ Yes ☐ No _____

d. metastasis: _____

_____

Spelled correctly? ☐ Yes ☐ No _____

e. Estradiole receptor assay: _____

_____

Spelled correctly? ☐ Yes ☐ No _____

f. projesterone receptor assay: _____

_____

Spelled correctly? ☐ Yes ☐ No _____

g. radiation therapy: _____

_____

Spelled correctly? ☐ Yes ☐ No _____

h. adjuvent: _____

_____

Spelled correctly? ☐ Yes ☐ No _____

i. chemotherapy: _____

_____

Spelled correctly? ☐ Yes ☐ No _____

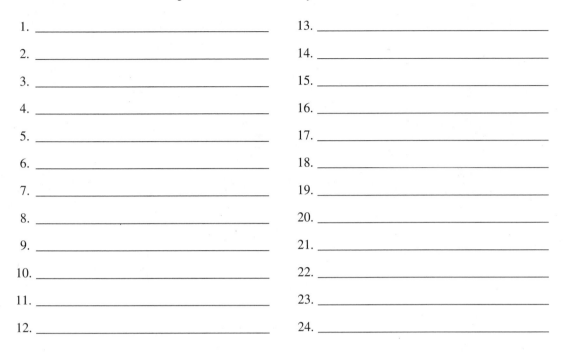

Listen to the section on your audiotape cassette that corresponds to this chapter and write the terms below. Be careful to spell each term correctly.

1. _____

2. _____

3. _____

4. _____

5. _____

6. _____

7. _____

8. _____

9. _____

10. _____

11. _____

12. _____

13. _____

14. _____

15. _____

16. _____

17. _____

18. _____

19. _____

20. _____

21. _____

22. _____

23. _____

24. _____

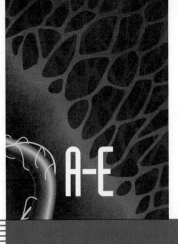

A-E

Appendices

APPENDIX A
Pharmacology

Pharmacology is the study of drugs and their effects on the body. Because drug treatment is so central to the practice of medicine, it is essential to be familiar with pharmacologic terms and the types of drugs used to treat disease. This appendix provides a glossary of commonly used pharmacologic terms and tables of major classes of drugs organized by body system.

additive effect. Drug interaction in which the combination of two or more drugs produces an effect that is equal to the sum of their individual effects.

adverse effect. Any undesired drug effect.

aerosol. Drug solution suspended in a fine mist for inhalation.

anaphylactic reaction (AN-uh-full-**LACK**-tick). Extreme, life-threatening allergic reaction to a drug or other foreign substance.

antidote. Substance that neutralizes or counteracts the effects of a drug or poison.

bioavailability. The amount of a drug that reaches the bloodstream and is available to the tissues.

chemotherapy. Drug treatment.

clearance. Removal of a drug (or other substance) from the blood.

contraindication. Any condition that makes it unwise to use a particular drug or line of treatment in a particular patient.

dosage. Size, frequency, and number of doses of a drug to be administered to a patient.

dose. The amount of a drug to be taken at a time.

efficacy. Effectiveness.

enteral. By way of the small intestine; route of administration of tube feeding.

formulation. Drug manufactured according to a prescribed method.

generic. Drug marketed under its public, nonproprietary name rather than as a trademarked product.

iatrogenic effect (eye-AT-troe-**JEN**-nick). Effect that occurs as a result of medical treatment.

idiosyncratic effect (ID-ee-oh-sin-**KRAT**-ick). Effect that occurs in a particularly sensitive individual, but is not generally expected to occur.

indication. Condition for which the U.S. Food and Drug Administration has approved a drug for use.

infusion. Introduction of fluid into a vein.

inhalation. The act of breathing in air; route of administration for drugs in gas, vapor, or aerosol form.

injection. Use of a syringe to introduce fluid into the body.

instillation. Drop by drop administration of a fluid into an orifice (the eyes, ears, or nose).

intra-arterial. Within an artery, as in the injection of a drug into an artery.

intra-articular. Within a joint, as in the injection of a drug into a joint.

intradermal. Within the skin, as in the injection of a drug into the skin

intramuscular. Within a muscle, as in the injection of a drug into a muscle.

intrathecal (in-truh-THEE-kull). Within the subarachnoid space, as in the injection of a drug into the spinal column.

intravaginal. Within the vagina, as in the insertion of a cream or suppository into the vagina.

intravenous. Within a vein, as in the injection of a drug into a vein.

metabolite. Product of metabolism; breakdown product; a drug metabolite may be active or inactive.

oral. By mouth, as in the administration of a drug by mouth.

palliative treatment (PAL-lee-uh-tiv). Therapy designed to relieve symptoms rather than to treat the underlying disease.

parenteral (per-EN-ter-ull). By any route other than through the digestive tract, as in the administration of a drug by injection or suppository.

pharmacodynamics. Study of the effects of drugs on the body.

pharmacokinetics. Study of what happens to drugs as they pass through the body, including the rate and extent of their accumulation in and clearance from the blood and tissues.

pharmacology. Study of drugs and their effects on the body.

placebo (pluh-SEE-boe). Inactive substance (e.g., a "sugar pill").

potency. Strength, as measured by the amount of drug required to produce a certain level of effect.

receptor. Cell surface molecule that initiates or inhibits a biological activity when occupied by a drug or chemical.

rectal. By way of the rectum, as in the insertion of a cream or suppository into the rectum.

resistance, drug. The ability of a microorganism to withstand the effects of a drug, rendering treatment ineffective.

side effect. Undesirable and/or nontherapeutic effect of a drug.

subcutaneous. Under the skin, as in the injection of a drug into the subcutaneous tissue under the skin.

sublingual. Under the tongue, as in the administration of a drug by placing it under the tongue.

synergistic effect (sin-ner-JISS-tick). Drug interaction in which the combination of two or more drugs produces an effect that is greater than the sum of their individual effects.

syringe. Tubular instrument used to inject fluid into or withdraw fluid from the body.

therapeutic. Pertaining to treatment; having a beneficial effect.

therapeutic range. The range of concentrations within which a drug produces the desired clinical effect without producing excessive adverse effects.

tolerance. Phenomenon in which larger and larger drug doses must be administered to achieve the same effect.

topical. On the surface, as in the application of a drug on the skin.

toxicity. The harmful or poisonous effects of a drug.

toxicology. Study of harmful substances and their effects on the body.

trade name. The manufacturer's commercial, proprietary name for a product; drugs may be referred to by their trade names or by their generic names.

transdermal. Across the skin, as in the administration of a drug through a patch placed on the skin.

vitamin. Chemical that is required for growth and normal functioning.

Thousands of drugs are available to treat hundreds of types of disorders. To make your introduction to these drugs manageable, the following table lists the major types of therapeutic agents by body system and drug class. Since some agents act on multiple body systems, some drug classes are listed in more than one category.

Body System	Class	Therapeutic Action
CARDIOVASCULAR	**anti-anginals** (beta blockers, calcium channel blockers, nitrates, vasodilators)	improve blood flow through the heart to alleviate angina
	anti-arrhythmics (beta blockers, calcium channel blockers, cardiac glycosides, quinidines)	restore normal heart rhythms by altering cardiac conduction or the heart's response to electrical impulses
	antihyperlipidemics	reduce cholesterol levels
	antihypertensives (ACE inhibitors, alpha/beta blockers, beta blockers, calcium channel blockers, diuretics, vasodilators)	reduce blood pressure
	cardiotonics (digitalis and other cardiac glycosides)	increase the force of heart muscle contractions in the treatment of heart failure
BLOOD	**anti-anemia drugs** (iron, vitamins)	promote hematopoiesis; increase iron stores
	anticoagulants (aspirin, heparin, warfarin)	prevent abnormal clotting
	antihyperuricemics (allopurinol, probenecid, sulfinpyrazone)	lower uric acid levels, thereby alleviating symptoms of gout
	fibrinolytics/thrombolytics	dissolve abnormal clots
	hemostatics (coagulation factors, vitamin K)	stop excessive bleeding

Body System	Class	Therapeutic Action
Lymph/Immune	**allergens**	administered in increasing doses to treat allergy
	immunosuppressants (corticosteroids, cyclosporine, cytotoxic agents, monoclonal and polyclonal antibodies)	suppress immune reactions to prevent graft rejection or to slow autoimmune disease
	vaccines	induce immunity to infectious micro-organisms or their toxins
Respiratory	**antitussives** (antihistamines, expectorants, mucolytics)	relieve cough and/or loosen sputum to facilitate coughing
	bronchodilators (anticholinergics, sympathomimetics, xanthines)	open airways to facilitate breathing
	decongestants	relieve nasal congestion
Digestive	**antacids** (aluminums, bicarbonates, calciums, magnesiums)	neutralize stomach acids to relieve indigestion, heartburn, and peptic ulcer symptoms
	antidiarrheals (bulking agents, narcotics)	slow intestinal activity or absorb water from stools
	anti-emetics (anticholinergics, antihistamines, phenothiazines)	relieve nausea and vomiting by suppressing the vomiting reflex or by relaxing stomach muscles
	antiflatulents	prevent or relieve flatulence
	antispasmodics (anticholinergics, belladonna)	relieve symptoms of irritable bowel by relaxing intestinal smooth muscles
	anti-ulcer drugs (antibiotics, histamine-2 receptor antagonists)	reduce secretion of gastric acid or inhibit bacterial growth, allowing ulcer to heal
	cathartics/laxatives/purgatives (bulking agents, enemas, fecal softeners, lubricants, saline, stimulants)	relieve constipation and promote defecation by increasing bulk, stimulating intestinal contraction, softening the feces, or drawing fluid into the feces

Body System	Class	Therapeutic Action
	emetics	induce vomiting
	enzymes/digestants	aid digestion of malabsorbed nutrients
URINARY	**urinary alkalinizers**	inhibit stone formation by reducing urine acidity
NERVOUS PSYCHOTROPICS:	**anesthetics** (generals, locals)	reduce or eliminate sensation in the whole body or in a particular region
	anticonvulsants/anti-seizure drugs (barbiturates, benzodiazepines, carbamazepine, hydantoins, succinamides, valproic acid)	prevent and treat seizures
	antiparkinson drugs (anticholinergics, dopamine agonists, levodopa)	reduce symptoms of Parkinson's disease
	anti-anxiety drugs/tranquilizers (benzodiazepines, beta blockers)	relieve symptoms of anxiety
	antidepressants (MAO inhibitors, serotonin reuptake inhibitors, tricyclics)	relieve depression
	antimanic drugs (lithium, some anticonvulsants)	reduce symptoms of mania
	neuroleptics/antipsychotics (butyrophenones, phenothiazines, thioxanthenes)	reduce symptoms of psychoses
	stimulants (amphetamines, caffeine)	increase alertness
SEDATIVES:	**hypnotics** (barbiturates, nonbarbiturates)	promote calmness and sleep
	anti-anxiety drugs	see psychotropics

Body System	Class	Therapeutic Action
ENDOCRINE	**antithyroid agents**	inhibit production of thyroid hormones
	hormones (androgens, anti-diuretics, estrogens, glucocorticoids, gonadotropins, gonadotropin-releasing hormones, growth hormones, hypocalcemics, insulin, progestogens, somatostatin, thyroid hormones)	treat endocrine disorders and problems related to hormone deficiency
	hyperglycemics (diazoxide, glucagon)	increase blood sugar levels by countering the effects of insulin
	hypoglycemics	lower blood sugar levels by increasing insulin production
REPRODUCTIVE	**contraceptives** (oral progesterones and estrogens, progestogen injections and implants)	prevent pregnancy by preventing ovulation and thickening cervical mucus
	fertility drugs (clomiphene, gonadotropin hormones)	increase male/female fertility by various mechanisms
	hormone replacement	increase male/female hormone levels to correct deficiencies and to treat menopausal symptoms, breast/prostate cancer, or abnormal uterine bleeding
	uterine contractants (oxytocics, prostaglandins)	increase uterine contractions to induce/facilitate childbirth
	uterine relaxants	decrease uterine contractions to prolong gestation
SKELETAL/ MUSCULAR	**anti-inflammatory agents** (corticosteroids, non-steroidal anti-inflammatory drugs)	relieve arthritic and muscular pain by reducing inflammation
	muscle relaxants (diazepam and other centrally-acting agents, dantrolene, neuromuscular blocking agents)	relieve muscle spasm by reducing neural stimulation of muscle contraction or by directly blocking muscle contraction

Body System	Class	Therapeutic Action
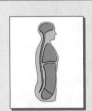 **SKIN**	**antipruritics** (corticosteroids, emollients)	relieve itching
	antiseptics	prevent infection by destroying microorganisms
	astringents	promote drying, thereby reducing perspiration and promoting healing
	keratolytics (acids, salicylic acid, sulfur)	loosen and remove excess keratin
ONCOLOGY	**antineoplastics** (alkaloids, alkylating agents, antibiotics, antimetabolites, steroids)	treat cancer by inhibiting the growth of cancer cells
BODY AS A WHOLE	**analgesics** (narcotics/opiates, non-steroidal anti-inflammatory drugs, salicylates)	relieve pain by blocking prostaglandin production or pain impulses
	anti-infectives/antimicrobials (antibacterials/antibiotics [aminoglycosides, cephalosporins, macrolides, penicillins, quinolones, sulfonamides, tetracyclines], antifungals, antiparasitics, antivirals)	treat infections by inhibiting the growth of or killing infectious microorganisms
	antipyretics (acetaminophen, aspirin)	reduce fever

APPENDIX B
Physicians and Allied Health Professionals

The field of medicine involves a wide array of trained professionals, including many types of physician specialists, non-physician healthcare providers, nurses, and paraprofessionals. The major types of physicians and allied health professionals are listed in this appendix. You may find it useful to study the list as a whole or you can use the list as a reference. The entries are presented in an alphabetized, glossary-style format for easy reference.

allergist. Physician specializing in the diagnosis and treatment of allergies.

anesthesiologist. Physician specializing in the administration of anesthetics, substances that produce a temporary loss of sensation.

anesthetist. Physician or nurse who administers anesthetics.

audiologist. Person specializing in the identification, evaluation, and non-surgical treatment of hearing disorders.

cardiologist. Physician specializing in diseases of the heart.

cardiovascular surgeon. Physician specializing in the surgical treatment of heart and vascular conditions.

chiropractor. Person who specializes in the treatment of disorders by physically manipulating the vertebral column.

colorectal surgeon. Physician specializing in the surgical treatment of disorders of the colon and rectum.

dentist. Person specializing in the diagnosis and treatment of diseases of the teeth.

dermatologist. Physician specializing in the diagnosis and treatment of skin conditions.

electroencephalographic technologist. Person trained to run electroencephalograms (EEGs).

emergency medical technician. Person trained to provide emergency care to sick or injured patients being transported to a hospital.

emergency medicine specialist. Physician specializing in the treatment of trauma and sudden (emergency) medical conditions.

endocrinologist. Physician specializing in diseases of the endocrine system.

epidemiologist. Physician or other person specializing in studying factors that affect the frequency and distribution of disease.

family practitioner. Physician who provides comprehensive medical care for individuals of all ages, often for all members of the families they serve.

gastroenterologist. Physician specializing in diseases of the digestive organs, especially the stomach and intestines.

general practitioner. Primary care physician who provides ongoing, comprehensive medical care and office treatment.

general surgeon. Physician specializing in the use of a wide variety of surgical techniques to treat disease.

geriatrician. Physician specializing in the treatment of elderly individuals.

gerontologist. Physician or other person who specializes in the treatment of elderly individuals.

gynecologist. Physician specializing in disorders of the female reproductive system.

hematologist. Physician specializing in diseases of the blood.

histologic technician. Person trained to prepare tissue samples for examination by a physician or pathologist.

histologist. Physician or other person specializing in the study of tissues.

homeopath. Person who specializes in alleviating symptoms by administering small quantities of substances that would cause the symptoms if given in larger doses.

immunologist. Physician specializing in diseases related to the functioning of the immune system.

infectious disease specialist. Physician specializing in the diagnosis and treatment of infectious diseases.

internist. Physician specializing in the diagnosis and treatment of a wide range of diseases in adults; often provides primary care.

licensed practical nurse. Nurse who is trained to provide basic care for patients under the supervision of a physician or registered nurse.

medical assistant. Person who performs routine administrative and clinical tasks under the direction of a physician.

medical laboratory technician. Person trained to perform routine laboratory tests under the supervision of a technologist, therapist, or physician.

medical technologist. Person trained in the theory and practice of complex as well as routine clinical laboratory procedures.

medical transcriptionist. Person who transcribes medical dictation describing patients' histories and care.

midwife. Person trained to provide information and care throughout pregnancy, supervise labor and delivery, and provide postpartum care.

naturopath. Person who uses natural substances (vitamins, light, heat, etc.) to treat illness.

neonatologist. Physician specializing in the care of infants from birth to 4 weeks of age.

nephrologist. Physician specializing in diseases of the kidneys.

neurologist. Physician specializing in neurologic diseases that are treated by non-surgical techniques.

neurosurgeon. Physician specializing in neurologic diseases that are treated surgically.

nuclear medicine physician. Physician specializing in the use of radioactive materials to diagnose and treat disease.

nuclear medicine technologist. Person trained to perform nuclear medicine procedures under the supervision of a physician.

nurse practitioner. Registered nurse trained to provide health services under the supervision of a physician.

nursing assistant. Person who performs routine patient care tasks under the supervision of a registered nurse.

obstetrician. Physician specializing in pregnancy, labor, childbirth, and medical care during the immediate postpartum period.

occupational therapist. Person who specializes in the rehabilitation of people disabled by illness or injury, usually with the goal of helping them regain sufficient muscular control to perform routine tasks.

oncologist. Physician specializing in the diagnosis and treatment of tumors.

ophthalmologist. Physician specializing in diseases of the eye.

optician. Person trained to grind lenses to fill prescriptions for corrective eyeglasses.

optometrist. Doctor of optometry; person trained and licensed to test visual acuity and to prescribe corrective lenses, but not to prescribe drugs or perform surgical procedures.

oral surgeon. Physician specializing in surgical procedures of the mouth.

orthodontist. Dentist with advanced training in the straightening of teeth and the correction of certain jaw disorders.

orthopedic surgeon. Physician specializing in surgical treatment of diseases of the bones and joints.

osteopath. Doctor of osteopathy; physician specializing in the treatment of disorders by ensuring proper formation and alignment of the muscles and bones as well as by traditional methods.

otolaryngologist. Physician specializing in diseases of the head and neck, especially the ears and respiratory system.

otorhinolaryngologist. Physician specializing in diseases of the ears, nose, and throat; also called an ear, nose, and throat specialist (ENT).

paramedic. Person trained to provide emergency care to patients being transported to a hospital; usually has more training than an emergency medical technician.

pathologist. Physician specializing in the diagnosis of disease by means of clinical and laboratory studies of tissues and cells.

pediatrician. Physician specializing in the treatment of children.

periodontist. Dentist specializing in the treatment of diseases affecting the structures that support the teeth, such as the gums.

pharmacist. Person professionally trained to prepare and dispense drugs.

physiatrist. Physician specializing in the rehabilitation of individuals debilitated by illness or injury.

physical therapist. Person who specializes in the treatment of muscle injuries and other disorders by physical methods such as exercise and massage.

physician's assistant. Person trained to perform certain functions of a physician, such as history taking and routine tests and treatment.

plastic surgeon. Physician specializing in the surgical repair or reconstruction of organs or other parts of the body.

podiatrist. Doctor of podiatric medicine; person specializing in the diagnosis and treatment of foot disorders.

proctologist. Physician specializing in diseases of the rectum and anus.

psychiatrist. Physician specializing in mental, emotional, and behavioral disorders.

psychologist. Doctor (PhD) who specializes in the non-medical treatment of emotional disorders.

pulmonologist. Physician specializing in diseases of the lungs.

radiation oncologist. Physician specializing in the use of radiation to diagnose and treat tumors, especially cancers.

radiation therapy technologist. Person trained to deliver courses of radiation treatment prescribed by a radiologist.

radiologic technologist. Person trained to perform diagnostic tests involving radiation and to deliver courses of radiation treatment.

radiologist. Physician specializing in the use of radioactive materials, radiation, and other imaging techniques to diagnose and treat disease.

registered nurse. Nurse who is registered and licensed to provide information and care to patients.

respiratory therapist. Person trained in the treatment, management, and care of patients with respiratory disorders.

respiratory therapy technician. Person trained to provide routine treatment for patients with respiratory disorders under the supervision of a respiratory therapist.

rheumatologist. Physician specializing in diseases of the joints.

sports medicine specialist. Physician specializing in fitness and in the prevention and treatment of sports-related (muscle and bone) injuries.

surgeon. Physician specializing in general surgery or the surgical treatment of disorders of particular body systems.

surgeon's assistant. Physician's assistant trained to perform certain procedures under the supervision of a surgeon.

surgical technologist. Person who assists surgeons and others during surgery.

thoracic surgeon. Physician specializing in surgical procedures involving organs of the chest (i.e., the heart and lungs).

urologist. Physician specializing in disorders of the urinary system and the male reproductive system.

vascular surgeon. Physician specializing in surgical procedures involving the vasculature.

APPENDIX C
Abbreviations by Body System

The following are lists of commonly used medical abbreviations organized by body system. They are written here as they most often appear in medical documents. According to individual preferences, these abbreviations may also appear in other forms: with or without periods, and with upper or lower case letters. As you use these lists, note also that some abbreviations have more than one meaning. In these cases, you must decipher the abbreviations according to the context in which they are used.

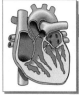

Cardiovascular System

Afib	atrial fibrillation		**HT**	hypertension
AMI	acute myocardial infarction		**LDL**	low-density lipoprotein
AS	aortic stenosis		**LVEDP**	left ventricular end-diastolic pressure
ASHD	arteriosclerotic heart disease		**LVEF**	left ventricular ejection fraction
AV	atrioventricular		**LVH**	left ventricular hypertrophy
BBB	bundle branch block		**MI**	myocardial infarction
BP	blood pressure		**MS**	mitral stenosis
CABG	coronary artery bypass graft		**MVP**	mitral valve prolapse
CAD	coronary artery disease		**nitro**	nitroglycerine
cath	catheterization		**P**	pulse
CCU	coronary care unit		**PAC**	premature atrial contraction
CHD	coronary heart disease		**PAT**	paroxysmal atrial tachycardia
CHF	congestive heart failure		**PTCA**	percutaneous transluminal coronary angioplasty
chol	cholesterol			
CPR	cardiopulmonary resuscitation		**PVC**	premature ventricular contraction
CV	cardiovascular		**PVD**	peripheral vascular disease
CVD	cardiovascular disease		**S-A**	sinoatrial
DOE	dyspnea on exertion		**SVT**	supraventricular tachycardia
DVT	deep vein thrombosis		**Trig**	triglycerides
ECG	electrocardiogram		**Vfib**	ventricular fibrillation
EKG	electrocardiogram		**VLDL**	very low-density lipoprotein
HDL	high-density lipoprotein		**VSD**	ventricular septal defect
HR	heart rate		**VT**	ventricular tachycardia

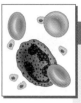

Blood

AHF	antihemophilic factor
ALL	acute lymphocytic leukemia
AML	acute myelocytic leukemia
baso	basophils
CBC	complete blood count
CLL	chronic lymphocytic leukemia
CML	chronic myelogenous leukemia
crit	hematocrit
diff	differential
eosins	eosinophils
ESR	erythrocyte sedimentation rate
Fe	iron
Hb	hemoglobin
Hct	hematocrit
Hgb	hemoglobin
Ht	hematocrit
lymphs	lymphocytes
lytes	electrolytes
MCH	mean corpuscular hemoglobin
MCHC	mean corpuscular hemoglobin concentration
MCV	mean corpuscular volume
mono	monocyte
PCV	packed cell volume
PMN	polymorphonuclear leukocyte; neutrophil
poly	polymorphonuclear leukocyte; neutrophil
pro time	prothrombin time
PT	prothrombin time
PTT	partial thromboplastin time
RBC	red blood cell; red blood count
Rh	Rhesus factor
sed rate	erythrocyte sedimentation rate
seg	polymorphonuclear leukocyte; neutrophil
TT	thrombin time
WBC	white blood cell; white blood count

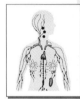

Lymphatic and Immune Systems

Ab	antibody
AFB	acid-fast bacilli
Ag	antigen
AIDS	acquired immune deficiency syndrome
ax	axillary
AZT	azidothymidine
EBV	Epstein-Barr virus
ELISA	enzyme-linked immunosorbent assay
HIV	human immunodeficiency virus
Ig	immunoglobulin
LE	lupus erythematosus
PCP	*Pneumocystis carinii* pneumonia
SLE	systemic lupus erythematosus

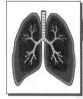

Respiratory System

A&P	auscultation and percussion
ABG	arterial blood gases
ARDS	adult respiratory distress syndrome
ARF	acute respiratory failure
broncho	bronchoscopy
CF	cystic fibrosis
CO_2	carbon dioxide
COLD	chronic obstructive lung disease
COPD	chronic obstructive pulmonary disease
CPR	cardiopulmonary resuscitation
CXR	chest x-ray
DOE	dyspnea on exertion
DPT	diphtheria, pertussis, tetanus (vaccination)
EENT	eyes, ears, nose, and throat
ENT	ears, nose, and throat
FEF	forced expiratory flow
FEV	forced expiratory volume
LRI	lower respiratory infection
O_2	oxygen
P&A	percussion and auscultation

PFTs	pulmonary function tests		**TB**	tuberculosis
R	respiration		**TLC**	total lung capacity
RDS	respiratory distress syndrome		**trach**	tracheostomy
resp	respirations		**URI**	upper respiratory infection
SOB	shortness of breath		**VC**	vital capacity
T&A	tonsillectomy and adenoidectomy			

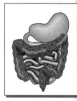

Digestive System

ALK	alkaline phosphatase		**IVC**	intravenous cholangiography
alk phos	alkaline phosphatase		**LFTs**	liver function tests
ALT	alanine transaminase (formerly SGPT)		**NG tube**	nasogastric tube
			OCG	oral cholecystography
AST	aspartic acid transaminase (formerly SGOT)		**PKU**	phenylketonuria
			PU	peptic ulcer
BaE	barium enema		**SGOT**	serum glutamic oxalacetic transaminase (AST)
BE	barium enema			
BM	bowel movement		**SGPT**	serum glutamic pyruvic transaminase (ALT)
GB	gallbladder			
GI	gastrointestinal		**TPN**	total parenteral nutrition
HCl	hydrochloric acid		**UGI**	upper gastrointestinal
IBD	inflammatory bowel disease			

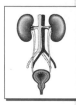

Urinary System

ADH	anti-diuretic hormone		**IVP**	intravenous pyelography
ARF	acute renal failure		**KUB**	kidneys, ureters, and bladder
BUN	blood urea nitrogen		**PD**	peritoneal dialysis
CAPD	continuous ambulatory peritoneal dialysis		**RP**	retrograde pyelography
			RU	routine urinalysis
cath	catheter; catheterization		**UA, U/A**	urinalysis
CRF	chronic renal failure		**U/O**	urinary output
cysto	cystoscopic examination		**urol**	urology
ESRD	end-stage renal disease		**UTI**	urinary tract infection
GFR	glomerular filtration rate		**VCUG**	voiding cystourethrography

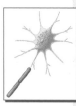

Nervous System

ACh	acetylcholine		**CSF**	cerebrospinal fluid
ALS	amyotrophic lateral sclerosis (Lou Gehrig's disease)		**CVA**	cerebrovascular accident
			DSM	*Diagnostic and Statistical Manual of Mental Disorders*
ANS	autonomic nervous system			
CNS	central nervous system		**EEG**	electroencephalogram
CP	cerebral palsy		**Em**	emmetropia

ICP	intracranial pressure
LP	lumbar puncture
MAO	monoamine oxidase
MRI	magnetic resonance imaging
MS	multiple sclerosis

NE	norepinephrine
PET	positron emission tomography
PNS	peripheral nervous system
Psych	psychiatry
TIA	transient ischemic attack

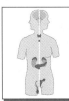

Endocrine System

ACTH	adrenocorticotropic hormone
ADH	anti-diuretic hormone
BMR	basal metabolic rate
DI	diabetes insipidus
DM	diabetes mellitus
FBS	fasting blood sugar
FSH	follicle-stimulating hormone
GH	growth hormone
GTT	glucose tolerance test
IDDM	insulin-dependent diabetes mellitus

LH	luteinizing hormone
MSH	melanocyte-stimulating hormone
NIDDM	non-insulin-dependent diabetes mellitus
PTH	parathyroid hormone
RAIU	radioactive iodine uptake
RIA	radioimmunoassay
T_3	triiodothyronine
T_4	thyroxine (tetraiodothyronine)
TSH	thyroid-stimulating hormone

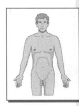

Male Reproductive System

BPH	benign prostatic hypertrophy
FTA-ABS	fluorescent treponemal antibody absorption test
GC	gonococcus; gonorrhea
GU	genitourinary
HSV	herpes simplex virus
NGU	nongonococcal urethritis

NSU	nonspecific urethritis
STD	sexually transmitted disease
TUR	transurethral resection
TURP	transurethral resection of the prostate (prostatectomy)
VD	venereal disease
VDRL	Venereal Disease Research Laboratory (or its syphilis test)

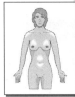

Female Reproductive System

AB	abortion
AFP	alpha fetoprotein
CPD	cephalopelvic disproportion
CS	cesarean section
CVS	chorionic villus sampling
Cx	cervix
D&C	dilation and curettage
D&E	dilation and evaluation
DES	diethylstilbestrol
EDD	expected date of delivery
ERT	estrogen replacement therapy

FHS	fetal heart sounds
FHT	fetal heart tones
FSH	follicle-stimulating hormone
G	pregnant (gravida)
GC	gonococcus; gonorrhea
Grav. 1, 2, 3	first, second, third pregnancy
GU	genitourinary
GYN	gynecology
HCG	human chorionic gonadotropin
IUD	intrauterine device
LH	luteinizing hormone

LMP	last menstrual period
multip.	multipara; multiparous
NB	newborn
NGU	nongonococcal urethritis
NSU	nonspecific urethritis
OB	obstetrics
OB/GYN	obstetrics and gynecology
OC	oral contraceptive
Pap	Papanicolaou smear

Para 1, 2, 3	having 1, 2, 3 live births
PID	pelvic inflammatory disease
PMS	premenstrual syndrome
STD	sexually transmitted disease
TSS	toxic shock syndrome
UC	uterine contractions
vag	vaginal
VD	venereal disease

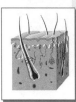

Skeletal and Muscular Systems

ALS	amyotrophic lateral sclerosis (Lou Gehrig's disease)
C1 - C7	cervical vertebrae (numbers 1-7)
DJD	degenerative joint disease
EMG	electromyography; electromyogram
Fx	fracture
L1 - L5	lumbar vertebrae (numbers 1-5)
LP	lumbar puncture
MG	myasthenia gravis

NSAID	non-steroidal anti-inflammatory drug
OA	osteoarthritis
Ortho	orthopedics
RA	rheumatoid arthritis
RF	rheumatoid factor
ROM	range of motion
S1 - S2	first, second sacral vertebra
T1 - T12	thoracic vertebrae (numbers 1-12)
THR	total hip replacement

Skin

bx	biopsy
Derm.	dermatology
exc	excision
I&D	incision and drainage

ID	intradermal
SC	subcutaneous
subcu	subcutaneous
subq	subcutaneous

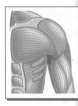

Special Senses: The Eyes

Acc	accommodation
Astigm	astigmatism
c. gl.	corrected (with glasses)
EOM	extraocular movement
ET	esotropia
IOP	intraocular pressure
myop	myopia
OD	right eye (oculus dexter)
Ophth	ophthalmic; ophthalmology

OS	left eye (oculus sinister)
OU	each eye (oculus uterque); both eyes (oculus unitas)
PERRLA	pupils equal, regular, and reactive to light and accommodation
REM	rapid eye movement
s. gl.	without correction (without glasses)
VA	visual acuity
VF	visual field

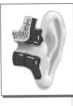

Special Senses: The Ears

AC	air conduction	**ENT**	ear, nose, and throat
AD	right ear (auris dexter)	**HD**	hearing distance
AS	left ear (auris sinister)	**NCL**	normal conversational level
BC	bone conduction	**OM**	otitis media
BOM	bilateral otitis media	**TM**	tympanic membrane
dB	decibel		

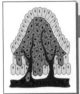

Oncology

AFP	alpha fetoprotein	**ERA**	estradiol receptor assay
ALL	acute lymphocytic leukemia	**5-Fu**	5-fluorouracil
AML	acute myelocytic leukemia	**Ga**	gallium
ara-C	cytosine arabinoside	**mets**	metastases
bx	biopsy	**MOPP**	nitrogen mustard, Oncovin, prednisone, procarbazine
Ca, CA	cancer; carcinoma	**MTX**	methotrexate
CEA	carcinoembryonic antigen	**POMP**	prednisone, Oncovin, methotrexate, 6-mercaptopurine
chem	chemotherapy		
chemo	chemotherapy	**PR**	partial response
CLL	chronic lymphocytic leukemia	**prot**	protocol
CMF	Cytoxan, methotrexate, 5-fluorouracil	**PSA**	prostate-specific antigen
CML	chronic myelogenous leukemia	**TNM**	tumor, nodes, and metastases
CR	complete response	**VPB**	Velban, cisplatin, bleomycin
DNA	deoxyribonucleic acid	**XRT**	radiation therapy
ER	estrogen receptor		

Pharmacology/General

a.c.	before meals (ante cibum)	**hs**	at bedtime (hora somni)
ABC	aspiration, biopsy, cytology	**hypo**	hypodermic
ad lib	as desired (ad libitum)	**I&O**	intake and output
AP	anteroposterior	**i.m., IM**	intramuscular
aq	water; aqueous (aqua)	**inj**	injection
b.i.d., BID	twice a day (bis in die)	**IU**	international unit
bx	biopsy	**i.v., IV**	intravenous
CAT	computerized axial tomography	**lap**	laparotomy
CT	computerized tomography	**MRI**	magnetic resonance imaging
D/C	discontinue	**NPO**	nothing by mouth (non per os)
Dx	diagnosis	**NSAID**	non-steroidal anti-inflammatory drug
exc	excision	**od**	every day (omnis die)
FU, F/U	follow-up	**OTC**	over the counter
FUO	fever of undetermined origin	**paren**	parenteral
gr	grain	**path**	pathology
gtt	drops (guttae)	**p.c.**	after meals (post cibum)

PDR	*Physicians' Desk Reference*	**RIA**	radioimmunoassay
PET	positron emission tomography	**Rx**	prescription; treatment
PO, po	by mouth (per os)	**sig**	label (signa)
PP	after a meal (post prandial)	**stat**	immediately (statim)
p.r.n.	when needed (pro re nata)	**supp**	suppository
q.d.	every day (quaque die)	**tab**	tablet
q.h.	every hour (quaque hora)	**t.i.d., TID**	three times a day (ter in die)
q.i.d.	four times a day (quater in die)	**UK**	unknown
q.n.s.	quantity not sufficient	**ung**	ointment
q.o.d.	every other day	**VS**	vital signs
q.o.h.	every other hour	**YOB**	year of birth
rad	radiation absorbed dose		

APPENDIX D
Alphabetical Abbreviations

The following is an alphabetical list of the abbreviations found in *Appendix C: Abbreviations by Body System*, as well as many additional medical abbreviations. It is provided so that you will be able to look up unfamiliar abbreviations quickly and easily. In a few cases, you may find that an abbreviation you are looking up has more than one meaning; when this happens, you will need to decipher its meaning according to the context in which it is used.

A

A&P	auscultation and percussion
AB	abortion
Ab	antibody
ABC	aspiration, biopsy, cytology
ABG	arterial blood gases
AC	air conduction
a.c.	before meals (ante cibum)
Acc	accommodation
ACh	acetylcholine
ACTH	adrenocorticotropic hormone
AD	right ear (auris dexter)
ADH	anti-diuretic hormone
ADL	activities of daily living
ad lib	as desired (ad libitum)
AFB	acid-fast bacilli
Afib	atrial fibrillation
AFP	alpha fetoprotein
Ag	antigen
AHF	antihemophilic factor
AIDS	acquired immune deficiency syndrome
ALK	alkaline phosphatase
alk phos	alkaline phosphatase

ALL	acute lymphocytic leukemia
ALS	amyotrophic lateral sclerosis (Lou Gehrig's disease)
ALT	alanine transaminase (formerly SGPT)
AMA	American Medical Association
AMI	acute myocardial infarction
AML	acute myelocytic leukemia
ANS	autonomic nervous system
AP	anteroposterior
aq	water; aqueous (aqua)
ara-C	cytosine arabinoside
ARDS	adult respiratory distress syndrome
ARF	acute renal failure; acute respiratory failure
AS	aortic stenosis; left ear (auris sinister)
ASA	aspirin
ASHD	arteriosclerotic heart disease
AST	aspartic acid transaminase (formerly SGOT)
Astigm	astigmatism
AV	atrioventricular
ax	axillary
AZT	azidothymidine

B

BaE	barium enema
baso	basophils
BBB	bundle branch block
BC	bone conduction
BE	barium enema
b.i.d., BID	twice a day (bis in die)
BM	bowel movement
BMR	basal metabolic rate
BOM	bilateral otitis media
BP	blood pressure
BPH	benign prostatic hypertrophy
BR	bed rest
broncho	bronchoscopy
BUN	blood urea nitrogen
bx	biopsy

C

C	Celsius; centigrade
c	with (cum)
C1 - C7	cervical vertebrae (numbers 1-7)
CA	chronological age; cancer; carcinoma
Ca	calcium; cancer; carcinoma
CABG	coronary artery bypass graft
CAD	coronary artery disease
CAPD	continuous ambulatory peritoneal dialysis
CAT	computerized axial tomography
cath	catheter; catheterization
CBC	complete blood count
CC	chief complaint
cc	cubic centimeter
CCU	coronary care unit
CDC	Centers for Disease Control
CEA	carcinoembryonic antigen
CF	cystic fibrosis
c. gl.	corrected (with glasses)
CHD	coronary heart disease
chem	chemotherapy
chemo	chemotherapy
CHF	congestive heart failure
chol	cholesterol

CLL	chronic lymphocytic leukemia
cm	centimeter
CMA	certified medical assistant
CMF	Cytoxan, methotrexate, 5-fluorouracil
CML	chronic myelogenous leukemia
CNS	central nervous system
CO$_2$	carbon dioxide
COLD	chronic obstructive lung disease
contra	against
COPD	chronic obstructive pulmonary disease
CP	cerebral palsy
CPD	cephalopelvic disproportion
CPR	cardiopulmonary resuscitation
CR	complete response
CRF	chronic renal failure
crit	hematocrit
CS	cesarean section
CSF	cerebrospinal fluid
CT	computerized tomography
CV	cardiovascular
CVA	cerebrovascular accident
CVD	cardiovascular disease
CVS	chorionic villus sampling
Cx	cervix
CXR	chest x-ray
cysto	cystoscopic examination

D

d	day
D&C	dilation and curettage
D&E	dilation and evaluation
dB	decibel
DC	doctor of chiropractic
D/C	discontinue
DDS	doctor of dental surgery
Derm.	dermatology
DES	diethylstilbestrol
DI	diabetes insipidus
diag	diagnosis
diff	differential
dil	dilute
disch	discharge
DJD	degenerative joint disease

dl	deciliter
DM	diabetes mellitus
DMD	doctor of dental medicine
DNA	deoxyribonucleic acid
DO	doctor of osteopathy
DOA	dead on arrival
DOB	date of birth
DOE	dyspnea on exertion
DPT	diphtheria, pertussis, tetanus (vaccination)
DRG	diagnosis-related group
DSM	*Diagnostic and Statistical Manual of Mental Disorders*
DT	delirium tremens
DVT	deep vein thrombosis
Dx	diagnosis

E

EBV	Epstein-Barr virus
ECG	electrocardiogram
EDC	estimated date of confinement
EDD	expected date of delivery
EEG	electroencephalogram
EENT	eyes, ears, nose, and throat
EKG	electrocardiogram
ELISA	enzyme-linked immunosorbent assay
Em	emmetropia
EMG	electromyography; electromyogram
ENT	ear, nose, and throat
EOM	extraocular movement
eos	eosinophils
eosins	eosinophils
ER	emergency room; estrogen receptor
ERA	estradiol receptor assay
ERT	estrogen replacement therapy
ESR	erythrocyte sedimentation rate
ESRD	end-stage renal disease
ET	esotropia
et	and
etiol	etiology
exc	excision

F

F	Fahrenheit
FBS	fasting blood sugar
FDA	Food and Drug Administration
Fe	iron
FEF	forced expiratory flow
FEV	forced expiratory volume
FH	family history
FHS	fetal heart sounds
FHT	fetal heart tones
5-Fu	5-fluorouracil
FP	family practitioner
FSH	follicle-stimulating hormone
FTA-ABS	fluorescent treponemal antibody absorption test
FU, F/U	follow-up
FUO	fever of undetermined origin
Fx	fracture

G

G	pregnant (gravida)
g	gram
Ga	gallium
GB	gallbladder
GC	gonococcus; gonorrhea
GFR	glomerular filtration rate
GH	growth hormone
GI	gastrointestinal
gm	gram
GP	general practitioner
gr	grain
Grav. 1, 2, 3	first, second, third pregnancy
GTT	glucose tolerance test
gtt	drops (guttae)
GU	genitourinary
GYN	gynecology

H

h	hour
Hb	hemoglobin
HCG	human chorionic gonadotropin

HCl	hydrochloric acid
Hct	hematocrit
HD	hearing distance
HDL	high-density lipoprotein
Hg	mercury
Hgb	hemoglobin
HIV	human immunodeficiency virus
H₂O	water
HR	heart rate
hr	hour
hs	at bedtime (hora somni)
HSV	herpes simplex virus
HT	hypertension
Ht	hematocrit
Hx	history
hypo	hypodermic
Hz	Hertz

I

I&D	incision and drainage
I&O	intake and output
IBD	inflammatory bowel disease
ICP	intracranial pressure
ICU	intensive care unit
ID	intradermal
IDDM	insulin-dependent diabetes mellitus
Ig	immunoglobulin
i.m., IM	intramuscular
inj	injection
IOP	intraocular pressure
IQ	intelligence quotient
IU	international unit
IUD	intrauterine device
i.v., IV	intravenous
IVC	intravenous cholangiography
IVP	intravenous pyelography

K

K	potassium
kg	kilogram
KUB	kidneys, ureters, and bladder

L

L	liter; left
l	liter
L1 - L5	lumbar vertebrae (numbers 1-5)
lap	laparotomy
lat	lateral
lb	pound
LDL	low-density lipoprotein
LE	lupus erythematosus
LFTs	liver function tests
LH	luteinizing hormone
LLQ	left lower quadrant
LMP	last menstrual period
LP	lumbar puncture
LPN	licensed practical nurse
LRI	lower respiratory infection
lt	left
LUQ	left upper quadrant
LVEDP	left ventricular end-diastolic pressure
LVEF	left ventricular ejection fraction
LVH	left ventricular hypertrophy
LVN	licensed vocational nurse
lymphs	lymphocytes
lytes	electrolytes

M

MAO	monoamine oxidase
MCH	mean corpuscular hemoglobin
MCHC	mean corpuscular hemoglobin concentration
MCV	mean corpuscular volume
MD	medical doctor
mets	metastases
MG	myasthenia gravis
mg	milligram
µg, mcg	microgram
MI	myocardial infarction
ml	milliliter
mm	millimeter
mono	monocyte
MOPP	nitrogen mustard, Oncovin, prednisone, procarbazine

MRI	magnetic resonance imaging
MS	mitral stenosis; multiple sclerosis
MSH	melanocyte-stimulating hormone
MTX	methotrexate
multip.	multipara; multiparous
MVP	mitral valve prolapse
myop	myopia

N

Na	sodium
NB	newborn
NCL	normal conversational level
NE	norepinephrine
NED	no evidence of disease
neg	negative
NG tube	nasogastric tube
NGU	nongonococcal urethritis
NIDDM	non-insulin-dependent diabetes mellitus
nitro	nitroglycerine
NPO	nothing by mouth (non per os)
NSAID	non-steroidal anti-inflammatory drug
NSU	nonspecific urethritis

O

O_2	oxygen
OA	osteoarthritis
OB	obstetrics
OB/GYN	obstetrics and gynecology
OC	oral contraceptive
OCG	oral cholecystography
OD	doctor of optometry; right eye (oculus dexter)
od	every day (omnis die)
OM	otitis media
Ophth	ophthalmic; ophthalmology
OR	operating room
Ortho	orthopedics
OS	left eye (oculus sinister)
os	mouth
OT	occupational therapy
OTC	over the counter

OU	each eye (oculus uterque); both eyes (oculus unitas)
oz	ounce

P

P	phosphorus; pulse
P&A	percussion and auscultation
PA	posteroanterior
PAC	premature atrial contraction
Pap	Papanicolaou smear
Para 1, 2, 3	having 1, 2, 3 live births
paren	parenteral
PAT	paroxysmal atrial tachycardia
path	pathology
p.c.	after meals (post cibum)
PCP	*Pneumocystis carinii* pneumonia
PCV	packed cell volume
PD	peritoneal dialysis
PDR	*Physicians' Desk Reference*
PE	physical examination
Ped, Peds	pediatrics
PERRLA	pupils equal, regular, and reactive to light and accommodation
PET	positron emission tomography
PFTs	pulmonary function tests
PH	past history
pH	hydrogen ion concentration
PI	present illness
PID	pelvic inflammatory disease
PKU	phenylketonuria
PM	after death (post mortem); physical medicine
PMN	polymorphonuclear leukocyte; neutrophil
PMS	premenstrual syndrome
PNS	peripheral nervous system
PO	postoperative
PO, po	by mouth (per os)
poly	polymorphonuclear leukocyte; neutrophil
POMP	prednisone, Oncovin, methotrexate, 6-mercaptopurine
pos	positive
post-op	postoperative

PP	after a meal (post prandial)
PR	partial response
pre-op	pre-operative
prep	prepare
p.r.n.	when needed (pro re nata)
prot	protocol
pro time	prothrombin time
PSA	prostate-specific antigen
Psych	psychiatry
PT	physical therapy; prothrombin time
pt	patient
PTCA	percutaneous transluminal coronary angioplasty
PTH	parathyroid hormone
PTT	partial thromboplastin time
PU	peptic ulcer
PVC	premature ventricular contraction
PVD	peripheral vascular disease

Q

q	every (quaque)
q.d.	every day (quaque die)
q. 2h.	every two hours (quaque secunda hora)
q.h.	every hour (quaque hora)
q.i.d.	four times a day (quater in die)
q.m.	every morning (quaque mane)
q.n.	every night (quaque nocte)
q.n.s.	quantity not sufficient
q.o.d.	every other day
q.o.h.	every other hour

R

R	respiration; right
RA	rheumatoid arthritis
rad	radiation absorbed dose
RAIU	radioactive iodine uptake
RBC	red blood cell; red blood count
RDS	respiratory distress syndrome
REM	rapid eye movement
resp	respirations
RF	rheumatoid factor

Rh	Rhesus factor
RIA	radioimmunoassay
RLQ	right lower quadrant
RMA	registered medical assistant
RN	registered nurse
R/O	rule out
ROM	range of motion
ROS	review of systems
RP	retrograde pyelography
RU	routine urinalysis
RUQ	right upper quadrant
Rx	prescription; treatment

S

s	without (sine)
S1 - S2	first, second sacral vertebra
S-A	sinoatrial
SC	subcutaneous
sec	second
sed rate	erythrocyte sedimentation rate
seg	polymorphonuclear leukocyte; neutrophil
s. gl.	without correction (without glasses)
SGOT	serum glutamic oxalacetic transaminase (AST)
SGPT	serum glutamic pyruvic transaminase (ALT)
sig	label (signa)
SLE	systemic lupus erythematosus
SOB	shortness of breath
sp. gr.	specific gravity
ss	half
staph	staphylococcus
stat	immediately (statim)
STD	sexually transmitted disease
strep	streptococcus
subcu	subcutaneous
subq	subcutaneous
supp	suppository
surg	surgery
SVT	supraventricular tachycardia
Sx	symptoms

T

T	temperature
T1 - T12	thoracic vertebrae (numbers 1-12)
T_3	triiodothyronine
T_4	thyroxine (tetraiodothyronine)
T&A	tonsillectomy and adenoidectomy
tab	tablet
TB	tuberculosis
THR	total hip replacement
TIA	transient ischemic attack
t.i.d., TID	three times a day (ter in die)
TLC	total lung capacity
TM	tympanic membrane
TNM	tumor, nodes, and metastases
TPN	total parenteral nutrition
TPR	temperature, pulse, respiration
trach	tracheostomy
Trig	triglycerides
TSH	thyroid-stimulating hormone
TSS	toxic shock syndrome
TT	thrombin time
TUR	transurethral resection
TURP	transurethral resection of the prostate (prostatectomy)
Tx	treatment; traction

U

U	unit
UA, U/A	urinalysis
UC	uterine contractions
UGI	upper gastrointestinal
UK	unknown
umb.	navel (umbilicus)
ung	ointment
U/O	urinary output
URI	upper respiratory infection

urol	urology
UTI	urinary tract infection
UV	ultraviolet

V

VA	visual acuity
vag	vaginal
VC	vital capacity
VCUG	voiding cystourethrography
VD	venereal disease
VDRL	Venereal Disease Research Laboratory (or its syphilis test)
VF	visual field
Vfib	ventricular fibrillation
VLDL	very low-density lipoprotein
VPB	Velban, cisplatin, bleomycin
VS	vital signs
VSD	ventricular septal defect
VT	ventricular tachycardia

W

WBC	white blood cell; white blood count
w/o	without
wt	weight

X

x, X	multiplied by
XRT	radiation therapy

Y

y/o	years old
YOB	year of birth
yr	year

APPENDIX E
Glossary of Word Elements

The following is a dictionary-style listing of the word elements presented throughout this book: prefixes, suffixes, and combining forms are all included in a single, alphabetized list. You can use this appendix to look up the definition of an unfamiliar or forgotten word element quickly and conveniently.

A

-a	condition
a-	without; not
ab-	away from
abdomin/o	abdomen
-ac	pertaining to
acoust/o	sound
acr/o	extremity (arm or leg)
ad-	toward; near
aden/o	gland
adenoid/o	adenoids
adip/o	fat
adren/o	adrenal glands
agglutin/o	clumping
-al	pertaining to
albumin/o	albumin
-algesia	sensitivity to pain
-algia	pain
aliment/o	food; nutrient
alveol/o	alveolus
-alysis	separation into components; analysis
ambly/o	dull; dim

amni/o	amnion (amniotic sac)
amphi-	both sides; double
an-	without; not
an/o	anus
ana-	without; not
andr/o	male
angi/o	vessel
aniso-	unequal
ankyl/o	crooked; stiff
ante-	before (in time); forward
anter/o	front
aort/o	aorta
append/o	appendix
aque/o	water
-ar	pertaining to
-arche	beginning
arteri/o	artery
arteriol/o	arteriole
arthr/o	joint
articul/o	joint
-ary	pertaining to
-assay	test; measure
-asthenia	weakness

-ated	subjected to; having
atel-	incomplete
ather/o	fatty substance
-ation	process
atri/o	atrium
audi/o	hearing
aur/o	external ear
auto-	self
ax/o	axon

B

bacteri/o	bacteria
balan/o	glans penis
bas/o	basic; alkaline
bi-	two
bi/o	life
bil/i	bile; gall
-blast	immature cell
blast/o	immature
blephar/o	eyelids
brady-	slow
bronch/o	bronchus

bronchiol/o	bronchiole
bucc/o	cheek
burs/o	bursa

C

-capnia	carbon dioxide
carcin/o	cancer
-carcinoma	malignant epithelial tumor
cardi/o	heart
caud/o	tail
cauter/o	burn; heat
cec/o	cecum
-cele	hernia; area of swelling
-centesis	puncture
cephal/o	head
cerebell/o	cerebellum
cerebr/o	cerebrum
cervic/o	cervix; neck
cheil/o	lip
chem/o	chemical; drug
chol/e	bile; gall
choledoch/o	common bile duct
chondr/o	cartilage
chori/o	chorion
choroid/o	choroid
chrom/o	color
chromat/o	color
chym/o	to pour
cili/o	ciliary body; eyelashes
circum-	around
-clasia	to break
-clast	cell that breaks
clon/o	turmoil
coagul/o	clotting
cochle/o	cochlea
col/o	colon; large intestine
colp/o	vagina
conjunctiv/o	conjunctiva
contra-	against; opposite side
cor/o	pupil

corne/o	cornea
coron/o	heart; crown
cortic/o	cortex; outer layer
crani/o	skull
crin/o	secrete
cry/o	cold
crypt/o	hidden
-cusis	hearing
-cuspid	tapered; pointed
cutane/o	skin
cycl/o	ciliary body
-cyesis	pregnancy
cyst/o	bladder; cyst; sac
cyt/o	cell
-cyte	cell

D

dacry/o	tear duct
dactyl/o	finger or toe
de-	down; lack of; loss of
dendr/o	dendrite
dent/i	teeth
derm/o	skin
-derma	skin
dermat/o	skin
-desis	to bind together
di-	two
dia-	through; across
-diastasis	separation
dipl/o	double; twice
dis-	apart; away from
dist/o	distant
dors/o	back
duoden/o	duodenum
-dynia	pain
dys-	abnormal; painful; difficult

E

-e	condition
-eal	pertaining to

ec-	out; away from
echo-	returned sound
-ectasis	expansion; dilation
-ectomy	surgical removal
-edema	swelling
electr/o	electricity
em-	in; inside
-ema	condition
embol/o	embolus
embry/o	embryo
-emesis	vomiting
-emia	blood condition
en-	in; surrounded by
encephal/o	brain
endo-	inside; within; inward
endometri/o	endometrium
enter/o	small intestine
eosin/o	red; dawn; rosy
epi-	on; over; above; outer
epididym/o	epididymis
episi/o	vulva
erythr/o	red
-esis	condition
esophag/o	esophagus
-esthesia	feeling; sensation
eu-	good; normal
ex-	out; away from
exo-	outside

F

fasci/o	fascia
fec/o	feces
fet/o	fetus
fibr/o	fiber; fibrous
flex/o	to bend
fove/o	fovea

G

galact/o	milk
ganglion/o	ganglion

gastr/o	stomach
-genesis	production of
-genic	producing
genit/o	reproductive
gest/o	gestation
gestat/o	gestation
gingiv/o	gum
glauc/o	gray
gli/o	glia
-globin	protein
glomerul/o	glomerulus
gloss/o	tongue
glyc/o	sugar; glucose
gon/o	genitals
gonad/o	gonads
goni/o	angle
-gram	record
granul/o	granules
-graph	recording instrument
-graphy	recording
gravid/o	pregnancy
-gravida	pregnant woman
gyn/o	woman; female
gynec/o	woman; female

H

hem/o	blood
hemat/o	blood
hemi-	one-half
hepat/o	liver
herni/o	hernia; protrusion through a tissue; rupture
hetero-	different
hidr/o	sweat
hist/o	tissue
homeo-	unchanging; same
homo-	same
hormon/o	hormone
hydr/o	water; hydrogen
hyper-	excessive
hypo-	under; reduced
hypophys/o	pituitary

hypothalam/o	hypothalamus
hyster/o	uterus

I

-ia	condition
-iasis	condition
-ic	pertaining to
-ical	pertaining to
-iferous	producing
-ile	pertaining to
ile/o	ileum
immun/o	immune; protected
in-	not; without
-in	substance
infer/o	lower; below
inguin/o	groin
inter-	between; among
intra-	within; inside
-ior	pertaining to
ipsi-	same; same side
ir/o	iris
irid/o	iris
-is	forms noun from root word
-ism	condition
iso-	equal; same
-ist	specialist
-itis	inflammation

J

jejun/o	jejunum

K

kerat/o	cornea; hard; horn-like
keton/o	ketones
-kinesia	movement; motion
kym/o	wave; quaver
kyph/o	humpback

L

labi/o	lip
labyrinth/o	inner ear
lacrim/o	tear
lact/o	milk
-lalia	speech; babbling
lapar/o	abdomen
laryng/o	larynx
later/o	side
lei/o	smooth
-lepsy	seizure
leuk/o	white
-lexia	word; phrase
ligament/o	ligament
lingu/o	tongue
lip/o	fat
-lith	stone
lith/o	stone
lob/o	lobe (of an organ)
loc/o	place
-logy	study of
lord/o	curve; swayback
lumb/o	loin; waist
-lunar	moon-shaped
lux/o	to slide
lymph/o	lymph
-lysis	dissolution; separation; destruction
-lytic	destroying; dissolving

M

macr/o	large
macro-	large
-malacia	softening
mamm/o	breast
mast/o	breast
mastoid/o	mastoid process
medi/o	middle
mediastin/o	in the middle; mediastinum
medull/o	medulla; inner layer

-megaly	enlargement	nucle/o	nucleus	pancreat/o	pancreas
melan/o	black	nulli-	none	papill/o	optic disk; nipple-like protrusion
men/o	menstruation	nyct/o	night		
mening/e	membranes; meninges			-para	to bear (a child); to bring forth
menstru/o	menstruation	**O**		para-	beside; beyond
-mentia	thinking	o/o	ovum; egg	parasympath/o	parasympathetic nervous system
mesencephal/o	midbrain	ocul/o	eye		
meta-	transfer; change	odont/o	teeth	parathyroid/o	parathyroid glands
-meter	measuring instrument	-oid	resembling	-paresis	partial paralysis
metr/o	uterus	olig/o	scanty; few	-partum	childbirth; labor
-metry	measurement	-oma	tumor; growth	-pathy	disease
mi/o	less; smaller	onc/o	tumor; mass	pelv/i	pelvis
micr/o	small	onych/o	nail	-penia	deficiency
micro-	small	oophor/o	ovaries	-pepsia	digestion
mio-	less; smaller	ophthalm/o	eye	per-	through
-mnesia	memory	-opia	vision	peri-	around; surrounding
mono-	one; single	-opsia	vision		
morph/o	shape	opt/o	eye	perine/o	perineum
multi-	many	or/o	mouth	peritone/o	peritoneum
mut/a	genetic change	orch/o	testes	phac/o	lens
my/o	muscle	orchi/o	testes	phag/o	eat; swallow
myc/o	fungus	orchid/o	testes	phak/o	lens
-mycosis	fungal infection	-orexia	appetite	pharyng/o	pharynx
mydr/o	widen; enlarge	orth/o	straight	-phasia	speech
myel/o	bone marrow; spinal cord	-ory	pertaining to	phe/o	brown; dark; dusky
		osche/o	scrotum		
myelin/o	myelin	-ose	having the qualities of	-phil	love; attraction
myos/o	muscle			phleb/o	vein
myring/o	eardrum	-osis	condition	-phonia	sound; voice
myx/o	mucus	oste/o	bone	phot/o	light
		ot/o	ear	phren/o	diaphragm
N		-otia	condition of the ear	-phylaxis	protection
nas/o	nose			-physis	to grow
nat/o	childbirth	-ous	pertaining to	pil/o	hair
ne/o	new	ov/o	ovum; egg	pineal/o	pineal gland
necr/o	death; corpse	ovari/o	ovaries	pituit/o	pituitary
neo-	new	ovul/o	ovum; egg	plas/o	growth; development
nephr/o	kidney	ox/o	oxygen		
neur/o	nerve; nerve tissue	-oxia	oxygen	-plasia	formation; growth condition
neuron/o	neuron				
neutr/o	neutral	**P**		-plasm	growth; development
noct/o	night	palat/o	palate	-plasty	surgical repair
normo-	normal	pan-	all	-plegia	paralysis
				pleur/o	pleura
				-pnea	breathing

pneum/o	lung; air	respir/o	breathing	spermat/o	spermatozoa
pneumon/o	lung; air	retin/o	retina	sphygm/o	pulse
-poiesis	formation	retro-	backward; behind	spir/o	breathing
-poietic	forming	rhabd/o	striated; skeletal	splen/o	spleen
poli/o	gray matter (in the nervous system)	rheumat/o	watery flow	spondyl/o	vertebrae
		rhin/o	nose	squam/o	scale-like
poly-	many	-rrhage	excessive flow; profuse discharge of blood	-stalsis	contraction
pont/o	pons			staped/o	stapes
-porosis	becoming porous or less dense			-stasis	stopping; standing still
		-rrhagia	excessive flow; profuse discharge of blood		
post-	after (in time or place)			-stenosis	narrowing
				sthen/o	strength
poster/o	back	-rrhaphy	suture; stitch	-stigma	point
-prandial	relating to a meal	-rrhea	discharge	-stitial	to set; to be situated
pre-	before (in time or place)				
				stomat/o	mouth
presby-	old age	**S**		-stomy	surgical opening
primi-	first			sub-	under; beneath
pro-	before (in time); in front of	salping/o	fallopian tube	sud/o	sweat
		sacr/o	lower back	super/o	upper; above
proct/o	anus; rectum	sarc/o	flesh; muscle	supra-	above
prostat/o	prostate gland	-sarcoma	malignant connective tissue tumor	sympath/o	sympathetic nervous system
proxim/o	near				
pseudo-	false			syn-	together; united
psor-	itching	scler/o	sclera	synapt/o	synapse
psor/o	itching	-sclerosis	hardening	synov/o	synovial fluid; synovial membrane
-ptosis	drooping; falling; prolapse	scoli/o	crooked; bent		
		-scopy	visual examination		
pulmon/o	lungs				
pupill/o	pupil	scot/o	darkness		
py/o	pus	seb/o	sebum	**T**	
pyel/o	renal pelvis	semi-	one-half; partly		
pylor/o	pylorus; pyloric sphincter	semin/o	semen	tachy-	fast
		sept/o	dividing wall	-taxia	muscular coordination
pyr/o	fever; fire; heat	sial/o	saliva		
		sialaden/o	salivary gland	ten/o	tendon
		sider/o	iron	tend/o	tendon
Q		sigmoid/o	sigmoid colon	tendin/o	tendon
		sin/o	sinus; sinus cavity	-tension	tautness; blood pressure
quadri-	four	-sis	condition		
		som/a	body	test/o	testes
		somat/o	body	testicul/o	testes
R		somn/i	sleep	thalam/o	thalamus
		-somnia	sleep	thec/o	sheath; covering
radi/o	radioactivity	son/o	sound waves	-therapy	treatment
rect/o	rectum	-spasm	sudden contraction	thorac/o	chest; thorax
ren/o	kidney	sperm/o	spermatozoa		

thromb/o	clot
thym/o	thymus
thyr/o	thyroid
thyroid/o	thyroid
toc/o	childbirth
-tochia	childbirth; labor
tok/o	childbirth
tom/o	section; layer; cut; incision
-tomy	surgical incision
ton/o	tension; pressure
tonsill/o	tonsils
-toxic	poisonous
trache/o	trachea
trans-	through; across
tri-	three
-tripsy	crushing
-trophic	nourishment; growth
-trophy	nourishment; growth
-tropic	turning; changing; acting upon
tympan/o	eardrum

U

ultra-	beyond
ultrason/o	ultrasound; very high frequency soundwaves
-um	thing; structure
umbilic/o	navel
un-	not
uni-	one
ur/o	urine; urea
ureter/o	ureter
urethr/o	urethra
-uria	urine condition
uter/o	uterus
uve/o	uvea
uvul/o	uvula

V

vagin/o	vagina
valvul/o	valve

vas/o	vessel; vas deferens
vascul/o	vessel
ven/o	vein
ventr/o	belly; belly-side
ventricul/o	ventricle
venul/o	venule
-version	turning
vertebr/o	vertebrae
vesic/o	bladder; blister; vesicle
vesicul/o	seminal vesicles
vestibul/o	vestibular apparatus
viscer/o	internal organs
vitre/o	glass
vulv/o	vulva

X

xen/o	strange; foreign
xer/o	dry

Answer Key

1. b, c, a, d

2. a. vascul/itis
   RW/S
   inflammation of the blood vessels
   b. brady/cardi/a
   P/RW/S
   condition characterized by a slow heart-beat (slow heart condition)
   c. cardi/o/vascul/ar
   RW/CV/RW/S
   pertaining to the heart and blood vessels
   d. immun/o/logy
   RW/CV/S
   the study of immunity (or immune reactions)
   e. nephr/itis
   RW/S
   inflammation of a kidney
   f. arthr/itis
   RW/S
   inflammation of a joint

3. o

4. a. keep
   b. drop
   c. keep

5. a. nephro/toxic
   b. nephr/itis

   c. pyelo/nephr/itis
   d. laryng/ectomy
   e. laryngo/scopy
   f. oto/laryngo/logy

1. d, f, b, a, e, c

2. a. -ated = subjected to; having
   b. -genic = producing
   c. -oid = resembling
   d. -ose = having the qualities of

3. a. conjunctiv*ae*
   b. test*es*
   c. ov*a*
   d. alveol*i*

4. d, b, a, g, f, e, c

5. a. different
   b. the same
   c. normal
   d. good
   e. one
   f. two (double)
   g. many
   h. half
   i. same
   j. same

6. b, d, e, a, c

7. a. dia-
   b. per-
   c. trans-

8. a. toward
   b. before
   c. under
   d. inside
   e. after
   f. before
   g. outer
   h. beneath
   i. backward

9. a. before (in time); in front of
   b. out; away from
   c. away from
   d. in; surrounded by
   e. against; opposite side
   f. first
   g. same; same side
   h. out; away from
   i. apart; away from
   j. in; inside

3

1. a, h, d, g, b, e, f, c

2. condition

3. a. pain
   b. swelling
   c. destroying; dissolving
   d. fungal infection
   e. poisonous
   f. nourishment; growth

4. b, c, d, a

5. a. abnormal; painful; difficult
   b. all
   c. false
   d. incomplete
   e. new
   f. unequal
   g. without; not
   h. fast

6. a. enlargement
   b. inflammation
   c. old age
   d. discharge
   e. slow
   f. without
   g. not
   h. not

7. a. narrowed
   b. Myosclerosis; osteomalacia
   c. excessive; reduced
   d. small; large

8. d, g, h, b, c, a, e, f

9. a. returned sound
   b. measurement
   c. visual examination
   d. ultrasound (very high frequency sound waves)
   e. record
   f. recording instrument

10. b, c, a

11. a. splenectomy
    b. angioplasty
    c. lobotomy
    d. cholecystectomy
    e. colostomy
    f. arthroplasty
    g. tympanostomy

1. a. body
   b. nucleus
   c. cell
   d. body
   e. tissue
   f. fat
   g. internal organs
   h. flesh; muscle

2. a. the body is standing erect, with the arms at the side and the palms facing forward
   b. lying face up
   c. lying face down
   d. lying down

3. a. frontal (coronal)
   b. transverse (horizontal or cross-sectional)
   c. sagittal (median) or midsagittal

4. a. pertaining to something farther from the point of interest; proximal
   b. pertaining to something inside; external
   c. pertaining to something close to the surface; deep
   d. pertaining to something away from the center; central

5. b, a, c, a, c, b, a, c

6. b, d, a, c, e

7. a. belly; belly-side
   b. back
   c. middle
   d. head
   e. tail
   f. near
   g. distant
   h. chest
   i. abdomen
   j. pelvis
   k. skull
   l. extremity (arm/leg)
   m. finger or toe
   n. groin
   o. navel
   p. loin; waist
   q. stomach
   r. cartilage

8. a. cranial (dorsal)
   b. spinal (dorsal)
   c. thoracic (ventral)
   d. abdominopelvic (ventral)

9. a. cranial cavity

   b. thoracic cavity
   c. spinal cavity
   d. abdominopelvic cavity
   e. abdominopelvic cavity
   f. thoracic cavity

10. a. right upper quadrant
    b. right lower quadrant
    c. left upper quadrant
    d. left lower quadrant

11. a. right hypochondriac
    b. right lumbar
    c. right inguinal
    d. epigastric
    e. umbilical
    f. hypogastric
    g. left hypochondriac
    h. left lumbar
    i. left inguinal

12. a. infero/medi/al
    below/middle/pertaining to
    pertaining to a location below and toward the middle

    b. antero/poster/ior
    front/back/pertaining to
    pertaining to the front and back

    c. dorso/ventr/al
    back/belly/pertaining to
    pertaining to the front and back

    d. antero/super/ior
    front/above/pertaining to
    pertaining to a location above and toward the front

    e. somato/megaly
    body/enlargement
    enlargement of the body (an unusually large body)

    f. dactyl/edema
    finger or toe/swelling
    swelling of the fingers or toes

    g. abdomino/thorac/ic
    abdomen/chest/pertaining to
    pertaining to the abdomen and chest

h. cyto/genic
cell/producing
producing cells

a. *vertical plane dividing the body into left side and right side*
no; sagittal plane

b. *horizontal plane dividing the body into upper and lower portions*
no; transverse plane

c. *pertaining to a location toward the front (i.e., the front ligament)*
no; anterior

d. *pertaining to a location toward the side (i.e., the side meniscus)*
yes

e. *pertaining to a location toward the middle (i.e., the middle meniscus)*
yes

f. *pertaining to a location toward the back (i.e., the back of the middle meniscus)*
yes

g. *pertaining to a location toward the front and middle (i.e., an incision in the middle of the front part of the knee)*
yes

h. *pertaining to a location toward the front and side (i.e., an incision on the side of the front part of the knee)*
no; anterolateral

1. frontal plane
2. transverse plane
3. sagittal plane
4. ventral
5. dorsal
6. medial
7. lateral
8. cephalic
9. caudal
10. proximal
11. distal
12. parietal
13. thoracic cavity
14. abdominopelvic cavity

15. cranial cavity
16. spinal cavity
17. hypochondriac
18. epigastric
19. lumbar
20. umbilical
21. inguinal
22. hypogastric

5

1. d, b, e, c, f, a

2. c, e, g, f, b, d, a

3. a. ventricle   f. vessel
   b. vessel   g. valve
   c. venule   h. embolus
   d. artery   i. vein
   e. pulse   j. fatty substance

4. e, c, f, b, g, d, a

5. a, d, g, e, c, f, b, h

6. a. electro/cardio/graphy
   electricity/heart/recording
   recording of electrical activity in the heart

   b. vaso/spasm
   vessel/sudden contraction
   sudden contraction of a blood vessel

   c. valvulo/plasty
   valve/surgical repair
   surgical repair (or replacement) of a valve

   d. endo/card/itis
   within/heart/inflammation
   inflammation within the heart

   e. a/rrhythm/ia
   without/rhythm/condition
   irregularity in the heart beat

   f. veni/puncture
   vein/puncture
   puncture of a vein (with a needle)

g. phleb/itis
vein/inflammation
inflammation of a vein

h. angio/graphy
vessel/recording
x-ray recording of the blood vessels

i. angio/spasm
vessel/sudden contraction
sudden contraction of a blood vessel

j. ather/oma
fatty substance/growth
growth of a fatty deposit (in a blood vessel)

k. embol/ism
embolus/condition
condition of having an embolus (which obstructs a blood vessel)

l. thrombo/phleb/itis
clot/vein/inflammation
inflammation of a vein with development of a clot

m. thromb/osis
clot/condition
condition characterized by having a clot (which obstructs a blood vessel)

n. veno/graphy
vein/recording
x-ray recording of a vein

o. phlebo/tomy
vein/surgical incison
surgical incision into a vein

p. ventriculo/graphy
ventricle/recording
x-ray recording of a ventricle

7. a. arterio/sclerosis
b. hypo/tension
c. valvo/tomy
d. cardio/myo/pathy
e. aorto/stenosis
f. valvul/itis
g. peri/cardio/centesis
h. angio/plasty
i. hyper/tension

8. a. slow; fast
b. myocarditis; pericarditis
c. Infarction; coarctation
d. Cardiac arrest; myocardial infarction

9. a. essential
b. malignant
c. secondary
d. heart beat
e. narrower
f. Raynaud's phenomenon
g. varicose
h. Mitral valve prolapse
i. rheumatic fever
j. aneurysm
k. cardioversion
l. electrical signals (or impulses)

a. *use of a treadmill to measure a patient's cardiovascular response to exercise*
yes

b. *enlargement of the left ventricular wall, usually due to chronic hypertension*
no; left ventricular hypertrophy

c. *diagnostic procedure in which a tube is pushed through a blood vessel to the heart*
no; cardiac catheterization

d. *condition in which the heart's blood pumping ability is impaired, resulting in the backup of fluid in the lungs*
no; congestive heart failure

e. *any disease that impairs the coronary arteries' ability to deliver blood to the heart*
yes

f. *severe chest pain and feeling of suffocation due to inadequate blood flow to the heart muscle*
no; angina pectoris

g. *procedure in which a vein taken from the leg is grafted onto the heart to bypass an obstruction in a coronary artery*
yes

1. endocardium
2. myocardium
3. epicardium
4. pericardium
5. atria
6. ventricles
7. vasculature
8. arteries
9. arterioles
10. capillaries
11. venules
12. veins
13. coronary arteries
14. systole
15. diastole
16. ischemia
17. angina pectoris
18. myocardial infarction
19. bradycardia
20. tachycardia
21. cardiomyopathy
22. congestive heart failure
23. endocarditis
24. arrhythmia
25. fibrillation
26. left ventricular hypertrophy
27. rheumatic heart disease
28. mitral valve prolapse
29. arteriosclerosis
30. atherosclerosis
31. aneurysm
32. embolism
33. thrombosis
34. phlebitis
35. thrombophlebitis
36. Raynaud's phenomenon
37. angiography
38. echocardiography
39. electrocardiography
40. balloon angioplasty
41. coronary artery bypass graft
42. phlebotomy

6

1. g, f, e, b, a, c, d, h

2. a. clumping   e. lymph
   b. clotting   f. blood
   c. clot   g. blood
   d. granules   h. iron

3. c, a, b, d

4. e, f, c, b, a, d

5. a. thrombo/cyto/penia
      clot/cell/deficiency
      deficiency of clotting cells (thrombocytes)

   b. hemo/rrhage
      blood/excessive flow
      excessive bleeding

   c. a/plast/ic an/emia
      without/formation/pertaining to; without/
      blood condition
      *blood cell deficiency caused by a lack of
      blood cell formation*

   d. hemo/lytic an/emia
      blood/destroying; without/blood condition
      *blood cell deficiency caused by excessive
      blood cell destruction*

   e. erythro/cyte
      red/cell
      red cell (red blood cell)

   f. hemo/phil/ia
      blood/love; attraction/condition
      *blood condition characterized by excessive
      bleeding*

   g. leuk/emia
      white/blood condition
      *malignant blood condition characterized
      by excessive production of white cells*

6. a. leuko/penia
   b. hemo/globin
   c. poly/cyt/hem/ia
   d. myel/oma

a. *bruises (discolorations caused by leakage of blood under the skin due to injury)*
   no; ecchymoses

b. *any abnormality of the blood*
   no; blood dyscrasia

c. *group of routine blood tests including hemoglobin and red cell, white cell, and platelet counts*
   yes

d. *test measuring each type of white cell as percentage of the total number of leukocytes*
   no; differential

e. *test measuring the amount of hemoglobin in the blood*
   yes

f. *test measuring the number of red cells in the blood*
   yes

g. *test measuring the number of white cells in the blood*
   yes

h. *use of a needle to extract bone marrow for examination and evaluation*
   no; bone marrow biopsy

i. *intravenous administration of blood into a patient, usually to replace lost blood cells*
   yes

j. *procedure in which a patient's diseased bone marrow is destroyed, then replaced with healthy donor bone marrow*
   no; bone marrow transplantation

1. plasma
2. erythrocytes
3. hemoglobin
4. leukocytes
5. granulocytes
6. polymorphonuclear leukocytes
7. neutrophils
8. eosinophils
9. basophils
10. agranulocytes

11. lymphocytes
12. thrombocytes
13. platelets
14. coagulation
15. thromboplastin
16. prothrombin
17. thrombin
18. fibrinogen
19. fibrin
20. serum
21. albumin
22. anemia
23. hemolytic anemia
24. pernicious anemia
25. sickle cell anemia
26. blood dyscrasia
27. hemophilia
28. hemorrhage
29. leukemia
30. leukopenia
31. polycythemia
32. purpura
33. thrombocytopenia
34. hematocrit
35. differential
36. Coombs' test
37. erythrocyte sedimentation rate
38. partial thromboplastin time
39. prothrombin time
40. thrombin time

7

1. d, f, c, e, b, a

2. a. lymph
   b. lymph gland
   c. lymph vessel

3. b, d, c, a

4. d, a, c, b, e

5. a. adenoid/ectomy
   adenoids/surgical removal
   surgical removal of the adenoids

   b. a/splen/ia
   without/spleen/condition
   condition characterized by lack of a spleen

   c. lymph/angio/graphy
   lymph/vessel/recording
   x-ray recording of the lymph vessels

   d. lymph/oma
   lymph/tumor; growth
   tumor of the lymph tissues

   e. lymph/aden/oma
   lymph/gland/tumor; growth
   tumor of the lymph glands

   f. lymph/angi/oma
   lymph/vessel/tumor
   tumor of the lymph vessels

   g. lymph/edema
   lymph/swelling
   swelling of the lymph tissues

   h. tonsill/itis
   tonsils/inflammation
   inflammation of the tonsils

6. a. lympho/graphy
   b. lymph/adeno/graphy
   c. lymph/angio/graphy
   d. lymph/adeno/tomy
   e. lymph/angio/tomy
   f. lymph/angio/plasty
   g. lymph/aden/ectomy

7. a. tonsill/ectomy
   b. spleno/megaly
   c. lymph/aden/itis
   d. adenoid/itis
   e. splen/ectomy
   f. lympho/pathy
   g. lymph/adeno/pathy

   a. *any disease of the lymph glands*
   no; lymphadenopathy

   b. *enlargement of the spleen*
   yes

   c. *any malignant lymphatic disease except Hodgkin's disease*
   no; non-Hodgkin's lymphoma

   d. *x-ray recording of the lymph vessels after injection of a contrast agent*
   no; lymphangiography

   e. *surgical removal of the spleen*
   no; splenectomy

1. lymph
2. lymph vessels
3. lymph nodes
4. spleen
5. thymus
6. adenoids
7. palatine tonsils
8. lingual tonsils
9. adenoiditis
10. lymphedema
11. elephantiasis
12. lymphadenopathy
13. lymphadenitis
14. mononucleosis
15. lymphoma
16. Hodgkin's disease
17. splenomegaly
18. tonsillitis
19. lymphangiography
20. adenoidectomy
21. splenectomy
22. tonsillectomy

8

1. a. immune; protected
   b. "immune protein" that can react with and neutralize specific foreign substances
   c. eat; swallow
   d. "eating cell" that can engulf and digest foreign substances
   e. protection

2. d, c, a, b

3. b, c, d, a, e

4. a. immuno/suppression
   immune/suppression
   suppression of immune responses

   b. auto/immune
   self/immune
   having immune responses to oneself

   c. ana/phylaxis
   backward/protection
   extreme immune reaction that is harmful instead of helpful

   d. immuno/globulin
   immune/protein
   immune protein

   e. phago/cyte
   eat; swallow/cell
   cell that eats (engulfs) foreign matter

   f. phago/cyt/osis
   eat; swallow/cell/condition
   condition (process) of a cell engulfing foreign matter

   g. immuno/genic
   immune/producing
   producing immune responses

   h. immuno/comprised
   immune/compromised
   having compromised (ineffective) immune responses

5. a. vaccin/ation
   b. immuno/therapy
   c. hyper/sensitivity
   d. immuno/suppression
   e. immuno/logy
   f. immuno/hemato/logy
   g. immun/ization

   a. *disease caused by HIV infection and characterized by extreme immunodeficiency, with opportunistic infections and/or rare cancers*
   no; acquired immune deficiency syndrome

   b. *infection caused by pathogens that do not normally cause disease, but are able to take hold due to immunodeficiency*
   no; opportunistic infection

   c. *state in which the immune system is unable to respond adequately*
   yes

   d. *test used to screen blood for the presence of antibodies to HIV (or other viruses)*
   no; ELISA

   e. *test used to detect the presence of HIV DNA (or other viral DNA)*
   yes

1. phagocytes
2. neutrophils
3. macrophages
4. complement
5. antigen
6. B-cells
7. plasma cell
8. antibodies
9. immunoglobulins
10. T-cells
11. hypersensitivity
12. anaphylaxis
13. autoimmune disease
14. immunodeficiency
15. opportunistic infection
16. acquired immune deficiency syndrome
17. ELISA
18. Western blot
19. immunization
20. vaccination
21. immunosuppression
22. immunotherapy

9

1. b, d, a, c, e

2. a. pleura   d. trachea
   b. lung; air   e. nose
   c. oxygen   f. breathing

g. alveolus   j. mouth
h. bronchiole   k. bronchus
i. lobe (of the lung)

3. g, b, f, c, a, e, d

4. b, d, a, e, c

5. e, a, d, b, f, c

6. a. acute respiratory syndrome in children characterized by a barking cough
   b. serious acute bacterial infection characterized by sore throat and fever
   c. accumulation of air in the pleural space
   d. infection, usually of the lungs, caused by *Mycobacterium tuberculosis*
   e. loud course breathing sounds; sign of obstructed airway

7. a. tracheo/tomy
      trachea/surgical incision
      surgical incision in the trachea

   b. spiro/metry
      breathing/measurement
      measurement of breathing

   c. lob/ectomy
      lobe of the lung/surgical removal
      surgical removal of a lobe of a lung

   d. hyp/oxia
      reduced/oxygen
      condition of reduced oxygen (in the tissues)

   e. hyp/ox/emia
      reduced/oxygen/blood condition
      condition of reduced oxygen in the blood

   f. pneumon/ia
      lung/condition
      inflammation of one or both lungs

   g. dys/pnea
      difficult; painful/breathing
      difficult or painful breathing

   h. pharyng/itis
      pharynx/inflammation
      inflammation of the pharynx

   i. rhino/plasty
      nose/surgical repair
      plastic surgery of the nose

j. atel/ectasis
   incomplete/expansion
   incomplete expansion (of a lung)

k. pulmono/logy
   lungs/study of
   study of the lungs

l. bronch/itis
   bronchus/inflammation
   inflammation of the bronchi

m. rhin/itis
   nose/inflammation
   inflammation of the nose

n. laryngo/scopy
   larynx/visual examination
   visual examination of the larynx

o. pulmon/ary
   lungs/pertaining to
   pertaining to the lungs

p. pneumon/itis
   lung/inflammation
   inflammation of the lungs

q. endo/trache/al
   inside/trachea/pertaining to
   pertaining to inside the trachea

r. bronchi/ectasis
   bronchus/expansion
   expansion (dilation) of the bronchi

8. a. laryngo/plasty
   b. pneumon/ectasis
   c. pneumono/centesis
   d. tachy/pnea
   e. dys/pnea
   f. a/pnea
   g. pneumon/ectomy
   h. hyper/capnia

9. a. laryng/ectomy
   b. broncho/scopy
   c. tracheo/stomy
   d. thora/centesis
   e. laryng/itis
   f. pleur/itis
   g. trache/itis
   h. bronchiol/ar

a. *whistling sounds during expiration caused by narrowing of an airway*
yes

b. *respiratory condition characterized by obstruction of the bronchi*
no; asthma

c. *tests used to evaluate lung function*
yes

d. *crackling breath sounds heard with a stethoscope*
no; rales

e. *accumulation of fluid in the pleural space*
no; pleural effusion

f. *test used to identify bacteria present in a sample of coughed-up mucus*
yes

g. *tests measuring oxygen and carbon dioxide levels in an arterial blood sample*
yes

1. sinuses
2. pharynx
3. larynx
4. trachea
5. bronchi
6. bronchioles
7. alveoli
8. visceral pleura
9. parietal pleura
10. pleural space
11. atelectasis
12. bronchiectasis
13. cystic fibrosis
14. epistaxis
15. bronchitis
16. laryngitis
17. pharyngitis
18. rhinitis
19. diphtheria
20. pertussis
21. tuberculosis
22. emphysema
23. pneumoconiosis
24. pneumonia
25. pleuritis
26. pleural effusion
27. pneumothorax
28. empyema
29. asthma
30. rales
31. rhonchi
32. stridor
33. wheeze
34. sputum culture
35. spirometry
36. arterial blood gases
37. bronchoscopy
38. laryngoscopy
39. thoracentesis
40. rhinoplasty
41. tracheostomy
42. tracheotomy

10

1. a. col/o
   b. duoden/o
   c. enter/o
   d. ile/o
   e. jejun/o
   f. pancreat/o
   g. pharyng/o
   h. pylor/o
   i. rect/o

2. g, d, a, e, c, b, f

3. b, a, c, e, d, j, f, g, i, h

4. a. bile; gall
   b. gallbladder
   c. common bile duct
   d. bile vessel (duct)
   e. salivary gland
   f. anus
   g. cecum
   h. appendix
   i. mouth

5. b, d, c, e, a

6. a. elimination of loose, watery stools, often with increased frequency

b. condition involving outpouchings of the intestinal wall

c. protrusion of the upper part of the stomach through the diaphragm

d. abdominal pain, diarrhea, and constipation occurring without known disease

e. open sore on the membrane lining the stomach or intestine

f. heartburn

g. x-ray of the upper digestive organs following oral administration of barium sulfate

7. e, c, a, f, b, g, d

8. a. chole/lith/iasis
bile; gall/stone/condition
condition involving gallstones

b. hepato/megaly
liver/enlargement
enlargement of the liver

c. gastro/enter/itis
stomach/small intestine/inflammation
inflammation of the stomach and small intestine

d. stomat/itis
mouth/inflammation
inflammation of the mouth

e. sigmoido/scopy
sigmoid colon/visual examination
visual examination of the sigmoid colon (using a sigmoidoscope)

f. esophago/scopy
esophagus/visual examination
visual examination of the esophagus (using an esophagoscope)

g. ileo/stomy
ileum/surgical opening
creation of a surgical opening in the ileum

h. hemat/emesis
blood/vomiting
vomiting blood

i. gastr/itis
stomach/inflammation
inflammation of the stomach

j. ile/itis
ileum/inflammation
inflammation of the ileum

k. colo/stomy
colon; large intestine/surgical opening
surgical creation of an opening in the colon or large intestine

l. pancreat/itis
pancreas/inflammation
inflammation of the pancreas

m. choledocho/litho/tomy
common bile duct/stone/surgical incision
surgical incision in the common bile duct to remove gallstones

n. an/orexia
without/appetite
lack of appetite

o. gastro/intestin/al
stomach/intestines/pertaining to
pertaining to the stomach and intestines (digestive organs)

p. endo/scopy
inside/visual examination
visual examination inside (an organ)

9. a. col/itis

b. chol/angio/graphy

c. col/ectomy

d. chole/cyst/ectomy

e. gastro/col/itis

f. entero/colo/stomy

g. gastro/jejuno/stomy

h. gastro/entero/stomy

10. a. append/ectomy

b. dys/pepsia

c. hepat/itis

d. chole/cysto/graphy

e. enter/itis

f. hemorrhoid/ectomy

g. ileo/stomy

h. periton/itis

a. *unpleasant sensation in the stomach, usually with a feeling of the need to vomit*
yes

b. *yellow discoloration of the skin*
no; jaundice

c. *swollen veins in the lining of the anus*
no; hemorrhoids

d. *protrusion of a portion of an intestine through the lower abdominal wall*
no; inguinal hernia

e. *chronic liver disease involving destruction of liver cells*
no; cirrhosis

f. *tests measuring levels of liver enzymes (ALT, AST, and ALK) in the blood*
yes

g. *detection of radiation emitted by liver cells following injection of radioactive material*
yes

1. pharynx
2. esophagus
3. stomach
4. small intestine
5. duodenum
6. jejunum
7. ileum
8. large intestine
9. cecum
10. colon
11. rectum
12. anus
13. liver
14. gallbladder
15. common bile duct
16. pancreas
17. peritoneum
18. colitis
19. gastroenteritis
20. hepatitis
21. hepatomegaly
22. peritonitis
23. anorexia
24. emesis
25. dyspepsia
26. pyrosis
27. hiatal hernia
28. inguinal hernia
29. Crohn's disease
30. diverticulosis
31. cirrhosis
32. jaundice
33. cholelithiasis
34. hemorrhoids
35. gastrointestinal endoscopy
36. cholangiography
37. cholecystography
38. barium enema
39. stool guaiac
40. appendectomy
41. colostomy
42. ileostomy

II

1. e, c, a, d, b, f

2. a. ketones   d. kidney
   b. urine condition   e. urinary bladder
   c. urethra   f. albumin

3. a, d, b, f, g, c, e, h

4. f, b, e, i, d, j, c, k, g, a, h

5. a. an/uria
   without; not/urine condition
   condition of not producing urine

   b. nephr/ectomy
   kidney/surgical removal
   surgical removal of a kidney

   c. dys/uria
   painful; difficult/urine condition
   painful or difficult urination

   d. olig/uria
   scanty; few/urine condition
   scanty production of urine

e. litho/tripsy
stone/crushing
crushing of a stone (in the bladder or ure-thra)

f. uretero/stenosis
ureter/narrowing
narrowing of the ureters

g. hemat/uria
blood/urine condition
blood in the urine

h. ur/emia
urine; urea/blood condition
condition characterized by excessive amounts of urea in the blood

i. urethro/plasty
urethra/surgical repair
surgical repair of the urethra

j. bacteri/uria
bacteria/urine condition
bacteria in the urine

k. keton/uria
ketones/urine condition
excessive ketones in the urine

l. pyelo/plasty
renal pelvis/surgical repair
surgical repair of the renal pelvis

m. nephro/lith/iasis
kidney/stone/condition
kidney stone condition

n. nephro/sclerosis
kidney/hardening
hardening of kidney tissue

o. cysto/plasty
urinary bladder/surgical repair
surgical repair of the urinary bladder

p. poly/uria
many/urine condition
excretion of large volumes of urine

6. a. cysto/graphy
b. cysto/urethro/graphy
c. cyst/ectomy
d. albumin/uria
e. glycos/uria
f. nephr/itis

g. nephr/oma
h. nephro/pathy

7. a. cyst/itis
b. pyelo/graphy
c. cysto/lith
d. pyelo/nephr/itis
e. glomerulo/nephr/itis
f. noct/uria
g. urethr/itis
h. uretero/plasty

a. *physical, microscopic, or chemical exami-nation of the urine*
no; urinalysis

b. *presence of abnormally high protein levels in the urine*
no; proteinuria

c. *presence of blood in the urine*
yes

d. *surgical extraction of kidney tissue for mi-croscopic examination*
yes

e. *test measuring the amount of urea in the blood (or the urea level measured)*
no; blood urea nitrogen

f. *removal of toxic substances by draining waste products through a tube inserted into the peritoneal cavity*
no; peritoneal dialysis

g. *any kidney disease advanced enough that the kidneys cannot filter blood adequately*
yes

h. *surgical implantation of a donor kidney into a recipient*
yes

1. kidneys
2. urea
3. nephrons
4. glomerulus
5. Bowman's capsule
6. glomerular filtrate
7. renal pelvis

8. ureters
9. urinary bladder
10. urethra
11. nephropathy
12. nephrosclerosis
13. nephrolithiasis
14. glomerulonephritis
15. pyelonephritis
16. oliguria
17. diuresis
18. enuresis
19. nocturia
20. polyuria
21. uremia
22. cystitis
23. ureterostenosis
24. hydronephrosis
25. urethritis
26. catheterization
27. retrograde pyelography
28. intravenous pyelography
29. voiding cystourethrography
30. urinalysis
31. bacteriuria
32. pyuria
33. hematuria
34. proteinuria
35. glycosuria
36. ketouria
37. lithotripsy
38. ureteroplasty
39. hemodialysis
40. peritoneal dialysis

12

1. f, c, a, g, b, e, d

2. f, i, b, h, e, d, c, g, a

3. c, g, d, f, a, h, e, b

4. a. partial paralysis   f. ventricle
   b. nerve;   g. glia
      nerve tissue   h. sheath; covering
   c. hypothalamus   i. thinking
   d. brain   j. memory
   e. synapse

5. a. neuron/o   e. pont/o
   b. ganglion/o   f. medull/o
   c. ax/o   g. mening/e
   d. cerebr/o   h. parasympath/o

6. g, f, d, e, b, c, a

7. a. reversible disorder involving facial numbness or paralysis due to nerve dysfunction
   b. disorder in which brain damage at birth or during infancy leads to motor deficits
   c. hereditary disorder in which progressive brain cell loss leads to bizarre movements
   d. disorder in which progressive loss of motor neurons leads to muscular weakness
   e. progressive disorder in which hardening of myelin sheaths produces weakness
   f. chronic viral disease in which painful skin blisters form along the path of a nerve

8. a. an/esthesia
   without/feeling; sensation
   insensitivity to pain, heat, or other stimuli
   b. electro/encephalo/graphy
   electricity/brain/recording
   recording of electrical activity within the brain
   c. mening/itis
   meninges/inflammation
   inflammation of the meninges
   d. de/mentia
   without/thinking
   loss of the ability to think clearly
   e. sympath/ectomy
   sympathetic nervous system/surgical removal
   surgical removal of a portion of the sympathetic nervous system

f. a/taxia
without/muscular coordination
loss of muscular coordination

g. quadri/plegia
four/paralysis
paralysis of all four extremities

h. neur/itis
nerve/inflammation
inflammation of a nerve

i. a/kinesia
without/movement
without movement (inability to move)

j. lobo/tomy
lobe/surgical incision
surgical incision in a lobe (of the brain)

k. my/asthenia
muscle/weakness
muscle weakness

l. narco/lepsy
sleep/seizure
seizure-like attacks of sleep

m. para/plegia
beside/paralysis
beside paralysis (paralysis of the lower portion of the body)

n. par/esthesia
beside/sensation
beside sensation ("pins and needles" sensation)

o. somn/ambul/ism
sleep/walking/condition
sleepwalking

p. lamin/ectomy
layer/surgical removal
surgical removal of a layer (a vertebra)

9. a. myelo/graphy
   b. neur/oma
   c. encephal/itis
   d. neuro/tomy
   e. myel/itis
   f. neur/algia (also neuro/dynia)
   g. gli/oma
   h. neuro/blast/oma

a. *paralysis affecting the left or right side of the body*
no; hemiplegia

b. *inability to produce or understand spoken language*
yes

c. *loss of consciousness resulting from diminished blood flow to the brain*
no; syncope

d. *temporary loss of function due to a transient decrease in the blood supply to the brain*
no; transient ischemic attack

e. *behavioral manifestation of abnormal electrical activity in the brain*
no; seizure

f. *disorder in which abnormal electrical activity in the brain results in seizures*
no; epilepsy

g. *damage to brain tissue due to an interruption in the blood supply (a stroke)*
yes

h. *x-ray of the head following injection of a contrast agent to visualize the cerebral vasculature*
no; cerebral angiography

i. *use of magnetic waves to produce a detailed image of the brain*
yes

1. neuron
2. dendrites
3. axon
4. myelin sheath
5. cerebrum
6. thalamus
7. hypothalamus
8. brainstem
9. cerebellum
10. spinal cord
11. meninges
12. cerebrospinal fluid
13. intrathecal
14. aphasia

15. ataxia
16. paresthesia
17. hemiparesis
18. hemiplegia
19. paraplegia
20. quadriplegia
21. neuralgia
22. sciatica
23. meningitis
24. encephalitis
25. cerebrovascular accident
26. transient ischemic attack
27. syncope
28. epilepsy
29. Alzheimer's disease
30. Parkinson's disease
31. cerebral palsy
32. multiple sclerosis
33. myasthenia gravis
34. cerebral angiography
35. electroencephalography
36. magnetic resonance imaging
37. lumbar puncture
38. neurotomy
39. laminectomy
40. trephination

13

1. h, d, b, g, e, a, c, f

2. a. secrete   f. gland
   b. gonads   g. adrenal glands
   c. thyroid   h. pituitary
   d. pancreas   i. parathyroid glands
   e. pineal gland

3. c, b, f, a, d, h, e, g

4. h, e, g, a, c, f, d, b

5. a, g, h, d, f, c, b, e

6. a. enlargement of the thyroid due to a dietary iodine deficiency
   b. tumor of the islets of Langerhans in the pancreas
   c. excessive growth of part or all of the body due to overproduction of growth hormone
   d. tumor, usually benign, of the adrenal medulla with increased hormone production
   e. acidification of the blood and urine due to improper metabolism of fats

7. a. adrenal/ectomy
      adrenal glands/surgical removal
      surgical removal of the adrenal glands
   b. thyro/megaly
      thyroid/enlargement
      enlargement of the thyroid gland (goiter)
   c. ex/ophthalm/os
      out/eye/condition
      protrusion of the eyeball
   d. hyper/gonad/ism
      excessive/gonads/condition
      overproduction of sex hormones by the gonads
   e. hyper/glyc/emia
      excessive/sugar/blood condition
      abnormally high levels of sugar (glucose) in the blood
   f. hypo/thyroid/ism
      under; reduced/thyroid/condition
      underactivity of the thyroid gland
   g. thyro/toxic/osis
      thyroid/poisonous/condition
      any toxic reaction due to overactivity of the thyroid gland (hyperthyroidism)
   h. hypophys/ectomy
      pituitary/surgical removal
      surgical removal of the pituitary gland
   i. pituitar/ism
      pituitary/condition
      any pituitary condition
   j. hyper/pituitar/ism
      excessive/pituitary/condition
      excessive pituitary activity

k. pan/hypo/pituitar/ism
all/under; reduced/pituitary/condition
reduced production of all pituitary hormones

l. acro/megaly
extremities/enlargement
enlargement of the extremities

m. aldosteron/ism
aldosterone/condition
condition involving high aldosterone levels

n. hypo/gonad/ism
under; reduced/gonads/condition
reduced production of sex hormones by the gonads

o. hypo/parathyroid/ism
under; reduced/parathyroid/condition
reduced parathyroid hormone production by the parathyroid

p. myx/edema
mucus/swelling
swelling due to the accumulation of mucus

8. a. pineal/ectomy
   b. thyroid/itis
   c. hyper/parathyroid/ism
   d. thym/ectomy
   e. aden/ectomy
   f. lob/ectomy
   g. hypo/glyc/emia

a. *enlargement of the thyroid gland*
   no; thyromegaly

b. *toxic reaction resulting from hyperthyroidism*
   yes

c. *surgical removal of the thyroid gland*
   no; thyroidectomy

d. *underactivity of the thyroid gland*
   no; hypothyroidism

e. *test used to assess thyroid function by measuring blood thyroxine levels*
   no; thyroxine (T_4) test

f. *test used to assess thyroid function by measuring blood TSH levels*
   yes

g. *administration of synthetic hormones to correct a hormone deficiency*
   yes

1. thyroid gland
2. parathyroid glands
3. adrenal glands
4. cortisol
5. aldosterone
6. androgen
7. epinephrine
8. norepinephrine
9. dopamine
10. pancreas
11. thymus
12. pineal gland
13. gonads
14. pituitary gland
15. thyroid-stimulating hormone
16. adrenocorticotropic hormone
17. luteinizing hormone
18. follicle-stimulating hormone
19. somatotropin
20. melanocyte-stimulating hormone
21. anti-diuretic hormone
22. hypothyroidism
23. hyperthyroidism
24. exophthalmos
25. thyromegaly
26. Graves' disease
27. thyrotoxicosis
28. pituitarism
29. acromegaly
30. Cushing's disease
31. diabetes insipidus
32. diabetes mellitus
33. ketoacidosis
34. aldosteronism
35. Addison's disease
36. pheochromocytoma
37. glucose tolerance test
38. radioactive iodine uptake test

39. adenectomy
40. hormone replacement therapy

14

1. e, a, f, b, d, c

2. a. testes   f. scrotum
   b. spermatozoa g. testes
   c. male   h. genitals
   d. testes   i. testes
   e. epididymis   j. semen

3. c, b, a, e, d

4. b, e, a, f, c, d

5. a. orchid/ectomy
      testes/surgical removal
      surgical removal of one or both testes

   b. crypt/orch/ism
      hidden/testes/condition
      condition characterized by hidden testes

   c. orchi/ectomy
      testes/surgical removal
      surgical removal of one or both testes

   d. an/orch/ism
      without/testes/condition
      condition characterized by the absence of one or both testes

   e. orch/itis
      testes/inflammation
      inflammation of the testes

   f. epididym/itis
      epididymis/inflammation
      inflammation of the epididymis

   g. trans/urethr/al prostat/ectomy
      through/urethra/pertaining to; prostate gland/surgical removal
      surgical removal of the prostate gland through the urethra

   h. a/zoo/sperm/ia
      not; without/animal life/spermatozoa/condition
      condition characterized by lack of spermatozoa

i. prostat/ic hyper/trophy
   prostate gland/pertaining to; excessive/growth
   excessive growth of the prostate gland

j. gyneco/mast/ia
   female/breast/condition
   condition of having female (enlarged) breasts

k. testicul/ar
   testes/pertaining to
   pertaining to the testes

l. orchido/plasty
   testes/surgical repair
   surgical repair of the testes

m. spermo/toxic
   spermatozoa/poisonous
   poisonous or damaging to the spermatozoa

n. testo/pathy
   testes/disease
   any disease of the testes

6. a. vas/ectomy
   b. balan/itis
   c. oligo/sperm/ia
   d. urethr/itis
   e. prostat/ectomy
   f. vesicul/itis
   g. oscheo/plasty

   a. *having undergone circumcision (removal of the prepuce or foreskin)*
      no; circumcized

   b. *infection of the genital skin and membranes by herpes simplex virus*
      no; herpes genitalis

   c. *chronic sexually transmitted infection characterized by skin lesions, flu-like symptoms, and eventually organ damage*
      no; syphilis

   d. *sexually transmitted infection, usually urethral, caused by Neisseria gonorrhoeae*
      no; gonorrhea

   e. *sexually transmitted infection, usually urethral, caused by Chlamydia trachomatis*
      no; chlamydia

f. *blood test used to determine if a person has been infected by the syphilis bacterium*
yes

g. *blood test used to determine if a person has been infected by the syphilis bacterium*
yes

1. testes
2. scrotum
3. spermatozoa
4. seminiferous tubules
5. epididymis
6. vas deferens
7. seminal vesicles
8. prostate gland
9. oligospermia
10. impotence
11. hydrocele
12. gynecomastia
13. epididymitis
14. prostatitis
15. benign prostatic hypertrophy
16. gonorrhea
17. chlamydia
18. herpes genitalis
19. syphilis
20. urethritis
21. phimosis
22. semen analysis
23. transurethral resection of the prostate
24. vasectomy

15

1. b, d, a, c, e, h, f, g

2. a. breast
   b. vagina
   c. uterus
   d. woman; female
   e. menstruation
   f. ovum; egg
   g. vulva
   h. ovaries
   i. uterus
   j. ovum; egg
   k. beginning
   l. turning
   m. ovum; egg

3. a. cervic/o
   b. endometri/o
   c. perine/o
   d. salping/o
   e. galact/o
   f. gon/o

4. f, g, a, d, b, e, c

5. a. mast/itis
   breast/inflammation
   inflammation of the breast

   b. oligo/meno/rrhea
   scanty; few/menstruation/discharge
   unusually light or infrequent menstruation

   c. pyo/salpinx
   pus/fallopian tube
   accumulation of pus in one or both fallopian tubes

   d. colpo/scopy
   vagina/visual examination
   visual examination of the vagina (using a colposcope)

   e. oophor/ectomy
   ovaries/surgical removal
   surgical removal of one or both ovaries

   f. ante/version
   forward/turning
   forward turning (tilting) of an organ

   g. dys/meno/rrhea
   pain/menstruation/discharge
   pain associated with menstruation

   h. leuko/rrhea
   white/discharge
   white discharge

   i. mast/ectomy
   breast/surgical removal
   surgical removal of a breast

   j. meno/rrhagia
   menstruation/excessive flow
   excessive menstrual flow

   k. oophor/itis
   ovaries/inflammation
   inflammation of one or both ovaries

   l. hyster/ectomy
   uterus/surgical removal
   surgical removal of the uterus

m. retro/version
backward/turning
tipping backward of an organ

n. galacto/cele
milk/hernia; swelling
swelling or cyst in a milk duct

o. lump/ectomy
mass/surgical removal
surgical removal of a mass or tumor

p. vagin/itis
vagina/inflammation
inflammation of the vagina

6. d, a, i, f, b, g, c, h, e

7. a. salping/ectomy
   b. episio/tomy (or vulvo/tomy)
   c. cervic/itis
   d. salping/itis
   e. a/meno/rrhea
   f. mammo/graphy
   g. mammo/plasty

a. *surgical procedure in which the endometrial lining is scraped away*
no; dilation and curettage

b. *presence of one or more fibrous cysts in the breast*
no; fibrocystic breast disease

c. *benign tumor of the smooth muscle of the uterus (fibroids)*
no; leiomyoma uteri

d. *growth of endometrial tissue outside the uterus*
no; endometriosis

e. *fluid-filled sac in the ovary*
yes

f. *visual examination of the organs in the abdominal cavity*
yes

1. ovaries
2. fallopian tubes
3. uterus
4. endometrium

5. cervix
6. vulva
7. mammary glands
8. amenorrhea
9. dysmenorrhea
10. endometriosis
11. ovarian cyst
12. oophoritis
13. salpingitis
14. pelvic inflammatory disease
15. cervicitis
16. vaginitis
17. candidiasis
18. Pap smear
19. mammography
20. laparoscopy
21. dilation and curettage
22. hysterectomy
23. oophorectomy
24. mastectomy

16

1. g, f, c, a, e, d, b

2. a. joint
   b. vertebrae
   c. tendon
   d. synovial fluid; synovial membrane
   e. tendon
   f. crooked; bent
   g. to bind together
   h. to break

3. a. crani/o
   b. chondr/o
   c. burs/o
   d. ligament/o
   e. lord/o
   f. myel/o
   g. kyph/o

4. a. bone cell
   b. skull
   c. breast bone
   d. joint
   e. tail bone
   f. joint

5. a. arthr/algia
   joint/pain
   joint pain

b. chondro/malacia
cartilage/softening
softening of the cartilage

c. kyph/osis
humpback/condition
condition characterized by a humpback posture

d. arthro/centesis
joint/puncture
puncture of a joint

e. synov/ectomy
synovial fluid; synovial membrane/surgical removal
surgical removal of a synovial membrane

f. burs/itis
bursa/inflammation
inflammation of the bursae

g. arthro/scopy
joint/visual examination
visual examination of a joint (using an arthroscope)

h. scoli/osis
crooked; bent/condition
condition characterized by a crooked or bent posture

i. ankyl/osis
crooked; stiff/condition
stiff condition (stiff joint)

j. ankyl/osing spondyl/itis
crooked; stiff/condition; vertebrae/inflammation
inflammation of the vertebrae with stiffness

k. osteo/myel/itis
bone/bone marrow/inflammation
inflammation of the bone and bone marrow

l. osteo/porosis
bone/becoming porous or less dense
disease in which the bones become porous

m. arthro/graphy
joint/recording
x-ray recording of a joint

n. arthro/clasia
joint/to break
the deliberate breaking of a joint

o. arthro/desis
joint/to bind together
the binding together of a joint

p. burs/ectomy
bursa/surgical removal
surgical removal of a bursa

q. osteo/tomy
bone/surgical incision
surgical incision in a bone

6. a. disease characterized by weakened, thickened, deformed bones

   b. inflammation of the joints caused by gout (abnormal uric acid metabolism)

   c. malformation of the spine due to congenital abnormalities in vertebra formation

   d. dislocation of a bone from its joint

   e. partial dislocation of a bone from its joint

   f. protrusion of a vertebral disk into the center of the vertebral column

   g. recording of radiation emitted by bone cells after injection of a contrast agent

7. e, a, f, d, c, b

8. a. synov/itis
   b. lord/osis
   c. cranio/tomy
   d. osteo/arthr/itis
   e. arthro/plasty
   f. arthr/ectomy
   g. osteo/malacia
   h. arthro/pathy

a. *joint pain*
   yes

b. *any disease of the joints*
   no; arthropathy

c. *chronic disease involving inflammation, pain, stiffness, and eventually deformity of affected joints*
   no; rheumatoid arthritis

d. *chronic disease involving destruction of articular cartilage and overgrowth of bone*
   yes

e. *test used to detect rheumatoid factor present in patients with rheumatoid arthritis*
no; rheumatoid factor test

f. *x-ray recording of the joints following injection of a contrast agent*
no; arthrography

1. cartilage
2. bone marrow
3. vertebrae
4. vertebral disks
5. arthrosis
6. synovial fluid
7. bursae
8. ligament
9. osteomyelitis
10. osteoporosis
11. Paget's disease
12. fracture
13. subluxation
14. arthritis
15. bursitis
16. rheumatoid arthritis
17. osteoarthritis
18. ankylosing spondylitis
19. spina bifida
20. herniated disk
21. bone scan
22. arthroscopy
23. arthrocentesis
24. arthroplasty
25. arthrodesis

17

1. e, b, d, c, a

2. a. muscle
   b. fiber; fibrous
   c. muscle fiber
   d. strength
   e. without strength (weakness)
   f. tendon
   g. fascia
   h. to bend
   i. tendon

3. d, a, e, h, g, f, c, b

4. d, c, a, e, b

5. a. tendo/plasty
   tendon/surgical repair
   surgical repair of a tendon

   b. my/algia
   muscle/pain
   muscle pain

   c. myos/itis
   muscle/inflammation
   inflammation of a muscle

   d. poly/myos/itis
   many/muscle/inflammation
   inflammation of many muscles

   e. tendin/itis
   tendon/inflammation
   inflammation of a tendon

   f. fascio/tomy
   fascia/surgical incision
   surgical incision in a fascia

   g. myo/diastasis
   muscle/separation
   separation of a muscle

   h. a/ton/ia
   not; without/tension/condition
   condition of having no muscle tension

   i. myo/rrhaphy
   muscle/suture; stitch
   suturing of a muscle wound

   j. teno/desis
   tendon/to bind together
   the binding of a tendon (to a bone)

   k. electro/myo/graphy
   electricity/muscle/recording
   recording of the electrical activity of muscle

6. a. myo/clonus
   b. myo/sarc/oma
   c. myo/pathy
   d. my/a/sthen/ia
   e. fasci/itis
   f. fascio/plasty
   g. fibro/my/algia

h. myo/malacia

7. a. my/oma
   b. myo/blast/oma
   c. myo/fibr/oma
   d. teno/plasty
   e. teno/myo/plasty
   f. myo/ton/ia

a. *muscle pain*
   yes
b. *rapid, uncontrollable twitching of a muscle or group of muscles*
   no; myoclonus
c. *surgical removal of muscle tissue for microscopic examination*
   yes
d. *wasting away or degeneration of muscle tissue*
   no; muscle atrophy
e. *test used to record the electrical activity of a muscle*
   no; electromyography
f. *group of hereditary diseases characterized by progressive muscle degeneration*
   no; muscular dystrophy

1. skeletal muscles
2. fasciae
3. tendon
4. smooth muscle
5. cardiac muscle
6. flexion
7. extension
8. abduction
9. adduction
10. pronation
11. supination
12. dorsiflexion
13. plantar flexion
14. rotation
15. circumduction
16. myalgia

17. dystonia
18. myoclonus
19. myositis
20. tendinitis
21. muscular dystrophy
22. electromyography
23. myotomy

18

1. c, e, d, b, f, a, g

2. a. skin   d. fat
   b. sweat   e. black
   c. skin   f. skin

3. c, a, d, b, e

4. a. thickening of the outer keratin-filled layers of skin due to excessive sun exposure
   b. inflammation and infection of all layers of the skin
   c. excessive body hair
   d. redness of the skin due to swelling of the capillaries
   e. smooth, slightly elevated area that is redder or paler than the surrounding skin
   f. contagious parasitic skin infection characterized by small, raised, itchy lesions

5. c, h, f, d, g, a, e, b, i

6. a. laceration; contusion
   b. Ecchymosis; petechia
   c. macule; papule
   d. Irrigation; debridement

7. a. dermat/itis
      skin/inflammation
      inflammation of the skin
   b. an/hidr/osis
      without/sweat/condition
      condition characterized by inadequate or no sweating

c. dermato/mycosis
skin/fungal infection
fungal infection of the skin

d. melan/oma
black/tumor
black tumor (arising from melanocytes)

e. chem/abrasion
chemical/scraping
use of chemicals to scrape away a layer of skin cells

f. erythro/derma
red/skin
redness of the skin

g. sebo/rrhea
sebum/discharge
excessive discharge (secretion) of sebum

h. psor/iasis
itching/condition
condition characterized by itching

i. kerat/osis
hard; horn-like/condition
any horny growth (on the skin)

j. seb/aceous cyst
sebum/pertaining to; cyst
sebum-filled cyst

k. derm/abrasion
skin/scraping
scraping of the skin (to remove lesions)

l. dermato/logy
skin/study of
study of the skin

m. sub/cutane/ous
under; beneath/skin/pertaining to
pertaining to beneath the skin

n. trans/derm/al
through; across/skin/pertaining to
pertaining to across the skin

o. intra/derm/al
within; inside/skin/pertaining to
pertaining to within the skin

8. a. lip/ectomy
b. lip/oma
c. hyper/hidr/osis
d. xero/derma

e. onycho/mycosis
f. kerato/lytic
g. hypo/hidr/osis

a. *lesion consisting of macules and papules (flat and raised spots)*
no; maculopapular lesions

b. *pus-filled vesicles or sacs within or just beneath the epidermis*
yes

c. *small spots on the skin that are colored or thickened, but not raised*
no; macules

d. *inflammatory skin condition characterized by redness, itching, and blisters*
no; eczema

e. *any of several skin diseases characterized by pus-producing lesions*
yes

f. *inflammation of the skin*
yes

g. *spreading bacterial infection in which abundant pus-producing vesicles form*
no; impetigo

1. epidermis
2. squamous epithelial cells
3. keratin
4. dermis
5. subcutaneous tissue
6. sebaceous glands
7. dermatitis
8. pruritis
9. urticaria
10. eczema
11. psoriasis
12. pustule
13. bulla
14. erythema
15. erythroderma
16. macule
17. papule
18. wheal

19. nevus
20. keratosis
21. actinic keratosis
22. ecchymosis
23. petechia
24. pyoderma
25. furuncle
26. carbuncle
27. impetigo
28. cellulitis
29. dermatomycosis
30. tinea
31. scabies
32. alopecia
33. hirsutism
34. seborrhea
35. sebaceous cyst
36. acne
37. skin biopsy
38. debridement
39. irrigation
40. cryosurgery

19

1. f, e, c, h, b, a, g, d

2. a. uvea
   b. eye
   c. pupil
   d. cornea
   e. vision
   f. eye
   g. iris
   h. lens
   i. conjunctiva
   j. vision
   k. glass
   l. dry

3. a. lacrim/o
   b. retin/o
   c. phot/o
   d. scot/o
   e. ambly/o
   f. cycl/o and cili/o
   g. scler/o
   h. dacry/o

4. b, f, c, h, a, g, e, d

5. a. nyct/al/opia
   night/blindness/vision
   reduced vision in dim light; night blindness

   b. fundo/scopy
   hollow interior/visual examination
   examination of the innermost structures of the eye

   c. ambly/opia
   dim; dull/vision
   dulled vision

   d. xer/ophthalm/ia
   dry/eye/condition
   dryness of the eyes

   e. hemi/an/opia
   half/without; not/vision
   blindness in one-half of the visual field

   f. aniso/cor/ia
   unequal/pupil/condition
   inequality in the size of the pupils

   g. tono/metry
   tension; pressure/measurement
   measurement of pressure within the eye

   h. blepharo/ptosis
   eyelids/drooping
   drooping of the eyelids

   i. a/metr/opia
   not; without/measure/vision
   vision problem caused by a refractive error

   j. a/stigmat/ism
   not; without/point/condition
   inability to focus on a point

   k. a/chromat/opsia
   not; without/color/vision
   without color vision (color blindness)

   l. dacryo/cyst/itis
   tear duct/sac/inflammation
   inflammation of a tear sac (lacrimal duct)

   m. gonio/scopy
   angle/visual examination
   examination of an angle (in the eye)

6. a. kerato/tomy
   b. ophthalmo/logy
   c. irid/ectomy
   d. irido/tomy
   e. irido/cycl/itis
   f. ophthalmo/scopy

g. dipl/opia

h. hyper/opia

7. a. kerat/itis

b. kerato/tomy

c. conjunctiv/itis

d. presby/opia

e. uve/itis

f. papill/edema

g. retino/pathy

h. scler/itis

8. a, g, e, d, b, i, f, h, k, c, j

a. *any disorder in which both eyes cannot be directed toward the same object*
no; strabismus

b. *dulled vision*
no; amblyopia

c. *test of visual acuity in which subject reads letters/numbers on a chart 20 feet away*
no; Snellen's chart

d. *farsightedness*
yes

e. *visual examination of the interior of the eye*
no; ophthalmoscopy

f. *the shining of light on the retina to determine if errors of refraction occur*
no; retinoscopy

g. *exercise program designed to restore normal coordination of eye muscles*
yes

1. cornea

2. uvea

3. miosis

4. mydriasis

5. lens

6. humor

7. retina

8. optic nerve

9. myopia

10. hyperopia

11. astigmatism

12. achromatopsia

13. amblyopia

14. strabismus

15. anisocoria

16. glaucoma

17. scotoma

18. cataract

19. diabetic retinopathy

20. ophthalmoscopy

21. fundoscopy

22. tonometry

23. orthoptic training

24. radial keratotomy

20

1. f, d, b, c, e, a

2. e, f, d, h, b, g, a, c

3. a. mastoid process

b. condition of the ear

c. hearing

d. vestibular apparatus

e. hearing

f. eardrum

g. external ear

4. a. myringo/tomy
eardrum/surgical incision
surgical incision in the eardrum

b. oto/plasty
ear/surgical repair
surgical repair of the ear (the outer ear)

c. audio/metry
hearing/measurement
measurement of hearing

d. tympan/ectomy
eardrum/surgical removal
surgical removal of the eardrum

e. oto/pyo/rrhea
ear/pus/discharge
discharge of pus from the ear

f. ana/cusis
without; not/hearing
without hearing (total deafness)

g. labyrinth/itis
inner ear/inflammation
inflammation of the inner ear

h. oto/dynia
ear/pain
pain in the ear; earache

i. ot/itis media
ear/inflammation; middle
inflammation of the middle ear

j. ot/itis externa
ear/inflammation; outer
inflammation of the outer ear

k. presby/cusis
old age/hearing
loss of hearing with age

l. myring/itis
eardrum/inflammation
inflammation of the eardrum

m. oto/sclerosis
ear/hardening
hardening of the ear (bone)

n. oto/mycosis
ear/fungal infection
fungal infection of the ear

5. a. mastoid/itis
   b. ot/itis
   c. oto/pathy
   d. tympan/ectomy or myring/ectomy
   e. tympano/stomy or myringo/stomy
   f. staped/ectomy
   g. labyrintho/tomy
   h. oto/scopy

6. a, k, e, g, i, b, d, f, c, j, h

a. *earache*
   yes

b. *discharge of pus from the ear*
   no; otopyorrhea

c. *visual examination of the ear using an otoscope*
   yes

d. *test measuring a patient's ability to hear different tones (hearing test)*
   no; audiometry

e. *surgical incision in the eardrum to drain fluid from the middle ear*
   no; myringotomy

1. auricle
2. external auditory meatus
3. tympanic membrane
4. ossicles
5. eustachian tube
6. cochlea
7. organ of Corti
8. vestibular apparatus
9. semicircular canals
10. auditory nerve
11. anacusis
12. conductive hearing loss
13. otosclerosis
14. sensorineural hearing loss
15. presbycusis
16. tinnitus
17. vertigo
18. otitis media
19. otopyorrhea
20. audiometry
21. otoscopy
22. myringotomy
23. cochlear implant
24. stapedectomy

21

1. a. tumor; mass
   b. tumor
   c. malignant epithelial tumor
   d. malignant connective tissue tumor
   e. growth; development

f. growth; development

g. chemical; drug

h. treatment

i. cold

j. burn; heat

k. immature

l. tissue

m. new

n. genetic change

o. cancer

2. a. Grading; staging

b. well differentiated; anaplastic

c. no; extensive

3. a, b, a, b, b, a, a, b, b, a, b, a

4. b, f, d, e, i, c, g, a, h

5. a. ring-shaped or circular

b. abnormal (but not clearly cancerous) in appearance; precancerous

c. having a large, soft consistency

d. containing dead tissue

e. having a hard, packed consistency

f. containing a thin, watery fluid

g. having an open lesion

h. confined to the site of origin

6. a. neo/plasm
new/growth; development
new growth (tumor)

b. anti/neo/plas/tic
against/new/growth; development/pertaining to
pertaining to acting against new growths or tumors

c. dys/plas/ia
abnormal/growth; development/condition
condition involving abnormal tissue development

d. ana/plas/ia
without; not/growth; development/condition
condition involving the absence of development

e. chemo/therapy
chemical; drug/treatment
drug treatment

f. cyto/toxic
cell/poisonous
poisonous or damaging to cells

g. electro/cauter/ization
electricity/burn; heat/process
process of using an electrical instrument to burn (destroy) tissue

h. laparo/tomy
abdomen/surgical incision
surgical incision in the abdomen

i. neuro/fibr/oma
nerve/fiber/tumor
tumor of nerve fibers (sheaths)

j. neuro/fibro/sarcoma
nerve/fiber/malignant connective tissue tumor
malignant tumor of nerve fibers (sheaths)

k. adeno/carcinoma
gland/malignant epithelial tumor
malignant epithelial tumor of glands

7. a. onco/genesis

b. carcino/genesis

c. histo/genesis

d. histo/logy

e. retino/blast/oma

f. neuro/blast/oma

g. lymph/oma

h. nephro/blast/oma

i. papillo/carcinoma

j. cholangio/carcinoma

8. a. angi/oma; angio/sarcoma

b. hem/angi/oma; hem/angio/sarcoma

c. lymph/angi/oma; lymph/angio/sarcoma

d. fibr/oma; fibro/sarcoma

e. leio/my/oma; leio/myo/sarcoma

f. rhabdo/my/oma; rhabdo/myo/sarcoma

g. oste/oma; osteo/sarcoma

h. chondr/oma; chondro/sarcoma

a. *removal of an entire tumor plus the surrounding normal tissue for examination*
   yes

b. *having a hard, packed consistency*
   no; scirrhous

c. *the condition of being without development (of being immature)*
   no; anaplasia

d. *spread of a tumor from the site of origin to another part of the body*
   yes

e. *test measuring the responsiveness of tumor cells to estrogen*
   no; estradiol receptor assay

f. *test measuring the responsiveness of tumor cells to progesterone*
   no; progesterone receptor assay

g. *use of ionizing radiation to destroy diseased tissue*
   yes

h. *assisting (as in therapy to assist a main mode of therapy)*
   no; adjuvant

i. *drug treatment*
   yes

1. carcinogenic
2. neoplasm
3. malignant
4. dedifferentiated
5. anaplasia
6. metastasis
7. grading
8. staging
9. in situ
10. scirrhous
11. dysplastic
12. diffuse
13. follicular
14. carcinoma
15. adenocarcinoma
16. sarcoma
17. leukemia
18. glioma
19. needle biopsy
20. excisional biopsy
21. chemotherapy
22. radiation therapy
23. exenteration
24. adjuvant therapy

Index

arterial blood gases, 115
arteries, 56
arteriosclerosis, 23, 61
arterioles, 56
arthralgia, 230
arthrectomy, 233
arthritis, 230
arthrocentesis, 232
arthroclasia, 233
arthrodesis, 233
arthrography, 232
arthropathy, 230
arthroplasty, 233
arthroscopy, 232
arthroses, 227
articular cartilage, 224, 228
articulations, 227
artificially acquired immunity, 100
ascending colon, 127
ascending spinal tracts, 162
asplenia, 91
asthma, 113
astigmatism, 275
ataxia, 24, 166
atelectasis, 24, 113
atheroma, 62
atherosclerosis, 62
atonia, 246
atria, 53
atrioventricular, 54
audiometry, 29, 291
auditory nerve, 288
auditory, 12
auricle, 285
autoimmune disease, 101
autonomic nervous system, 163
axial skeleton, 224
axon, 159
azoospermia, 199

B

B-cells, 99
bacteriuria, 148
balanitis, 199
balloon angioplasty, 66

barium enema, 133
barium swallow, 133
Bartholin's glands, 210
basal, 255
basal cell carcinoma, 258
basilar membrane, 287
basophils, 75
Bell's palsy, 166
benign, 299
benign prostatic hypertrophy, 199
biceps, 242
biceps femoris, 245
biceps muscle, 14
bicuspid valve, 57
bile, 128
biological therapy, 308
bleeding time, 80
blepharoptosis, 275
blind spot, 272
blood clotting, 76
blood dyscrasia, 78
blood pressure, 59
blood transfusion, 81
blood urea nitrogen, 148
body, 126
body cavity, 42
body plane, 40
body systems, 39
bone marrow, 222
bone marrow biopsy, 80, 307
bone marrow transplant, 81
bone scan, 232
Bowman's capsule, 142
bradycardia, 24, 62
brain, 160
brainstem, 161
breasts, 210
bronchi, 110
bronchiectasis, 113
bronchioles, 110
bronchitis, 113
bronchoscopy, 115
bruise, 59
bucca, 123
buccal cavity, 123
bulbourethral glands, 197
bulla, 258

bundle branches, 54
bundle of His, 54
burn, first-degree, 258
burn, second-degree, 258
burn, third-degree, 258
bursae, 228
bursectomy, 233
bursitis, 230

C

calcitonin, 180
cancellous bone, 224
candidiasis, 212
capillaries, 56
carbuncle, 258
carcinogenic, 12, 300
carcinoma, 301
cardiac, 12
cardiac arrest, 62
cardiac catheterization, 65
cardiac conduction system, 54
cardiac cycle, 59
cardiac muscle, 240
cardiac sphincter, 126
cardiologist, 11
cardiology, 11
cardiomyopathy, 62
cardioversion, 66
carotid ultrasound, 169
carpals, 225
cartilage, 222
cataract, 275
cataract surgery, 277
catheterization, 148
caudal 40, 41
CEA test, 307
cecum, 127
cell, 38
cell body, 159
cell-mediated immune response, 99
cellulitis, 258
central, 42
central nervous system, 160
cephalic, 40, 41
cerebellum, 161

glans penis, 197
glaucoma, 275
glia, 162
glioma, 167
globulins, 74
glomerular filtrate, 142
glomerulonephritis, 146
glomerulus, 142
glucagon, 182
glucocorticoids, 181
glucose tolerance test, 187
gluteus maximus, 245
glycosuria, 148
gonads, 183
gonioscopy, 277
gonorrhea, 199, 213
gouty arthritis, 230
graafian follicle, 207
grading, 304
grand mal, 167
granulocytes, 75
granuloma, 259
Graves' disease, 186
greenstick fracture, 230
growth hormone, 178
gums, 125
gynecomastia, 199

hair cells, 287
hair fibers, 256
hair follicle, 256
hair root, 212
hair shaft, 212
hard palate, 95
heart block, 63
hematemesis, 131
hematochezia, 131
hematocrit, 81
hematopoiesis, 74
hematuria, 148
hemianopia, 275
hemiparesis, 167
hemiplegia, 14, 167
hemispheres, 160

hemodialysis, 149
hemoglobin, 11, 74
hemolytic anemia, 79
hemophilia, 79
hemorrhage, 79
hemorrhoidectomy, 134
hemorrhoids, 131
heparin, 56
hepatic duct, 100
hepatitis, 131
hepatocyte, 11
hepatomegaly, 132
hepatotoxic, 24
herniated disk, 231
herniorrhaphy, 31
herpes genitalis, 200, 213
heteromorphic, 15
hiatal hernia, 132
hirsutism, 259
histamines, 56
histogenesis, 301
HIV-positive, 101
Hodgkin's disease, 91
homeostasis, 15
homotopic, 15
horizontal plane, 40
hormone replacement, 188
hormones, 178
humerus, 225
humoral immune response, 99
Huntington's chorea, 167
hydrocele, 200
hydronephrosis, 146
hyperglycemia, 25, 186
hypergonadism, 186
hyperhidrosis, 259
hyperopia, 275
hyperparathyroidism, 186
hyperpituitarism, 186
hypersensitivity, 101
hypertension, 63
hyperthyroidism, 23, 186
hypochondriac, left, 43
hypochondriac, right, 43
hypogastric, 44
hypogonadism, 186
hypoparathyroidism, 186

hypopharynx, 108
hypophysectomy, 188
hypotension, 63
hypothalamus, 16, 160
hypothyroidism, 25, 186
hypoxemia, 113
hypoxia, 113
hysterectomy, 215

ileitis, 132
ileocecal valve, 127
ileostomy, 31, 134
ileum, 127
ilium, 225
immune responses, 97
immunization, 102
immunodeficiency, 101
immunoglobulins, 99
immunosuppression, 102
immunotherapy, 102
impacted fracture, 231
impetigo, 259
impotence, 200
incisional biopsy, 261, 307
incus, 286
infarction, 63
inferior, 40, 41
inferior vena cava, 57
infundibular stalk, 178
inguinal hernia, 132
inguinal, left, 44
inguinal, right, 44
insertion, 241
in situ, 304
insomnia, 25
insulin, 182
insulinoma, 186
interatrial septum, 53
intermediate lobe, 180
internal, 42
interstitial fluid, 87
interstitial, 16
interventricular septum, 53
intrathecal, 162

intravenous, 17
intravenous pyelography, 148
involuntary muscles, 240
ipsilateral, 17
iridectromy, 277
iris, 270
iron-deficiency anemia, 79
irregular bones, 223
irridesis, 232
irrigation , 262
irritable bowel syndrome, 132
ischemia, 63
ischium, 225
isles of Langerhans, 182
isomorphic, 15
isthmus, 180

lacrimal apparatus, 273
laminectomy, 170
laparoscopy, 215
large bowel, 127
large intestine, 127
laryngectomy,115
laryngitis, 23, 113
laryngopharynx, 108
laryngoplasty, 115
laryngoscopy, 115
larynx, 109
lateral, 40, 41
left lower quadrant, 44
left upper quadrant, 44
left ventricular hypertrophy, 63
leiomyoma uteri, 213
lens, 271
lesion, 259
lethargy, 167
leukemia, 79
leukocytes, 74
leukopenia, 23, 79
leukorrhea, 213
LH, 180
ligaments, 228
lingual tonsils, 90
lipectomy, 262
lipocytes, 256
lipoma, 260
lips, 123
lithotripsy, 31, 149
liver, 128
liver function tests, 133
liver scan, 133
lobectomy, 115, 188
lobes, 110
lobotomy, 170
long bones, 223
loop of Henle, 143
lordosis, 231
Lou Gehrig's disease, 167
lumbar, left, 44
lumbar, right, 44
lumbar puncture, 170
lumbar vertebrae, 225
lumpectomy, 215
lungs, 110

luteinizing hormone, 180
luxation, 231
lymph, 87
lymph nodes, 88
lymph vessels, 88
lymphadenitis, 91
lymphadenopathy, 91
lymphangiography, 92
lymphangioma, 92
lymphedema, 22, 92
lymphocytes, 76
lymphoma, 23, 92
lynphedema, 22

osteoblast, 11
osteoblasts, 222
osteomalacia, 23, 231
osteomyelitis, 231
osteoporosis, 231
osteotomy, 233
otitis externa, 290
otitis media, 290
otodynia, 22, 290
otoliths, 288
otomycosis, 23, 290
otopathy, 290
otoplasty, 292
otopyorrhea, 23, 291
otosclerosis, 291
otoscopy, 291
oval window, 286
ovarian cyst, 214
ovaries, 183, 207
oviducts, 208
ovulation, 207
oxygenation, 57
oxytocin, 180

P

pacemaker, 54
Paget's disease, 231
palate, 125
palatine tonsils, 90
palpitation, 64
pancreas, 128, 182
pancreatic duct, 100
pancreatic islet, 182
pancreatitis, 132
panhypopituitarism, 25, 187
Papanicolaou test, 215
papilla, 256
papillary, 303
papillary carcinoma, 260
papilledema, 276
papilloma, 260
papillae, 125
papule, 260
paresthesia, 168
paralysis, 247

paraplegia, 168
parasympathetic nervous system, 163
parathyroid glands, 17, 181
parathyroid hormone, 181
parietal, 42
parietal lobe, 160
parietal peritoneum, 128
parietal pleura, 111
Parkinson's disease, 168
partial thromboplastin time, 81
passive immunity, 100
patella, 225
pectoralis major, 242
pelvic girdle, 225
pelvic inflammatory disease, 214
penile, 12
penile prosthesis, 201
penis, 197
peptic ulcer, 132
percutaneous, 17
pericardiocentesis, 65
pericarditis, 64
pericardium, 17, 53
peripheral, 42
perimetrium, 209
perineum, 210
periodontium, 125
periostitis, 231
periosteum, 224
peripheral nervous system, 162
peripheral vascular disease, 64
peristalsis, 126
peritoneal dialysis, 149
peritoneum, 128
peritonitis, 132
peritubular capillaries, 143
pernicious anemia, 79
pertussis, 114
petechia, 260
petit mal, 168
phagocytes, 98
phagocytic, 56
phalanges, 225, 227
pharyngeal tonsils, 90
pharyngitis, 114
pharynx, 108, 126

pheochromocytoma, 187
phimosis, 200
phlebitis, 64
phlebotomy, 66
photopigments, 271
phrenic, 111
pia mater, 162
pineal gland, 182
pinealectomy, 188
pinna, 285
pituitarism, 187
pituitary dwarfism, 187
pituitary gland, 178
plantar flexion, 242
plasma, 74
plasma cell, 99
platelets, 76
pleural space, 111
pleuritis, 114
plurual effusion, 114
PMNs, 75
pneumatic otoscopy, 291
pneumoconiosis, 114
pneumonia, 23, 114
pneumothorax, 114
PNS, 130
poliomyelitis, 168
polycythemia, 79
polymorphonuclear leukocytes, 75
polymorphonuclear, 14
polymyositis, 247
polypoid, 303
polyuria, 147
pons, 161
positron emission tomography, 170
posterior, 40, 41
posterior lobe, 180
postpartum, 17
postsynaptic, 159
prenatal, 17
prepuce, 197
presbycusis, 25, 291
presbyopia, 276
presynaptic, 159
primigravida, 17
progesterone, 183, 207
progesterone receptor assay, 308

prolactin, 180
prolapse, 17
pronation, 242
prone position, 39
prostatectomy, 201
prostate gland, 197
prostate-specific antigen test, 308
prostatitis, 200
proteinuria, 149
prothrombin time, 81
prothrombin, 74
proximal, 42
proximal tubule, 143
pruritus, 260
pseudocyesis, 25
psoriasis, 25, 260
PTH, 181
pubis, 225
pulmonary, 12
pulmonary artery, 57
pulmonary circulation, 57
pulmonary function tests, 115
pulmonary semilunar valve, 57
pulmonary veins, 57
pulp, 95
punch biopsy, 262
pupil, 270
Purkinje fibers, 54
purpura, 79
pustule, 260
pyelonephritis, 147
pyeloplasty, 149
pyloric sphincter, 126
pylorus, 126
pyoderma, 260
pyosalpinx, 214
pyrosis, 132
pyruria, 149

Q

quadriceps, 14
quadriceps femoris, 245
quadriplegia, 169

R

radial keratotomy, 278
radiation therapy 309
radioactive iodine uptake test, 187
radiography, 28
radioimmunoassay, 29, 188
radionuclide scan, 308
radius, 225
rales, 114
Raynaud's phenomenon, 64
reabsorption, 143
receptors, 159
rectum, 128
recumbent position, 39
red blood cells, 74
red blood count, 81
renal artery, 142
renal biopsy, 149
renal colic, 147
renal corpuscle, 142
renal cortex, 142
renal medulla, 142
renal pelvis, 142
renal transplantation, 149
renal tubule, 142
renal vein, 142
renin, 142
respiration, 106
retina, 271
retinal detachment, 276
retinitis pigmentosa, 276
retinopathy, 276
retinoscopy, 277
retrograde pyelography, 148
retroversion, 17, 214
Rh factor, 77
rheumatic heart disease, 64
rheumatoid arthritis, 231
rheumatoid factor test, 232
rhinitis, 114
rhinoplasty, 115
rhonchi, 114
ribs, 225
right lymphatic duct, 88
right lower quadrant, 44
right upper quadrant, 44

Rinne test, 291
rods, 271
rotation, 242
RPR test , 200, 215
rugae, 126

S

S-A node, 54
saccule, 288
sacrum, 225
sagittal plane, 40
saliva, 126
salivary glands, 126
salpingectomy, 216
salpingitis, 214
sarcoma, 301
sartorius, 245
scabies, 260
scapula, 225
sciatica, 169
scirrhous, 303
sclera, 269
scleritis, 276
scoliosis, 232
scotoma, 276
scrotum, 195
sebaceous cyst, 261
sebaceous glands, 256
seborrhea, 261
sebum, 256
secondary hypertension, 64
secretion, 143
seizure, 169
semen, 197
semen analysis, 201
semicircular canals, 288
semilunar, 15
seminal duct, 197
seminal vesicles, 197
seminiferous tubules, 196
seminoma, 200
sensorineural hearing loss, 291
septum, 108
serous, 303
serratus anterior, 245

tissue, 38
tomography, 28
tongue, 125
tonometry, 277
tonsillectomy, 92
tonsillitis, 92
tonsils, 90
toxic shock syndrome, 214
trachea, 109
tracheotomy, 31, 115
tracts, 161
transfused, 77
transient ischemic attack, 169
transurethral prostatectomy, 201
transurethral, 17
transverse colon, 127
transverse plane, 40
trapezius, 242
tremor, 169, 247
trephination, 170
triceps, 242
trichomoniasis, 214
tricuspid, 15
tricuspid valve, 57
triiodothyronine, 180
triiodothyronine uptake test, 188
trophic, 178
tropic, 178
TSH, 178
tubal ligation, 216
tuberculosis, 114
tumors, 299
tympanectomy, 292
tympanic membrane, 286
tympanocentesis, 244
tympanostomy, 292

U

ulcerating, 303
ulna, 225
ultrasonography, 28

umbilical, 44
unilateral, 15
unmyelinated, 25
uremia, 147
ureter, 143
ureteroplasty, 149
ureterostenosis, 24, 147
urethra, 144
urethritis, 147, 200
urethroplasty, 149
urinalysis, 29, 148
urinary bladder, 144
urinary meatus, 144
urinary retension, 147
urticaria, 261
uterine prolapse, 214
uterine tubes, 208
uterus, 208
utricle, 288
uvea, 269
uveitis, 277
uvula, 125

V

vaccination, 11, 102
vagina, 209
vaginitis, 214
valves, 40
valvotomy, 66
valvulitis, 64
valvuloplasty, 31, 66
varicose vein, 65
varicose, 12
vas deferens, 197
vasculature, 56
vasectomy, 201
vasopressin, 180
vasospasm, 24, 65
VDRL test, 201, 215
veins, 56
venae cavae, 57

venipuncture, 66
venography, 65
venous, 12
ventilation, 111
ventral, 40, 41
ventricles, 53, 162
ventriculography, 66
venules, 56
verrueous, 303
vertebrae, 224
vertebral column, 224
vertebral disks, 224
vertigo, 291
vesicles, 159
vestibular apparatus, 287
vestibulocochlear nerve, 288
villi, 127
visceral muscles, 240
visceral peritoneum, 128
visceral pleura, 111
vitamin D, 142
vitreous humor, 271
voiding, 144
voiding cystourethrography, 148
voluntary muscles, 240
vulva, 209

W

Western blot, 102
wheal, 261
wheeze, 114
white blood cells, 74
white blood count, 81

X

xenophthalmia, 231
xeroderma, 261
xerophthalmia, 277